BIOMEDICAL ODYSSEYS

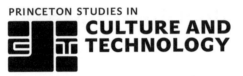

PRINCETON STUDIES IN
CULTURE AND TECHNOLOGY

PRINCETON STUDIES IN CULTURE AND TECHNOLOGY
Tom Boellstorff and Bill Maurer, series editors

This series presents innovative work that extends classic ethnographic methods and questions into areas of pressing interest in technology and economics. It explores the varied ways new technologies combine with older technologies and cultural understandings to shape novel forms of subjectivity, embodiment, knowledge, place, and community. By doing so, the series demonstrates the relevance of anthropological inquiry to emerging forms of digital culture in the broadest sense.

BIOMEDICAL ODYSSEYS

FETAL CELL EXPERIMENTS FROM CYBERSPACE TO CHINA

Priscilla Song

PRINCETON UNIVERSITY PRESS
PRINCETON AND OXFORD

Copyright © 2017 by Princeton University Press

Published by Princeton University Press, 41 William Street, Princeton, New Jersey 08540

In the United Kingdom: Princeton University Press, 6 Oxford Street, Woodstock, Oxfordshire OX20 1TR

press.princeton.edu

Jacket image courtesy of Shutterstock

All Rights Reserved

ISBN 978-0-691-17477-8
ISBN (pbk.) 978-0-691-17478-5

Library of Congress Control Number 2017933371

British Library Cataloging-in-Publication Data is available

This book has been composed in Adobe Minion and Adobe Heiti Std

Printed on acid-free paper ∞

Printed in the United States of America

10 9 8 7 6 5 4 3 2 1

TO MY FAMILY,

FOR ALL OF THE ODYSSEYS

WE HAVE UNDERTAKEN

AND FOR THOSE STILL TO COME

CONTENTS

ILLUSTRATIONS

ACKNOWLEDGMENTS

OVER A DECADE IN THE making, this book has accumulated debts across three continents and survived the deaths of many who contributed to its development during these long years. Above all, I am grateful to the many people who shared their life stories and biomedical odysseys with me, both online and offline. My biggest debt is to Chinese neurosurgeon Huang Hongyun for welcoming me into the everyday routines and inner workings of his neurosurgical enterprises in Beijing and Qingdao. With his permission and encouragement, I observed and often participated in department meetings and training procedures, clinical treatment and medical rounds, surgical operations, laboratory experiments, patient follow-up protocols, staff retreats and KTV singing sessions, and even family barbeques at his second home in New Jersey. Patients from around the world waited for months for a chance to consult him, yet he always made time to talk with me. My fieldwork would not have been possible without his appreciation for what the "study of humankind" (人类学 *rénlèi xué*, the literal Chinese translation for anthropology) could contribute to medical science.

I also thank the clinical, scientific, and administrative staff at the pseudonymous "New Century" Hospital Neurological Disorders Research and Treatment Center ("新世纪" 医院神经疾病研治中心 "Xīn Shìjì" Yīyuàn Shénjīng Jíbìng Yánzhì Zhōngxīn) in Beijing. Nurses, neurosurgeons, acupuncturists, physical therapists, laboratory technicians, scientists, patient coordinators, secretaries, and custodial workers all helped me navigate the complexities of the Chinese health care bureaucracy, tolerated the disruptions I created in their work routines, explained the intricacies of treatment protocols, shared lunches with me in the hospital canteen, compiled patient statistics to help my analyses, and endured my endless questions with patience and good humor through the years. In order to protect their confidentiality I will not thank them by name here, but they appear in the book under pseudonyms and in some cases English names they adopted to facilitate interactions with foreign patients. I am also grateful to neuroscientist Wise Young at Rutgers University and his China Spinal Cord Injury Network collaborators, who greatly enlarged my understanding of both the human and scientific dimensions of spinal cord injury, research, and treatment.

Over a hundred patients and their family members, caregivers, and friends shared their stories with me in Beijing, Qingdao, and Shenzhen. I analyzed the experiences of hundreds more who posted their experiences online. Members of the online CareCure Community deserve special mention. Their public discussions of living in the aftermath of spinal cord injuries and pursuing experimental therapies abroad animate the pages of this book. I respect their contributions by giving full acknowledgment of their authorship for their public commentaries; I have therefore linked back to every individual online post that I cite in this book. I am grateful to Cyrilla Fahlsing for giving me permission to feature her late husband Jeff Dunn's experiences; I share her hope that this book will help someone with ALS or others to learn more about this devastating condition. I am indebted to Oren Bersagel-Briese, Barb and Steve Byer, Geoff Gregory, Roger and Sandy Gullet, Leo Hallan, Gary and Wayne Janaszek, David Landewee, Jenet Langjahr, Doug McGuiness, Bob and Annie Naugle, Suzanne Poon, Helene and Claude Tougard, and Anil Yilmaz for helping at crucial junctures along the way to making this book a reality. I am unable to thank many more by their actual names, but I hope that the stories I record in the following pages offer an enduring testament to their fortitude, courage, and vital humanity.

It is not easy to write about the lives of people who are grappling with devastating disabilities and terminal illnesses. But the eloquence, deep reflection, and urgency with which many spoke have made me determined to do right by them. One of my cherished goals in writing this book is to overturn the simplistic caricature of desperate patients duped by medical charlatans in third-world countries; this narrative emerged far too often on the lips of American scientists quick to dismiss the experimental engagements of patients seeking care abroad. Contrary to these naysayers and Western media portrayals, the vast majority of people I met in Beijing and online often proved to be more expert than leading neurologists with Ivy League pedigrees and state-of-the-art laboratories. The politics and possibilities of knowledge production have shifted dramatically with the advent of new communication technologies, as I hope to show through the nuanced and complicated narratives of people who have sought experimental fetal cell therapies in China. I have tried to let them speak in their own words as much as possible throughout this book, because they describe their experiences better than any dry academic prose can. Some surprised me with their quirky humor, joking about dull drill bits in the operating theater and brain cells getting stuck to hospital pillows. Others brought tears to my eyes as they shared their fears, proclaimed their dreams, and reflected on all they stood to lose or gain. At the time, I had little to contribute beyond conversation, some translation help, and a brief period of camaraderie during their sojourns in China. Yet almost everyone I met generously answered my questions and shared their stories. In recognition of their contributions to this research, I plan to donate 100 percent of the royalties from this book to the Spinal Cord Injury Project at Rutgers University, which runs the CareCure website and supports research on neuroregeneration.

My anthropological engagement with regenerative medicine began at Harvard University the day after the twin towers of the World Trade Center collapsed. The intellectual and moral guidance of James (Woody) Watson, Arthur Kleinman, and Michael Herzfeld helped anchor my thinking about transnational connections and the role of technoscience in a transformed world. I thank Woody for urging me to think about the broader significance of China for the rest of the world (while always keeping my eye on the ball), Arthur for encouraging me to focus on what really matters, and Michael for reminding me to challenge the claims of a crass scientism that has often failed to keep pace with science itself. I also thank Ted Bestor, Steve Caton, Michael Fischer, Byron Good, Hugh Gusterson, Engseng Ho, Jim and Doreen Hogle, Sheila Jasanoff, Bruno Latour, Michael Sandel, Mary Steedly, Ezra Vogel, Kay Warren, Rubie Watson, Martin Whyte, and Susan Zawalich for fostering my intellectual growth in Cambridge. I am grateful to Douglas Melton at the Harvard Stem Cell Institute, who allowed me to audit his stem cell biology classes and spend a summer conducting anthropological fieldwork in his laboratory. I thrived on the intellectual engagement, friendship, and solidarity of colleagues in William James Hall, Dudley House, Tozzer Library, and the Widener stacks, especially Felicity Aulino, Marjan Boogert, Manduhai Buyandelger, Yao Chen, Joon Choi, Denise Ho, Karen Felzer, Vanessa Fong, Angela Garcia, Zongze Hu, Akin Hubbard, Rusaslina Idrus, Zahra Jamal, Jaesok Kim, Angela Lai, Geng Li, Megwen Loveless, Lilith Mahmud, Ernesto Martinez, Katrina Moore, Nicole Newendorp, Prista Ratanapruck, Saubhagya Shah, Miriam Shakow, Lindsay Smith, Maria Stalford, Wen-Ching Sung, and Sarah Wagner.

In Beijing, the Chinese Academy of Social Sciences (CASS) provided me with key institutional support during my first fieldwork stint from 2004 to 2007, including giving me the all-important *dānwèi* affiliation, securing my research visa, printing my business cards, and helping me conduct a large-scale survey of clinician attitudes. I am grateful for the help of my CASS mentor Yang Yiyin and deputy director Zhao Kebin. I am obliged to medical historian Zhang Daqing, who invited me to teach and learn from clinical and graduate students at Peking University's Health Sciences campus. Colleagues at Tsinghua University in Beijing (including Jing Jun, Guo Yuhua, and Zhang Xiaojun) and Fudan University in Shanghai (including Chen Honglin, Gao Yanning, Pan Tianshu, Shen Dingli, Shen Yifei, Yan Fei, Zhang Letian, Zhang Meiyin, and Zhu Jianfeng) provided an intellectual base for subsequent follow-up trips.

At Yale, Helen Siu and William Kelly launched me on my anthropological career first as an inquisitive undergraduate and subsequently as a colleague after I received my doctorate. Working with Zhang Jun, Ling Minhua, and Yang Meijian to organize the Chinese History and Anthropology Reading Group at Yale gave me an unparalleled opportunity to engage leading and emerging scholars in the field of China studies. Hugh Raffles subsequently provided an intellectual home for me at the New School for Social Research and the opportunity to teach a graduate seminar on the cultures of technoscience. In St. Louis, my colleagues in anthropology and East Asian studies at Washington University and in the broader region have provided a superb environment for incubating this book. I am indebted to John Bowen for reading every chapter of this book; his generous support and advice helped me overcome a perfectionist streak to get the manuscript out the door. Other St. Louis colleagues have offered intellectual engagement, social support, and crucial feedback, including Peter Benson, Susan Brownell, Geoff Childs, Rebecca Copeland, Talia Dan-Cohen, Elsa Fan, Linling Gao-Miles, Dan Giammar, Maris Gillette, Robert Hegel, Jean Hunleth, Jong Bum Kwon, Rebecca Lester, Zhao Ma, Stephanie McClure, Steven Miles, Laura Miller, David Morgan, Bruce O'Neill, Shanti Parkih, E. A. Quinn, Crickette Sanz, Carolyn Sargent, Lihong Shi, Rachel Slaughter, Glenn Stone, Brad Stoner, Kedron Thomas, Lori Watt, and James Wertsch. I want to thank my students at Harvard, New School, Washington University, and Yale for stimulating discussions and giving me opportunities to articulate the broader significance of my work, particularly Chelsey Carter, Carolyn Powers, Elyse Singer, Adrienne Strong, Xu Jing, and Zhang Chaoxiong.

I am deeply appreciative of the intellectual community of China anthropologists that Woody and Rubie Watson have fostered over the course of their careers. To my academic brothers and sisters in the House of Watson, our annual reunion meals at the American Anthropological Association meetings are always a source of inspiration and camaraderie in an often lone-wolf enterprise. I am also grateful for a wonderful community of mentors, colleagues, and friends working at the intersections of China studies and the anthropology of science, technology, and medicine. I thank in particular Nancy Chen, Susan Greenhalgh, Jing Jun, Arthur Kleinman, Matthew Kohrman, Lai Lili, Jennifer Liu, Anna Lora-Wainwright, Katherine Mason, Shao Jing, Jeanne Shea, Elanah Uretsky, Ayo Wahlberg, Zhang Li, Zheng Tiantian, and Zhu Jianfeng. Our intellectual exchanges have shaped my thinking immeasurably and their work has been an inspiration for my own. I am indebted to Margaret Sleeboom-Faulkner at the University of Sussex for her continued interest in my work, which has included inviting me several times across the Atlantic to share my work with European colleagues and participate in lively discussions with her Bionetworking in Asia consortium. I would also like to acknowledge the influence of Judith Farquhar's work on my thinking.

Over the years, this project has also benefited from the sharp eyes and generous spirit of many other colleagues around the world, including Sara Ackerman, Aren Aizura, Allison Alexy, Aditya Bharadwaj, Anna Boermel, Joe Bosco, Sean Brotherton, Liz Cartwright, Caroline Chen, Elana Chipman, Nicole Constable, Kimberly Couvson, Sienna Craig, Joe Dumit, Mei-Ling Ellerman, Matthew Erie, Adam Frank, Sarah Franklin, Joan Fujimura, Hugh Gusterson, Sherine Hamdy, Erik Harms, Angelique Haugerud, Seyoung Hwang, Marcia Inhorn, Beth Kangas, Jelena Karanovic, Sharon Kaufman, Jean Langford, Angela Leung,

Liu Shao-hua, Fuji Lozada, Zhiying Ma, Vera Mackie, Theressa MacPhail, Lenore Manderson, Karen Nakamura, Amy Ninetto, John Osburg, Prasanna Patra, Johanna Ransmeier, Hyeon-Ju Rho, Douglas Rogers, Achim Rosemann, Ellen Rubenstein, Shao Jing, Hilary Smith, Amy Speier, Stefan Sperling, Kaushik Sunder Rajan, Ling-Yun Tang, Charis Thompson, Wang Yu, Andrea Whittaker, Yan Yunxiang, and Everett Zhang. Thank you all for responding to various drafts or providing feedback to materials presented at conferences and workshops.

At Princeton University Press, I am deeply grateful to my editor, Fred Appel, for his unwavering enthusiasm, his responsiveness to my many queries, and his dedication to ensuring the highest-quality feedback for my work. Three brilliant and generous reviewers made invaluable contributions to this book. I am grateful that they have stepped forward at the end of this process so I can acknowledge them by name: Nancy Chen, Matthew Kohrman, and Mei Zhan. Their incisive suggestions, thoughtful engagement, and careful reading (twice over for Matthew and Mei) helped me immensely through major revisions of the book by overhauling my analytical framework, honing my arguments, and developing my thinking in new directions. Copyeditor Jennifer Backer's meticulous eye sharpened my prose and brought order to my sprawling citations. Sheila Bodell prepared the index. I appreciate the expertise and professionalism of Princeton's editorial, production, and marketing staff and would like to thank in particular Juliana Fidler, Thalia Leaf, and Brigitte Pelner for shepherding the book to publication and beyond.

Several institutions provided the financial support that made this decade-long project possible, including the National Science Foundation, the Andrew W. Mellon Foundation, the Foreign Language and Area Studies Program, Harvard University, and Washington University in St. Louis. Several individuals and organizations also contributed the images and material analyzed in this book. I thank Oikeat Lam in Singapore for designing many of the beautiful illustrations that grace this book; her creativity in visualizing the data in interesting ways and responsiveness to my exacting specifications are much appreciated. I am grateful to Doug Kanter for allowing me to feature his dramatic photographs of the fetal cell transplantation procedure. Carolyn Moffatt of the American Spinal Injury Association gave me permission to reprint the International Standards for Neurological Classification of Spinal Cord Injury. Jennifer Korman took my author photograph as part of her philanthropic project Headshots 4 Hunger. I am grateful to Susanne van den Buuse at the University of Amsterdam for correcting my rough translations of the Dutch blog excerpts. While all translations from Chinese into English are my own (unless otherwise noted), I am grateful to Lihong Shi, Leila Song, Yihhong Song, Xu Jun, Zhang Chaoxiong, and Zhang Yao for discussions on the idiosyncrasies of Chinese and English grammar and word choice as well as broader philosophical questions on cross-cultural medical ethics. Some materials in this book have been expanded from articles published in two journals: *Medical Anthropology* (Song 2010) and *New Genetics and Society* (Song 2011). I thank the editors and anonymous reviewers of these journals for pushing me to articulate my contributions to broader intellectual conversations in anthropology.

Finally, I want to recognize and honor my family for their steadfast support and encouragement. My parents, Leila and Yihhong, paved the path for me to higher education with their doctorates in polymer science and chemical engineering; I am proud to be the third Dr. Song in the family. I thank my brother, Berwin, for his expert writing and publishing advice from his perspective of leading the editorial helm of several magazines in China and Singapore. I am also grateful for the enthusiastic support of the Walline family from Lake Winola and Sacramento to Framingham and Ma'adi: Vera, David, Dorothy, Catherine, Wael, and Solomon are the best family anyone could choose to join. I am indebted to our honorary aunt Lu Baolian for taking care of us in Beijing and St. Louis and giving me the time I needed to complete this book.

I owe my biggest debt of gratitude to my husband, Joseph Walline. While I cannot do justice to the countless ways that he has supported me, I can at least enumerate a small selection to illustrate the depth of his commitment and the many sacrifices he has made to help me bring this book into being: reading every one of my drafts over the past two decades (although alas he is no longer the jargon detector he used to be and can operationalize analytical assemblages as well as any cultural anthropologist), pausing his medical school studies in Philadelphia to accompany me to the field in 2004–5 (and garnering a Fulbright award along the way to do so), moving halfway across the country for me to pursue my career, building the computer (with the help of Micro Center and online tutorials) upon which most of the revisions of this book have been typed, compiling the Chinese glossary and bibliography for the book, and relinquishing his spacious attic office to give me the distance and quiet from the hubbub of our family life to focus on my writing. Our daughters came into our lives during the odyssey of writing this book. Linnaea and Camellia have restructured my habits, reordered my priorities, and transformed my perspective (even giving me the visceral experience of paraplegia for a brief twelve hours following a spinal block for a cesarean section). Their love, joy, and renewed wonder for life remind me every day what matters most of all.

BIOMEDICAL ODYSSEYS

CHAPTER 1

INTRODUCTION

LIGHTS BLAZING AND SIRENS SCREAMING, the honor convoy of fire engines and ambulances launched Jeff Dunn[1] on his transnational quest for medical treatment. The thirty-three-year-old Colorado firefighter and his wife, Cyrilla, were bound for China's capital city, leaving their toddler son in safekeeping as they embarked on their biomedical odyssey. Jeff had been diagnosed a year earlier with amyotrophic lateral sclerosis (ALS), the same disease that had terminated the lives of American baseball star Lou Gehrig and allegedly China's revolutionary leader Mao Zedong.[2] ALS was a death sentence inexorably taking away the firefighter's ability to walk, talk, and ultimately breathe. Jeff's American doctors had told him that there was no cure for the disease that was destroying the motor neurons in his brain and spinal cord. All they could offer him was a bottle of Rilutek—the only FDA-approved treatment for ALS—that slowed the course of the neurodegenerative disease by a few months at a cost of thousands of dollars.[3] Jeff's doctors advised him to complete a last will and testament. They sent him home with a prescription for sleeping pills.

Jeff was now traveling six thousand miles from his home to seek an experimental therapy devised by a neurosurgeon in Beijing—and blogging each step of the way about the procedure that would transplant fetal olfactory bulb cells into the deteriorating corona radiata (white matter) of his brain. Jeff's fellow firefighters and paramedics had set up a blog on their official brigade website to raise awareness about their comrade's plight. Initially a way to solicit donations for Jeff to help him manage the fatal disease, the blog had now become Jeff's digital lifeline to his friends and family back home as he journeyed halfway around the world.

Jeff was not alone in his quest for treatment. Galvanized by the potential of fetal cells to regenerate damaged neurons and restore lost bodily functions, thousands of people from more than eighty countries have journeyed to China since 2001 to undergo experimental treatment. Despite the warnings of doctors and scientists back home, hundreds of people paralyzed by spinal cord injuries and brain damage have sought fetal cell transplantation in Beijing, including a teenager from California who had broken his back snowboarding, a middle-aged man from Istanbul who had fallen sixty feet down an empty elevator shaft, a young lawyer from the Philippines crippled in a motor vehicle accident, a salaryman from Japan struck down by a stroke, and a three-year-old girl from Romania born with cerebral palsy. Hundreds more suffering from neurodegenerative disorders like Jeff have staked their lives on this experimental therapy, including a golf pro from Florida trying to maintain his weakening grip, a newspaper columnist from Utrecht seeking more time with her family, a police officer from Belgium immobilized in a wheelchair, and a schoolteacher from Italy rendered speechless by ALS. I met these people and many more online and in Beijing, all with individual biographies of busy lives arrested by disease or injury.

This book is an ethnographic account of these biomedical odysseys, of why and how people like Jeff—and Derek, Nedim, Michael, Takeshi, Denisa, Doug, Loes, Patrick, and Maria—have entrusted their bodies to Chinese neurosurgeons operating on the cutting edge of experimental medicine. I invoke the metaphor of "cutting edge" in three distinct ways throughout the book: to suggest the latest advances in biomedical science, to focus attention on the embodied experiences of surgical intervention, and to allude to the borderline nature of experimental therapies occurring at the limits of ethics and legality. In a world in which technologies and risks are moving faster than our ethics and laws can keep pace, we need to take a closer look at what we mean by "cutting edge" medicine by examining the experiences of those on the front lines of these experimental developments.

The easy story here is the standard one of exploitation: of desperate patients duped by medical charlatans peddling false hope with their quack therapies. This is the story reiterated by journalists, international medical experts, and other outside critics—but challenged repeatedly by thousands of patients whose very lives are at stake and the Chinese neurosurgeons who have cared for them. This book follows these patients and clinicians from online discussion forums to Chinese hospital wards in order to understand the hopes, frustrations, and possibilities that experimental therapies offer those living with conditions deemed incurable. I bracket my own normative impulse and delve beneath headline news hyperbole in order to investigate the core issues from the diverse perspectives of the participants involved. What convinced Jeff to travel halfway around the world to undergo experimental surgery? What prompted his Chinese neurosurgeons to try out laboratory procedures on human patients? What motivated the Chinese clinic staff—nurses, neurologists, acupuncturists, scientific researchers, information technology specialists, patient coordinators, custodial workers—to work in this experimental setting? Focusing on the participants' perspectives is a necessary methodological and ethical position for studying such a fraught phenomenon in which the stakes are so high.

For people whose futures have been cut short by diagnoses of paralysis and degeneration, what does it mean to take their hopes seriously? Although some patients lived in suburban housing tracts while others inhabited crowded tenements, some were long retired while a few had barely begun life, some had never flown on an airplane before while others frequented business class lounges, they all shared similar stories of frustration from their fruitless encounters with the medical establishment back home. Written off by busy doctors and insurance companies, these patients and their families had turned to the Internet to pursue alternative possibilities. Through online discussion forums, email listservs, patient blogs, and other social media channels, they had discovered a new fetal cell transplantation surgery in Beijing. By undergoing an experimental procedure in a foreign country, each of these medical pioneers was seeking to overturn the prevailing medical consensus that had written them off as hopeless cases.

Facing the limits of conventional medicine and regulation in their home countries, they have not acquiesced to what others consider the inevitable: resignation, hopelessness, death. In the face of overwhelming neurological catastrophes, their hopes have oriented them to life. Their orientation toward a hopeful future is particularly significant given the expanding politics of resignation following in the wake of corporate capitalism around the world (Benson and Kirsch 2010). Instead of giving up, they have tried to maintain what philosopher Ernst Bloch (1986 [1959]) has described as the "not-yet," an orientation toward what has not yet come into being. Bloch's work focuses attention on the temporal dimensions of hope in generating desires about the future. I bring this inquiry specifically into the realm of Internet-mediated health, seeking to examine how the differential chronicity of illness experiences intersects with the temporal variability of digital communication technologies.

In the chapters that follow, I develop an anthropology of transnational regenerative medicine that documents how hope is produced and troubled both online and through physical encounters with experimental therapies transpiring on the fringes of biomedicine. By framing hope as an important affect organizing human engagements with "cutting edge" medicine, I seek to recast our understanding of the experimental in light of a changing political and moral economy in China that enables novel medical practices. I demonstrate how the production of hope is entangled in differences in ethical values, regulatory frameworks, and politico-economic histories that stoke border-crossing quests for regenerative medicine.

THEORIZING A NEW BIOLOGY OF HOPE

As technological innovations enable alternate futures and the processes of globalization accelerate contact between people in far-flung corners of the world, new social relations and subjectivities have emerged that extend far beyond the conventional dyad of the doctor-patient relationship. The new forms of social experience coalescing around biomedical technologies and therapies offer us a critical opportunity to explore the interactions between biological and cultural processes.[4] Researchers studying the social uses of DNA have high-lighted the new relationships and subjectivities engendered by genetic knowledge (Rabinow 1996, 1999; Simpson 2000; Novas and Rose 2000; Rapp, Heath, and Taussig 2001; Lee, Mountain, and Koenig 2001; Rose 2007; Wagner 2008; Sleeboom-Faulkner 2010; Montoya 2011; TallBear 2013).[5] But more than half a century after James Watson and Francis Crick discovered the chemical structure of DNA (in 1953) and over a decade since the completion of the Human Genome Project (in 2003), new modes of analysis are being devised as scientists move beyond sequencing DNA and identifying genes to integrating them with the cellular mechanisms of life. In his testimony supporting stem cell research before the U.S. Senate Committee on Health, Education, Labor and Pensions on September 5, 2001, Harvard biologist Douglas Melton (founding director of the Harvard Stem Cell Institute) urged senators to remember that "the unit of life is not DNA nor the gene, but rather the unit of life is the cell. . . . Whereas the last century of biology can be said to have focused on the gene and the sequence of DNA, I believe this century will see biologists come to understand and harness the unit of life: the cell, specifically stem cells" (Melton 2001). Social scientists working at the intersection of anthropology and science studies have examined the ramifications of these new cellular forms of life in the contexts of laboratory culture (Landecker 2007; Hogle 2010), animal cloning (Franklin 2007), and assisted conception (Franklin 2013).

As the cell displaces the gene as the central unit of analysis for both biomedical researchers and social scientists in the twenty-first century, we need to rethink how an alternative form of biological knowledge is reshaping human relations and futures.[6] Two decades ago, Paul Rabinow (1996, 1999) launched a deluge of exciting anthropological scholarship on the formation of new collectivities around shared genetic markers. But what different forms of biosociality emerge when we shift our analytical focus from deterministic "markers of identity" to dreams of "pluripotency"? As Aditya Bharadwaj notes in his comprehensive review of anthropological engagements with stem cells in the first decade of the new millennium, a proliferating body of anthropological work has begun to recognize the importance of "theoretically unpack[ing] and ethnographically illustrat[ing] cultures of stem cells both as a medium for gestating cellular form as well as a new medium for exploring ideas about life, knowledge, commerce, governance, and ethics" (2012, 304–5). Rather than the splintering of divergent interest groups along various genetic differences and restriction loci, I argue in this book that the hope embodied by emerging cellular therapies is rallying together disparate groups that may never have come into contact otherwise— from Beijing nurses and former mayors in South Dakota to Kuwaiti princes, Dutch grandmothers, and military-trained Chinese surgeons.

While the Human Genome Project engendered metaphors of a "master plan" or "the book of life" determining our identity (Nelkin and Lindee 2004 [1995]; Kay 2000; Fox Keller 2000), regenerative medicine in the twenty-first century offers a different outlook on human life.[7] Stem cell science and its application in regenerative medicine promise the exciting possibility of transforming our destinies. Endowed with the twin capacities of renewing themselves and differentiating into other cell types in the body (the scientific definition of "pluripotency"), stem cells have proliferated in scientific, economic, and social imaginations.[8] Described as "one of the most fascinating areas of contemporary biology" by the National Institutes of Health (2015), stem cells hold enormous potential for unlocking the secrets of embryonic development and for restoring diseased, damaged, or aging cells and tissues in the human body—the holy grail of the broader field of regenerative medicine. In a fact sheet intended to educate the public on the past, present, and future of regenerative medicine, the U.S. National Institutes of Health (2010) asks us to "imagine a world where there is no donor organ shortage, where victims of spinal cord injuries can walk, and where weakened hearts are replaced. This is the long-term promise of regenerative medicine." The power of the stem cell thus lies in its potential—from producing neurons to generating new organs and replacing failing body parts. As a creative entity with the capacity of transforming itself into seemingly endless possibilities, the stem cell can be understood as the biological instantiation of hope itself.

Hope has been a key analytic for social scientists who study biomedicine and biotechnology.[9] Drawing on her work on the culture of American clinical oncology, Mary-Jo DelVecchio Good suggests that the "political economy of hope" (Good et al. 1990) generated by biotechnology envelops all of us in a "biotechnical embrace" (Good 2001) that leads patients suffering from cancer to pursue experimental therapies and encourages nations to invest billions in medical research. Carlos Novas (2006) examines the "capitalization" of hope by analyzing the efforts of patient advocacy groups that have accelerated research initiatives for rare genetic disorders. Comparing the genomics research industry in the United States and India, Kaushik Sunder Rajan (2006) has articulated the "promissory horizon" of biotechnology as both a "therapeutic realization" on the level of personalized medicine and a "commercial realization" for corporate, academic, and state actors.[10] These approaches emphasize both the financial and affective dimensions of biotechnology by showing how hope in the possibility of a cure is linked to the public and private funding of research, the professional ambitions of scientist-clinicians, the business dreams of entrepreneurs, and the subjective experiences of patients and their families.[11]

The proliferation of clinics offering experimental stem and fetal cell therapies in China capitalizes on the biological potentiality to sell imagined futures in which damaged tissue may be regenerated, lost function may be regained, and previously irreparable organs may even heal themselves. For patients from North America and Europe, these new forms of experimental biomedicine circulating in China leverage their expectations of familiarity for biomedical treatment with the radical othering of a different cultural, legal, and ethical context to produce new horizons of hope. While pursuing the latest technological advances in regenerative medicine abroad, these patients simultaneously circumvent the legal restrictions and ethical qualms stymieing stem and fetal cell research in their home countries. These experimental fields of activity ultimately deepen our understanding of the political and moral economy of hope by illuminating the ways in which regenerative medicine intersects with technology, travel, and the political economies of health care and medical research in a global era.

THE GEOPOLITICS OF STEM CELL SCIENCE AND FETAL TISSUE RESEARCH

The biomedical odysseys documented in this book have been enabled by differing political climates, regulatory regimes, religious values, ethical controversies, and financial considerations in various countries. In Europe, a diverse regulatory continuum has ranged from the outright ban of research on embryos in Austria (Austrian Bioethics Commission 2009), to the criminalization of embryonic stem cell derivation within German borders but permission to import cell lines from other countries (Germany Federal Law Gazette 2002), to British authorization for creating human embryos for research purposes including cloning (United Kingdom 2008).[12] The Catholic Church has played a key role in exerting political pressure on European Parliament members to oppose the use of human embryos in medical science (Pontifical Academy for Life 2000; Minkenberg 2002; Salter and Salter 2007).

In the United States, advances in stem cell science have collided with political and religious controversies surrounding the moral status of the embryo. Although American researchers were the first to cultivate human embryonic stem cell lines successfully in 1998 (Thomson et al. 1998; Shamblott et al. 1998), the excitement surrounding the therapeutic potential of stem cell science ran headlong into President George W. Bush's 2001 executive order restricting federal funding for stem cell research involving the destruction of human embryos (Bush 2001). Although individual states—most notably California (Benjamin 2013; Thompson 2013)—tried to fill the gaps with state-level funding initiatives, the restrictive federal policies stoked fears of a "brain drain" of stem cell researchers to other countries with more welcoming policies (Kahn 2001; BBC 2001; Watt 2006; Longstaff et al. 2013; Thompson 2013).[13] Scientists have not been the only ones looking beyond American borders. The therapeutic potential of stem cells has conjured up previously unimaginable hope for suffering patients awaiting regeneration and repair of damaged body parts. Frustrated by regulatory restrictions and the slow pace of research, increasing numbers of American patients have decided to take matters into their own hands by traveling abroad to other countries such as China to obtain experimental fetal and stem cell therapies.

While pro-life lobbyists, religious fundamentalists, and "compassionate" conservatives have stymied stem cell research in the United States, the prospects for regenerative medicine look very different from the perspective of a country where abortion is a routine practice and where atheism itself is the reigning paradigm of the ruling party.[14] Responding to American religious and regulatory scruples constraining research on human embryos and fetuses, Chinese scientists and clinicians have leveraged a different ethical and legal terrain to offer experimental therapies not possible in the United States (Song 2011; Zhang 2012; Rosemann 2013; Sui and Sleeboom-Faulkner 2015).[15]

The practice of radically new and potentially dangerous therapeutic interventions in China has emerged at a particular historical moment, as a market-driven development agenda collides with the remnants of socialist ideology. From "serving the people" (为人民服务 *wèi rénmín fúwù*) to "getting rich is glorious" (致富光荣 *zhìfù guāngróng*), Chinese health care workers have found themselves caught between conflicting ideological slogans and institutional practices from different political eras. As the former emphasis on preventive medicine during Mao's era of collectivism has given way to a market-driven push for high-tech interventions and financial profitability, Chinese clinicians have faced increasing threats to their professional identities and their very livelihoods. These economic and political changes have heightened doctors' anxiety and sense of besiegement, but they have also enabled unparalleled opportunities for profit-making and success.[16] Accelerating privatization (Zhang and Ong 2008) and a growing sense of moral crisis (Kleinman et al. 2011) in the twenty-first century[17] are transforming entrepreneurial medicine in urban China on a transnational scale.

The Chinese party-state has sought to promote "scientific and technological modernization" (科学技术现代化 *kēxué jìshù xiàndàihuà*) as the engine for economic growth and its source of political legitimacy, encouraging scientists and clinicians to experiment with innovative medical therapies. The hype over stem cells and regenerative medicine has created new futures and careers for ambitious Chinese neurosurgeons and other health care professionals in China's urban metropolises. These urban clinicians interpret experimental medical interventions for foreign patients as their ticket to personal survival and professional success in an uncertain environment where increasingly profit-driven hospitals and restructured government priorities have left former state-employed medical workers to fend for themselves.

Differences in ethical values, regulatory frameworks, and politico-economic histories between China and other countries have enabled shrewd Chinese clinicians to attract patients from around the world. These transnational variations have opened up new promissory horizons for these clinicians and their foreign patients—who may not be willing or able to wait for the uncertain course of biomedical research to wind its way through years of animal testing and multistage clinical trials. Yet these same differences have also served as fodder for critique. Charis Thompson observes that the American scientific community has dismissed stem cell tourism as an "off-shore hazard to good science" marketed by "rogue" clinicians (2013, 118)—but she points out that "a rhetoric of

East versus West, or good versus bad science is much too crude and inaccurate (and, to many, offensive) to capture the geopolitics of the science or the ethics" (2013, 148). As ambitious Chinese clinicians have "surged ahead"[18] of their more constrained and cautious counterparts in North America and Europe, they have faced accusations of being charlatans who exploit desperate patients. Margaret Sleeboom-Faulkner and colleagues (2016, 241) have also challenged these "hackneyed" dichotomies, noting that the stark delineation between "bona fide science" and "snake oil traders" operates as a form of "boundary work" (Gieryn 1983) that establishes epistemic authority and claims scientific integrity for a small group of elite researchers while dismissing the rest. These suspicions must also be situated against broader anxieties about academic fraud (Lancet 2010; Economist 2013; Hvistendahl 2015) and contaminated foods and medicines (Chen 2014) plaguing intellectual and material production in China. Given these serious concerns, why have thousands of patients from around the world undergone experimental stem and fetal cell transplantation in China? My book takes on this question by following the science out of the lab and into hospital wards in order to examine the embodied dynamics and lived experience of clinical experimentation. I leverage an ethnographic perspective based on long-term, situated fieldwork to illuminate the stories and life trajectories of patients and clinicians on the front lines of regenerative medicine.

FETAL CELL EXPERIMENTS IN CHINA

The experimental fetal cell therapy sought by Jeff and thousands of other patients suffering from neurodegenerative conditions—and the central focus of this book—was developed by Dr. Huang Hongyun, a military-trained neurosurgeon based in Beijing. His experimental procedure involved injecting a suspension of cultured fetal cells around the area of neurological damage. The injected fetal cells were a special type of nerve support cell extracted from the olfactory bulbs of aborted human fetuses, a controversial source I will describe in more detail in subsequent chapters.[19] These olfactory ensheathing glial (OEG) cells had shown potential in laboratory experiments he had conducted as a postdoctoral researcher in the United States for restoring functional recovery in rats after spinal cord injury. Dr. Huang began testing this experimental therapy on Chinese patients with spinal cord injuries upon his return to the Naval General Hospital in Beijing in 2001. His initial clinical successes enabled him to move to a larger public hospital and eventually to set up his own regenerative medicine clinic based in a rehabilitation hospital in western Beijing.

Dr. Huang's experimental fetal cell therapy has garnered extensive attention from media outlets around the world, including China Central Television (CCTV 2002), the *Wall Street Journal* (Regalado 2004), *TIME* magazine (Forney 2004), the *New Zealand Herald* (Macbrayne and Rowan 2005), and the Madrid-based daily newspaper *ABC* (Mediavilla 2006), as well as prestigious scientific journals such as *Nature* (Cyranoski 2005) and the *New England Journal of Medicine* (whose editor-in-chief, Jeffrey Drazen, paid a personal visit to the Chinese neurosurgery clinic in March 2005). Many of these news reports emphasized the high hopes of patients, publishing glowing praise from the neurosurgeon's satisfied customers from around the world: "My husband's tremors ceased the day after surgery. He could shave by himself. He was ecstatic. My husband could barely talk, swallow or drink. Now he can do all of that," declared one American patient's wife to the Beijing bureau chief for Knight Ridder Newspapers, whose story was picked up by newspapers throughout North America (Johnson 2004). Other accounts portrayed the neurosurgeon with skeptical caution, suggesting that the procedure smacked of quackery: "Snake oil is not too strong a word," warned a disapproving neurologist at Northwestern University quoted in the *Chicago Tribune* (Lev 2004). Much of the media coverage oscillated between these extremes. As a journalist for London-based newspaper the *Guardian* proclaimed with biblical excess:

> They come to him in search of miracles. The lame, the sick and the dying; young and old; Christians from the US, Muslims from the Middle East, Buddhists from Japan, agnostics from Europe. Some have been in wheelchairs for years and believe he can help them walk; others are kept alive by respirators, yet hope he can make them breathe. The voiceless have heard he can bring them speech. The terminally ill seek nothing less than more life. In many cases doctors and friends advise them to stay at home, not to waste their money, and warn them of potential risks. For they come in search of one of the most pioneering—and controversial—medical procedures on the planet: the injection of cells from aborted foetuses into the brains and spines of the sick. And the object of their faith is a Chinese surgeon who spent many of his university years labouring as a peasant and is now conducting trial-and-error experiments on live subjects despite his research being rejected by the western medical establishment. (Watts 2004)

Dramatizing the life-and-death stakes of the controversial Chinese medical procedure, international media coverage tended to fluctuate between giddy talk of miracles and dire warnings about apocalyptic consequences. But the patients, caregivers, and medical professionals I met in the hallways of New Century Hospital avoided these sensational terms in describing their experiences. Most of the foreign patients preferred instead to speak about "small victories" and the incremental steps toward recovery they hoped to make: improvements in finger dexterity so they could grasp utensils and feed themselves; increased sensation in order to feel the touch of loved ones. This focus on the ordinary activities that their injuries and illnesses had disrupted rather than the sensational aspects of the procedure provided patients and their families with a practical framework for incorporating their extraordinary experiences in China into their everyday lives.

I follow these patients' lead by focusing on the everyday dimensions of hope that materialize in the grounded interactions of transnational biomedicine, from online debates about the efficacy of experimental fetal cell therapies to cross-cultural miscommunications on the operating table. Both patients and clinicians deploy hope in experimental medicine as a survival tactic to transcend the uncertainties threatening their lives and futures. The proliferation of high-tech therapies in China has become a fount of hope for patients worldwide suffering from conditions that have been written off as incurable in their home countries. But those who have entrusted their bodies to Chinese clinics such as New Century have had to reconcile the elusive promises of regenerative medicine with the corporeal experiences of undergoing experimental surgical procedures while navigating an unfamiliar health care system. Meanwhile, the allure of biotechnology and the globalization of medicine have also created new futures and careers for ambitious Chinese neurosurgeons and other health care professionals. The transformation of health care into a business, combined with an unpredictable regulatory landscape, has encouraged urban Chinese surgeons to experiment with lucrative biomedical interventions with uncertain therapeutic efficacy.

The Chinese fetal cell therapies I examine in this book can be considered experimental from both a biological and a regulatory perspective. On the biological level, Chinese clinicians are translating laboratory findings into novel forms of care as their foreign patients try out therapeutic innovations and develop new methods of self-tracking to monitor potential neurological change and functional recovery. This field of experimental activity in the biological realm is simultaneously accompanied by experimentation on the regulatory level as Chinese clinicians and their foreign patients engage in bureaucratic forms of practice that mitigate regulatory scrutiny and deflect charges of illegality. While Adriana Petryna (2009) maps out the contours of experimentality emerging from the opportunistic activities of pharmaceutical corporations offshoring their clinical trials industry to poorer countries, my ethnographic materials demand a different theoretical and ethical intervention on the experimental.[20] For people around the world with incurable neurodegenerative conditions who actively seek experimental cellular therapies in Beijing, the ethics, science, and politics underlying their transnational odysseys are not so clear-cut. As we will see in the following chapters, enterprising Chinese neurosurgeons and foreign health care seekers are coming together in new configurations and in new spaces, both online and in clinical settings in China's urban metropolises. Their encounters at the margins of medicine vividly capture the hopes engendered by new biomedical and communication technologies. By tracking these biomedical odysseys from cyberspace to China, my goal is to illuminate the moral, socioeconomic, and geopolitical fault lines of hope at the limits of medicine.

METHODOLOGY ON- AND OFFLINE

This book is based on a decade of ethnographic research on experimental stem and fetal cell therapies in China, including twenty-eight months of sustained fieldwork in Beijing conducted between 2004 and 2007 and several shorter research trips to various sites of experimental medicine in urban China carried out through 2015. The chapters that follow provide a detailed account of one of the most successful experimental regenerative medicine clinics to date: the New Century Hospital Neurological Disorders Research and Treatment Center in Beijing. Located in Shijingshan district on the western outskirts of China's capital city, this experimental neurosurgery clinic was housed in a former worker's sanatorium, hoping to become a state-of-the-art rehabilitation hospital. Typical of other state-owned health facilities in post-Deng China, New Century Hospital faced growing budget deficits at the beginning of the new millennium that encouraged hospital administrators to remake the neglected health facility into a profitable institution that could provide advanced medical services and new technologies to more lucrative patrons. Recruiting Dr. Huang Hongyun, the neurosurgeon sought out by Jeff and eventually thousands of other non-Chinese patients, to set up a regenerative medicine clinic played a key role in the hospital's revamped agenda.

The New Century Neurological Disorders Research and Treatment Center provided a crucial vantage point for researching the transnational dimensions of experimental medical treatment. Nearly two thousand people from more than eighty countries around the world have undergone Dr. Huang's fetal cell therapy procedure since 2001 (figure 1.1).[21] As a Chinese American anthropologist who spoke English and Mandarin fluently, I focused primarily on the experiences of the Chinese staff (including doctors, nurses, scientists, and administrative workers) and their English-speaking patients. With the help of dog-eared dictionaries, digital translation software, and interpreters, I also interacted with people of many other linguistic backgrounds seeking treatment in Beijing. By the time I started conducting my fieldwork, Dr. Huang had decided to focus almost exclusively on foreigners and treated very few Chinese patients at New Century Hospital. As I will explain later in the book, this focus on foreign patients reflected local institutional and financial motivations as well as larger geopolitical processes.

My ethnographic research methods at New Century Hospital included participant observation, formal and informal interviews, surveys, and textual analysis of medical and scientific documents. As other anthropologists who have worked intensively in clinical settings have illustrated so vividly (Garcia 2010; Livingston 2012), my work with the Chinese staff and foreign patients entailed forms of engagement that extended beyond the confines of a typical workday. I shared an office on the patient ward with a junior neurosurgeon and a neurologist, often keeping them company as they worked late into the night past their

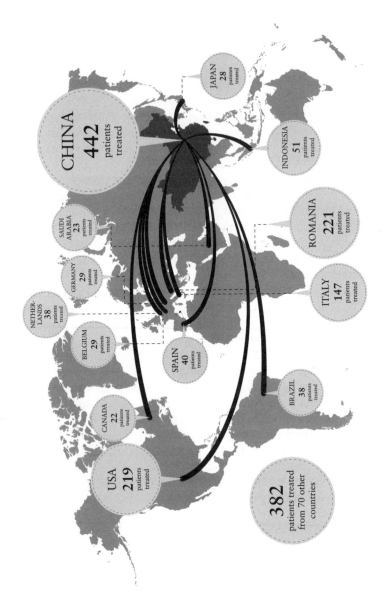

Figure 1.1. Geographic distribution of Chinese neurosurgeon Huang Hongyun's fetal cell therapy recipients by country of origin (map designed by Oikeat Lam).

scheduled hours. I lived in a two-room apartment in the hospital dormitory with the clinic's acupuncturist and the head cleaning woman, which enabled me to experience the dimensions of off-duty life for the clinic's employees. My proximity meant that I was called in at all hours to help nurses straighten out garbled "Chinglish" instructions to their foreign patients, plan impromptu shopping trips with foreign caregivers who had run out of snacks and entertainment options in the secluded hospital, coach administrative staff on their American pop culture know-how, place orders for digital pulse oximeters and mechanical ventilators, and edit research papers the clinical staff hoped to submit to prestigious international medical journals.

I complemented my research at New Century Hospital with shorter periods of participant observation at several other sites of elite high-tech medicine in China conducted between 2004 and 2015. These sites included the emergency department and "special needs" outpatient center at one of Beijing's most prestigious hospitals, a VIP treatment ward of a public hospital that was rented out to foreign businessmen in Shenzhen (China's first designated Special Economic Zone located just across the border from Hong Kong), an elite neurosurgery ward devoted to foreign patients at a for-profit hospital that eventually went bankrupt in Qingdao (another coastal city granted more flexibility by the central Chinese state in setting market-oriented economic policies), an orthopedic surgery department in Shanghai (my work there included accompanying surgeons on follow-up visits to patients with spinal cord injuries in the Zhejiang countryside), and the China Spinal Cord Injury Network (a consortium of medical centers in mainland China, Taiwan, and Hong Kong funded by the Hong Kong Spinal Cord Injury Fund and managed by the Clinical Trial Centre at Hong Kong University).

Online activities figured prominently in the experiences of the foreign patients and caregivers who journeyed to China for high-tech therapies. I quickly discovered that almost every foreign family who came to Beijing remained in constant contact with relatives, friends, and even strangers back home and throughout the world—via the Internet. They posted updates about their cross-cultural encounters to online discussion forums, uploaded digital videos that documented their post-surgical changes to journalists tracking their progress for viewers back home, and vented their frustrations about language barriers and hospital food on their personal blogs. Although their online activities often got bogged down by slow connection speeds or were even blocked by Chinese Internet filters (as with most popular blog-hosting services), many patients and caregivers spent more time in front of their computer screens during their sojourns in Beijing than they did hanging out with their hospital ward neighbors in the communal activity room.

As their mediated experiences bear witness, the Internet is playing an increasingly significant role in the lives of Americans grappling with challenging disabilities and terminal illnesses. The Pew Internet and American Life Project has tracked the "online health care revolution" since 2000, calculating in its inaugural report that 52 million American adults searched online for health information (Fox and Rainie 2000). These numbers more than tripled a decade later (Fox 2011). Another national poll monitoring online health behavior since 1998 calculated that these "cyberchondriacs" comprised 74 percent of the American adult population in 2011 (HarrisInteractive 2011).[22] Through the Internet, patients and their family members can obtain instant information on troubling symptoms from a variety of sources ranging from other patients' blogs to clinician-managed health websites, advocacy organizations' discussion forums, and pharmaceutical companies' social media accounts.

The Internet is not just a source of information, however; it is also a mediator of social experience. By broadening access to information on an unprecedented level and bringing people in far-flung corners of the world into contact with each other, the Internet creates opportunities for new forms of social engagement.[23] In the medical realm, ethnographers and digital media scholars have called attention to the Internet's role in transforming patients and their caregivers into active participants in the quest for health.[24] For example, people living with contested "sociomedical disorders" such as attention deficit hyperactivity disorder and chronic fatigue syndrome have taken control of their identities by sharing strategies online for dealing with medical bureaucracies unwilling to acknowledge their suffering (Dumit 2000, 2006). While living in a digitally mediated world can empower patients, it can also further entrench existing financial and technoscientific interests. The ability to access information online has intensified cancer patients' emotional attachment to high-technology treatment options, fueling the lucrative American oncology enterprise (Good 2001).

More recently, digital mediation in the health realm has encompassed a growing trend for individuals to engage in self-tracking and quantification practices. From wristband activity trackers such as FitBit to patient-networking websites such as PatientsLikeMe.com, these new forms of digital mediation are leveraging patient-generated data to drive therapeutic regimens and medical innovation. Olivia Banner (2014) observes that these digital practices of self-quantification transform contested subjective experience into legitimate statistical data. By tracking changes to their physical and mental states online, women living with fibromyalgia and other contested conditions generate hard evidence not so easily dismissed by skeptical medical professionals. Banner argues that this type of "informatic subjecthood" (2014, 199) is ultimately a Foucauldian project that transforms these women into biomedicalized subjects, encouraging a cybersociality that enmeshes them in biomedical discourses.

Whether emancipatory or hegemonic, these emergent forms of "biomediation" (Thacker 2004) warrant closer investigation as various biological conditions become increasingly refracted through digital modes of representation. As scholars of virtuality have noted, we must "disaggregate . . . the monolithic

medium called 'Internet'" (Miller and Slater 2000, 14) into its component technologies in order to understand the complex dynamics of mediation. What we
call the "Internet" serves as a convenient but obfuscating shorthand for an as-
semblage of technologies that enable but also constrain social action in particular ways. Seductive terms like the "World Wide Web" and "Information
Superhighway" make it all too easy to take the "global reach" of the Internet
for granted. But as Anna Tsing (2005) highlights with the metaphor of friction,
these connections do not happen seamlessly. In order to understand how "global
connections" emerge in practice, we need to take a closer look at how contingent
alliances and unstable interactions shape health-based cyberspace networks. A
key aspect of this analytical project involves understanding the form and function of specific digital technologies that underpin online activities, from web
browsers and email clients to online forum platforms and blogging software.
This approach dovetails with the "technological turn" characterizing studies of
the virtual (Nardi 2015), which examines how specific properties of different
technologies constrain and enable digital activity. These studies have also recognized the historical situatedness of these technologies, noting that the Internet
of today is different from the Internet of a decade ago (Karpf 2012; Nardi 2015).
As a loose collection of haphazardly connected nodes and affiliated technologies, the Internet enables a diversity of social practices, modes of representation,
and forms of interaction that must be situated in historical and technological
context.

Accounting for the online lives of my informants has demanded critical
innovations in ethnographic methodology and writing practices in order to
trace the emergence of new cultural forms and modes of biosociality online.
When I first began researching digital health practices, Mark Zuckerberg had
yet to launch Facebook. Although ethnographers were becoming interested in
the social implications and methodological challenges posed by Internet communication technologies (cf. Markham 1998; Hakken 1999; Heath et al. 1999;
Hine 2000; Miller and Slater 2000; Kendall 2002; Wilson and Peterson 2002;
Sveningsson 2003), many of the foundational ethnographies and handbooks on
virtual worlds and social media were yet to come (Taylor 2006; Boellstorff 2008;
Fielding, Lee, and Blank 2008; Gershon 2010; Nardi 2010; Boellstorff et al. 2012;
Horst and Miller 2012). The digitally mediated quests for experimental therapy
that I analyze in this book began in 2001, several years before the advent of
popular social media platforms such as Facebook in 2004, Twitter in 2006, and
Instagram in 2010. Without the existence of major social media platforms dominating the market, patients in the early 2000s leveraged a wide assortment of
online communication tools that I will examine in greater detail in the following
pages. Over the past decade, I have logged thousands of hours online participating in health discussion forums devoted to neurodegenerative conditions,
performing content analysis on the websites of hospitals and health regulatory
agencies, and studying the blogs of patients and caregivers who have chronicled

their experiences online. As I tracked the emergence of new cultural forms and modes of sociality online, the Internet became not only a crucial research tool but also a key subject in my ethnographic analysis.

The electronic archiving function of the Internet has given researchers unprecedented access to people's online lives—and raises critical questions about the ethical dilemmas of conducting research and representing others in a digital age. Although I observed some discussions about experimental medical treatments in China as they occurred online, the archiving function of many Internet discussion forums enabled me to reconstruct conversations and debates that happened earlier. My research in cyberspace often resembled more archival sleuthing than conventional ethnography. Unlike survey respondents and interviewees who actively agree to participate in research studies and sign consent forms acknowledging their status as research subjects, some of these online denizens became inadvertent participants in my after-the-fact study of their digitized activities. I struggled with conflicting obligations of research: Should I credit my sources as authors in their own right? Or should I disguise their identities in order to protect them as vulnerable subjects?

In navigating the ethical and methodological challenges of conducting research online, I have chosen to cite the source of materials that were posted in the public domain in order to give due credit to authors who wrote eloquent narratives and detailed explanations that they clearly put much time into crafting. Of course others typed out less careful replies, often in the heat of an impassioned debate. Site administrators of one of the main online health discussion forums I analyzed warned members that "everything posted on public forums such as CareCure can be seen by anybody and is often archived elsewhere on the Internet" (Young 2007). In my quotations of publicly accessible forum discussions, I have thus attributed this material to the online noms de plume under which members have posted their messages, rather than disguising them with additional pseudonyms.[25] Furthermore, I have reproduced quotations verbatim as they appeared online, without editing for grammar and spelling errors (with the exception of a few obvious typos that I corrected in order to improve readability). I also have kept the original punctuation and capitalization; quadriplegics using typing sticks controlled by their mouths often write in all lowercase letters since they can only press one key at a time. While some toil over multiple revisions of a single post, others dash off hasty replies in seconds, concerned more about getting their point across than following formal grammar rules. My goal is to capture the tenor of the online discussions as faithfully as possible in order to remind us of the embedded and embodied dimensions of Internet-mediated lived experience.

I recognize the fraught politics of knowledge production, in which my presence provides an additional degree of legitimacy to the experimental enterprises I describe in this book. Over the past decade, neurosurgeon Huang Hongyun has relished highlighting my institutional affiliations as an index for his own status. Although he always called me Little Song (小宋 Xiǎo Sòng) during private conversations and among his staff members, he enjoyed referring to me as his "American brand-name university Ph.D." (美国名牌大学博士 *Měiguó míngpái dàxué bóshì*) in front of visiting dignitaries—while toasting a municipal health official during a holiday banquet or shaking hands with a foreign scientist touring the facilities, for example. To resist being co-opted by other people's agendas, I have thus chosen to use a selective mix of actual names, online screen names, and pseudonyms for the institutions and clinicians I discuss in this book. This has also served as a strategic way to balance often conflicting norms of scholarly acknowledgment and the protection of my interlocutors' privacy. While determined readers may be able to deduce the identities of some of the pseudonymous individuals and institutions discussed in this book, I maintain the fiction of pseudonymity in order to keep their names from being indexed on search engines and out of general circulation. I do this for two important reasons: first, to avoid serving as an unwitting mouthpiece for these experimental clinics' marketing departments, and second, to provide the involved parties with plausible deniability. Given the renewed crackdown on corruption and the growing censorship dragnet implemented by Chinese president Xi Jinping, anthropologists and our interlocutors working in China face heightened stakes of disclosure.

ORGANIZATION OF THE BOOK

The chapters that follow tell a story of how people facing devastating disabilities and terminal illnesses around the world have sought fetal cell transplantation surgery from enterprising neurosurgeons in China.[26] As I have already begun to show, the conjunction of Internet-based communication technologies and market-driven health care reforms has enabled a global search for high-tech cures stretching from computer screens in Colorado to hospital wards in Beijing. Part 1 of this book, "Online Mediations," theorizes the digital mediation of health-seeking by exploring how and why American and European patients with spinal cord injuries and neurodegenerative diseases have pursued experimental fetal cell transplantation in Beijing. Over the next three chapters, I highlight the ways in which different Internet communication technologies have transformed patient activism in a transnational era.

Chapter 2, "Mobilizing the Paralyzed Online," traces the spatial and temporal dynamics of CareCure—an online discussion forum devoted to research and treatment for spinal cord injury (SCI). Created from a U.S. neuroscientist's experiment in caring and curing, the CareCure website links the scientific pursuit of the cure with the construction of a community for those living and dealing with SCI. The cybersociality engendered by CareCure has produced a new form of mobility that might otherwise be lost in the offline, visceral world of chronic paralysis. I demonstrate how this virtual forum has fostered a technologically mediated social movement of patients, families, researchers, and doctors who pursue experimental therapies for conditions considered incurable by conventional medicine.

Chapter 3, "Cyberanatomies of Hope," explores how the embodied dynamics of illness and chronicity shape online modes of health-seeking by comparing the experiences of people living with spinal cord injuries to those of people suffering from amyotrophic lateral sclerosis (ALS). As diverse biological conditions become increasingly mediated by digital modes of representation, these emergent forms of "biomediation" (Thacker 2004) catalyze new hopes and possibilities for those seeking to challenge orthodox prognoses and bodily limitations. While the chronic nature of SCI enables the formation of robust and stable online communities such as CareCure, the cybersociality cultivated by people living with the immediate threat of ALS is much more contingent and ephemeral. The kinds of social connections forged online in turn shape the forms of mobilization and digital pathways to experimental medicine.

Chapter 4, "Where the Virtual Becomes Visceral," explores how the online and offline experiences of illness and mobilization converge and collide on the operating table and in the corridors of Huang's experimental neurosurgery clinic in Beijing. I follow the digitally mediated trajectories of several American and European patients who underwent experimental fetal cell transplantation, providing ethnographic insight into their embodied experiences of transnational health-seeking. By comparing these distinctive digital pathways to experimental biomedicine, the chapters in part 1 illuminate how dynamics of illness and chronicity map onto patterns of endurance and ephemerality that characterize different forms of digital technology. I ultimately show how various modes of mediation open up alternative horizons of hope for those facing incurable neurological catastrophes.

Part 2 of this book, "Chinese Experiments," shifts perspective to consider these transnational encounters from the standpoint of the Chinese clinicians. I examine how urban medical entrepreneurs have responded to the proliferating political uncertainties and economic anxieties in a complex regulatory landscape where rules are flexibly interpreted and arbitrarily enforced. The experimental forms of health care that they practice are turning China's urban medical system into a laboratory for entrepreneurial tactics.

Chapter 5, "Medical Entrepreneurs," examines how changes in the political economy of health care have encouraged enterprising Chinese clinicians to experiment with lucrative biomedical interventions for foreign patients. I follow the career trajectory of New Century Hospital's lead neurosurgeon, Dr. Huang Hongyun, and contrast his experiences with those of other clinicians in order to illustrate the ethnographic contours of medical entrepreneurialism in urban China. Recounting their struggles to balance individual interests, professional ethics, and global ambitions, I demonstrate how the pursuit of high-tech therapies by medical entrepreneurs is not just about making money but also about professional ambitions and nationalistic pride—a cultural phenomenon I frame as technonationalism.

Chapter 6, "Borderline Tactics," takes a closer look at the institutional practices that have enabled medical entrepreneurs such as Huang to survive and even thrive in the fluctuating regulatory regime of China's emergent "market socialism." Rather than producing better modes of governance, formal regulation has encouraged experimental practices that circumvent administrative oversight. Facing increasing challenges to their professional identities and their very livelihoods, Huang and his compatriots deploy myriad borderline tactics ranging from exploiting bureaucratic loopholes to capitalizing on technological advances in order to evade government scrutiny and attract new patients. These experimental forms of health care are pushing the limits of medical practice as they remake the boundaries between public and private, legal and illegal, ethical and unethical.

Part 3 of this book, "Heterogeneous Evidence," focuses attention on the ethics and epistemology of clinical experimentation. The transition from laboratory bench to hospital bed is happening at an accelerated pace in post-Deng China, with increasing numbers of new treatments being tested on patients. Researchers and regulators in the United States and Europe have lambasted Chinese practitioners for moving too quickly into human therapies without subjecting their treatments to the rigors of evidence-based medicine. These Chinese clinicians are being framed as charlatans preying upon the desperation of patients by detractors who critique them for failing to produce proof in the form of placebo-controlled clinical trials. I provide ethnographic insight on how New Century clinicians and patients are interpreting signs of evidence, negotiating standards of proof, and resolving questions of efficacy in the transnational realm of experimental medicine. Chapter 7, "Seeking Truth from Facts," investigates how Chinese neurosurgeons are navigating the line between quackery and gold standard. I examine these Chinese clinicians' efforts to develop viable alternatives to the hegemonic discourse of randomized controlled trials. Chapter 8, "i-Witnessing," focuses on foreign patients' methods of assessing whether the experimental procedure worked. The forms of knowledge they produce both on- and offline offer a poignant challenge to what counts as expertise and data in the quest for "evidence" in experimental medicine.

The epilogue reflects on the ways in which the biomedical odysseys documented in the book open up important questions about the contours of experimentality and the proliferating hopes generated by transnational regenerative medicine. I return to the metaphor of "cutting edge" in order to illuminate how the experiences of Chinese neurosurgeons and their foreign patients deepen our understanding of the multiple and material ways in which hope transforms technology, travel, and the political economies of health care and medical research in a digitally mediated world.

PART I

ONLINE MEDIATIONS

_____

PLANET PARALYZED

A THREAD EXCERPT FROM CARECURE, an online discussion forum devoted to spinal cord injury:

MORGAN: Yo, like I dont want to kill nobody's enthusiasm, but all you people's putting in your little dippy comments and all, like I thought we was gonna get a blow by blow account of the man over in Beijing and instead alls we get is one after the other insipid little comments from y'all standin on the sidelines and gawkin. Lets not water this thread down and get all like distracted with empty nothings. Gimminy, his experience be more important than everybody's effin 2 cents. Just my 2 cents. (2003a)

JMUBLUEDUCK: it's called encouragement & support, Morgan. He needs it more than we need *this single thread* to only deliver news for us to us. (2003c)

MORGAN: Hey jumbledick, all's I'm sayin is this is the most interestin shit to happen to Carecure in years and especially this thread and yet we gotta weed through all this fluff. I'm just sayin let the man speak and report, IF HE WANT TO. If he don't, cool, but I be urgent and livin and dyin over every one of his reports. I don't think he need nobody's encouragement, jumbledick, he way past encouragement, he done do it!!! Jumbledick: name says it all. (2003b)

CURT LEATHERBEE: Hey [CJO], hope you are feeling better, Happy Birthday!!! Ignore Morgan, he is having a bad hair day. ☺ (2003f)

CAROL: ☺ Morgan I certainly understand how very interested you are in hearing [CJO]'s reports. But, I am asking you please, please let's keep this thread positive, without insults or name calling. If you want to vent your frustrations just start a new topic, that way no one, especially [CJO], will have to weed through the negativity. (2003)

GLOMAE: morgan, where the hell planet are you from? this thread is as much for support as information. if you don't want to read the support being sent then just go to the progress thread. (2003a)

MORGAN: Yo, I didnt realize I was bein an ass. Im sorry, CJO and y'all, I'm just like itching to get the eff outta this chair and I'm hangin on every word this cat says and yeah, I am havin a bad hair day, a bad life, like. I from the same planet you from, Glo, planet paralyzed. But I ain't here to fight with nobody, I'm just effin tired, big time. I'll just crawl back into my hole now and go away till Huang calls me. Damn if I wanted to piss anybody off, not my intention, I'm just achin for positives from Huangs procedure. Aching. But yo, I'm sorry, I aint into name-callin and shit, tho you like gotta think like my dyslexic ass do, I just read his name all effed up and stuff and damn if it dont come out all "jumbledick." Hey, to me I think thats funny, but hell you can call me what you like, I just dont want to be called "paralyzed" no mo. So I'll eat some crow and say "sorry, no mo" and let my man CJO say it all. Still dont think the boy need no encouragement, tho, true, we all need support. (2003c)

JMUBLUEDUCK: hehe, well that was a new one . . . glad I've got thick skin. I confess I even smiled at it. But geez, am I that wrong in defending the right to encourage this guy who ventures to the complete opposite end of the world into completely uncharted territory? the news will still come out either way . . . so calm down & be patient. (2003d)

GLOMAE: it's cool MORGAN i feel your pain brotha and if you were over there we'd be crowding this thread with support for you cuz that's how CC [CareCure] is we are like a big extended FAMILY. lol gloria all is forgiven. (2003b)

Conversation excerpted from the CareCure thread "Beijing—CJO's Big Trip" (*http://sci.rutgers.edu/forum/showthread.php?18117-Beijing-CJO-s-Big-Trip, accessed January 11, 2017*)

CHAPTER 2

MOBILIZING THE PARALYZED ONLINE

I FIRST MET LEO IN April 2006 at the New Century Neurological Disorders Research and Treatment Center in Beijing. Although this was our first face-to-face encounter, we had corresponded via email for over a year. Paralyzed from the chest down in a motorcycle accident in 1976, the fifty-year-old American had been a tireless advocate for disability rights for nearly three decades. He had even served as the mayor of his hometown in South Dakota, after successfully campaigning for improved social services. A few years earlier, however, he had discovered CareCure, an Internet discussion forum devoted to research and treatment for spinal cord injury. Online information about scientific breakthroughs and promising therapies overturned the medical dogma he had been taught—that adult nerve cells in the brain and spinal cord were incapable of regenerating. As a Chinese nurse helped him peel a banana, Leo explained, "I was actively involved in leadership roles in national disability organizations, but CareCure opened my eyes. Information was being stifled—it was a matter of job security for the disability advocates; they weren't doing anything about finding a cure for paralysis . . . I never had a clue that researchers were working on the problem, that it wasn't a matter of if, but when." Unlike the static newsletters published by disability organizations he had been used to reading, CareCure's dynamic debates and active conversations infused him with excitement over dramatic new possibilities. He turned to me, still incredulous: "On CareCure, leading researchers answered questions from me—Leo from South Dakota."

These digitally mediated discussions on CareCure ultimately led Leo to undergo fetal cell transplantation surgery in Beijing: "Rats were walking. . . . Enough of the rats. Let's get it on! I was reading about results from China, but [the disability advocates] wouldn't believe me. I knew I had to come over here and show them. They had to see a living example that return was possible. I couldn't wait to go up and shake their hands. Guess what, guys? I can feel that now." Huang's experimental procedure helped Leo regain sensation in his arms, something that he had not felt in the thirty years since his injury. "It took me a while to raise the money," Leo noted, but generous donations from family, community supporters back home, and sympathetic online compatriots enabled him to become the fifteenth foreign patient (and 391st patient overall) to receive the experimental procedure in April 2004. Leo was now back in Beijing two years later at the invitation of Dr. Huang, who paid for the South Dakotan's return trip in order to conduct a follow-up assessment. In addition to participating in the clinic's post-surgical evaluation study, Leo had agreed to endure another arduous thirty-hour journey to Beijing in order to consider the possibility of launching his own patient support service for foreigners seeking the experimental Chinese therapy. Leo declared: "This has been an opportunity to make liars out of what the doctors told me, that I would be paralyzed for life. The Internet is bringing all this together. It's the most powerful tool of the cure movement." For Leo, CareCure revolutionized his life, transforming him from disability advocate to cure crusader.

As Leo explained to me during his return trip to Beijing, digital communication technologies are playing an increasingly significant role in the lives of Americans grappling with catastrophic disabilities and terminal illnesses. In this chapter, I first offer a brief genealogy of online health forums in the United States in order to provide historical grounding for how an alternative mode of patient-driven knowledge production has arisen through digital mediation. I then dissect the digital architecture of the CareCure forum in order to show how the underlying structure and function of the technological platform create a novel form of sociality. The spatial and temporal dimensions of online interaction play an important role in shaping the dynamics of community formation for this group of people living with spinal cord injuries. In the second half of the chapter, I examine how this emergent cybersociality has catalyzed what Leo describes as the "cure movement"—a technologically mediated social movement of patients, families, researchers, and clinicians who pursue experimental treatments for conditions considered incurable by conventional medicine. For those living on "Planet Paralyzed," the cybersociality engendered by online patient forums such as CareCure produces alternative practices of mobility that might otherwise be lost in the offline, visceral world of physical paralysis. Instead of languishing in isolation, CareCure members have the opportunity to investigate and even contribute to the latest advances in spinal cord injury research and treatment through their participation in the online forum. CareCure members' pursuit of fetal cell therapy in China offers one of the most profound examples of how cybersociality mobilizes new hopes and possibilities for those seeking to challenge previous limitations and boundaries. I explore how this mobility is predicated upon a tension between the familiarity of biomedicine and a radical othering of China's politico-ethical environment.

FROM ST. SILICON'S HOSPITAL TO E-COMMERCE DREAMS:
A BRIEF HISTORY

Online health discussion forums such as the CareCure website originated with earlier experiments in community computing known as electronic bulletin board systems (BBS). Popular in the 1980s before commercial Internet access became widely available in the United States, these networks consisted of a centralized computing terminal that accepted incoming calls from users who dialed into the system using modem-equipped personal computers. Once connected, users could retrieve information stored on the main terminal or leave their own messages for other users to read. Unlike Internet-based discussion forums, a dial-up BBS served a localized "catchment area." Users generally lived within the same geographic vicinity, since access required calling a local phone line connected directly to the central terminal.

American health professionals recognized the potential of these interactive information and communication systems early on. Tom Grundner, then an assistant professor in the Department of Family Medicine at Case Western Reserve University in Cleveland, set up one of the earliest computer bulletin board systems in 1984 as an experiment in community health education (Grundner and Garrett 1986). Laypeople could use their personal computers to call "St. Silicon's Hospital and Information Dispensary" and anonymously ask medical questions, which would be answered by a physician within twenty-four hours. With administrative support from the university, financial and equipment donations from regional telecommunications companies, and political support from municipal and state officials (Neff 1995), Grundner later expanded "St. Silicon's Hospital" into a full-fledged "electronic city" with a post office, library, government center, courthouse, school, and public square (which featured kiosks, polling booths, "cafés" for chatting, and even a "speakeasy lounge"). The renamed Cleveland Free-Net was the earliest and most successful example of community computing, attracting tens of thousands of people living in northeast Ohio (including this anthropologist as a middle school student) who could participate in the online city for the cost of a local phone call.

While St. Silicon's Hospital was predicated on a conventional model of health education in which expert physicians enlightened uninformed patients, the growing community fostered by the Cleveland Free-Net demonstrated the importance of computer-mediated communication in empowering laypeople to draw upon each other for knowledge, advice, and experience. Rather than relying on doctors for guidance and advice, patients and their families actively utilized these new telecommunication technologies to share information about their conditions, compare notes on potential treatments, obtain multiple opinions, and pursue alternative therapies.[1]

The Cleveland Free-Net developed during a time when the Internet was not yet a major business platform, but its alternative model of knowledge production has continued to flourish in the dot-com era of the 1990s and beyond.[2] The idea for an Internet startup company devoted to the spinal cord injury community initially arose from the partnership of New York–based neuroscientist Wise Young and business executive Mark Pinney, the wheelchair-bound CEO of an Internet publishing company. With high hopes of capitalizing on electronic commerce to support spinal cord injury research, the two men launched a website called SpineWire in 1999 at the peak of the Internet dot-com boom. The founders envisioned an accessible online interface that would provide the latest news and information on research, treatment, and lifestyle issues for people with spinal cord injury. SpineWire featured a popular discussion forum that provided users with the opportunity to discuss research on restoring function after spinal cord injury or chat with the SpinalNurse—the online moniker for a group of professional nurses hired to answer health-related questions on the forum. The linchpin of the site was an online store selling medical supplies and aids for daily living whose profits would be used to support research efforts selected by the website's users:

> The company would donate 10% of its revenues to non-profit organizations (including research laboratories) that would be chosen by the consumers when they made purchases. The theory was that this would provide a strong incentive for people to buy from the site and at the same time generate significant revenues for research. The radical idea was that the consumers would choose the research. (Wise Young 2001a)

In other words, the SpineWire project sought to connect the SCI community with research efforts through the mechanism of the market.

Although SpineWire successfully provided news updates and established a vibrant community-based discussion forum, developing a viable online store that provided a catalog of appealing products and enabled secure financial transactions turned out to be a significant challenge that required more extensive resources. With the backing of venture capitalists, the popular SCI online forum thus merged with another Internet startup company called CanDo.com in order to establish a broader platform for e-commerce transactions (CanDo.com 2000a). Seeking to make CanDo a more lucrative prospect, these new cyberspace entrepreneurs sought to expand the initial focus from spinal cord injuries to a more general disability portal to attract a broader audience. Sam Maddox, the editor of SpineWire's online newsletter, described the merger as a global alliance with the potential to encompass anyone with health concerns:

> If you think of SpineWire as a distinct nation—a bustling culture of people, resources and services for those concerned with spinal-related disabilities, then think of CanDo as a virtual globe—full of interactive communities and solutions for people anywhere in the world concerned with any type of chronic health issue. (Maddox 2000)

Whereas the original SpineWire homepage highlighted news and information ranging from the latest stem cell research advances to wheelchair basketball statistics, the revamped CanDo site took an explicit consumer-oriented approach to helping people with disabilities that emphasized their purchasing power. The new homepage offered "solutions for life with disability" by encouraging users to "shop thousands of products" from wheelchair umbrellas to featherweight aluminum reachers (CanDo.com 2000b). While some found this "handicapitalism" empowering compared with earlier understandings of people with disabilities as "charity cases" or "regulatory burdens" (Prager 1999), the crass commercialization of disability alienated others. In a review featuring disability-oriented websites to celebrate the tenth anniversary of the Americans with Disabilities Act, a *USA Today* columnist contrasted CanDo's "product-based solutions" approach with the heartfelt camaraderie she observed on another website for people affected by disabilities (Holmes 2000).

Although over twenty thousand people were visiting CanDo's online discussion forum by 2001, the modest e-commerce revenues they generated fell far short of the several million dollars that venture capitalists had invested in the project (Wise Young 2001a). Focused on the bottom line rather than community building, the new investors deemed the website a liability and decided to liquidate the company. They unilaterally took the CanDo website offline in June 2001, deleting hundreds of gigabytes of user-contributed content.

Losing the online home(page) of their virtual community was even more worrying for users than having their information erased, however. Wise Young, the neuroscientist who had helped establish the original SpineWire, captured the distress of the community that had formed around the website:

> It is hard for me to bear. In the last few hours, many people have been posting their farewells to each other on the forums, leaving their email addresses so that they can remain in touch. It is like a boat sinking and everybody is getting into his or her lifeboat, desperately hugging each other and exchanging goodbyes. (Wise Young 2001a)

The shuttering of the SpineWire/CanDo project offers a cautionary tale to temper the often overblown promises of an Internet-enabled utopian future. While the Internet has democratized access to information, the broken links and bankrupt enterprises that have followed in its wake pose significant challenges to community building and political mobilization. Information from around the world can be accessed instantaneously through the Internet, but it can disappear just as easily—as the demise of SpineWire so painfully underscored for its members. Although the failure suggests the fragility of online communities built upon corporate whims, the emotional response of participants over the loss of their website underscores the important role that this virtual community played in their lives.

Burned by the fallout from the dot-com bust, neuroscientist Wise Young restarted the SCI community website on a Rutgers University Internet server in 2001. Its reincarnation as the "CareCure Community," hosted by a tenured professor at a major research university on a nonprofit basis, has given the new community more institutional stability than other Internet sites created, maintained, and hosted by private individuals or companies.[3]

CareCure—the website that inspired Leo to travel from South Dakota to Beijing for experimental treatment—has become the most extensive site on the Internet devoted to research and treatment for spinal cord injury. With tens of thousands of registered members who have collectively posted nearly two million messages since 2001, CareCure links together people with SCI and their caregivers, health professionals, and researchers.[4] In the following section, I take a closer look at the digital architecture of the CareCure website in order to understand the process of virtual community formation.

CYBERSOCIALITY: THE DIGITAL ARCHITECTURE OF CARECURE

The role of media technologies in creating new collectivities is hardly a new phenomenon. In his classic book on the rise of nationalism, Benedict Anderson (1991) analyzed the crucial role of print capitalism in establishing the "imagined political community" of the modern nation-state. As booksellers and newspaper printers across the New World and Europe sold cheap popular editions printed in vernacular languages, they created mass readerships that became aware of being part of a widespread but inherently limited community of fellow readers who shared a common print-language. Web-based discussion forums such as CareCure enable a very different configuration of language, imagination, and community building, however. Unlike static books and newspapers, Internet forums permit their far-flung readers to become active participants in multiple ongoing dialogues. This constant interaction (or even just the possibility of interaction) enabled by new digital technologies plays a crucial role in moving from the imagined national linkages emphasized by Anderson to the transnational cybersociality enabled by CareCure.

To understand how CareCure effected a transformation from an informational website into a bona fide community transgressing time and space, we need to take a closer look at how its electronic architecture shapes users' engagement with online content and patterns their social interactions.[5] This approach takes up Miller and Slater's call to "disaggregate . . . the monolithic medium called 'Internet'" (2000, 14) and enables us to evaluate just how "World Wide" the Web is for those living with paralysis. CareCure members participate in the online spinal cord injury forum by visiting the site's address on the World Wide Web at http://sci.rutgers.edu/ (figure 2.1). As a web-based forum, Care-Cure provides a communal "meeting place" for users to interact with each other in a publicly accessible location.[6] CareCure members read and write messages while logged onto the website, starting new discussion topics or responding to old ones. By collecting, displaying, and archiving members' messages in a singular and publicly accessible location, the CareCure website creates an enduring record of ongoing conversations that ultimately spatializes hope for its participants.

Only registered community members can post, but anyone with an Internet connection can sign up for a free membership or browse the discussions without enrolling. The open registration system allows people to create their own member identities. While some opt to use their actual names, others invent more fanciful personalities—ranging from CapnGimp and CrazyCracker to Wheeliecoach and Zillazangel. Thus users can decide upon the level of anonymity, disclosure, and veracity with which they feel comfortable. Individuals can also sign up for more than one CareCure account, potentially creating multiple online personas to represent themselves. Furthermore, more than one individual may use the same account, which sometimes happens with families who log in from the same computer. Thus CareCure member names do not necessarily represent distinct individuals. Since member profiles on CareCure are self-reported and optional, it can be difficult to get precise demographic information about the actual people creating the online accounts. But my ethnographic research suggests that the active membership is consistent with the demographics of spinal cord injury more broadly. According to the National Spinal Cord Injury Statistical Center (2016), the estimated annual incidence of SCI in the United States is approximately 12,000 new cases each year (or 40 cases per million population). The most common cause is motor vehicle crashes, followed by acts of violence (primarily gunshot wounds), falls, and sporting activities. Not surprisingly, more than half of SCIs occur among young adults in the sixteen- to thirty-year-old age group, and over 80 percent are men. The participants in the discussion threads I monitored consisted primarily of men with SCI, as well as their caregivers and family members.

The nature and extent of participation vary widely among members. An analysis of CareCure site statistics reveals that only a subset of the registered members actively contributes to the discussions. For example, a snapshot analysis of the forum taken on January 11, 2017, shows that 19 members had posted more than 10,000 messages each, 292 members had posted between 1,000 and 9,999 messages, and 1,120 members had posted between 100 and 999 messages; 26,642 members had posted fewer than 10 messages each, including 11,961 who signed up for accounts but had not posted any messages at all.[7] Still other users read messages but never register or write their own posts—these "lurkers" make use of the information without revealing their presence or becoming participants in the community. Some visitors might be more aptly characterized as "stumblers" who accidentally come across the CareCure site after being directed to a specific posting through a hyperlinked referral from another website or a search engine.

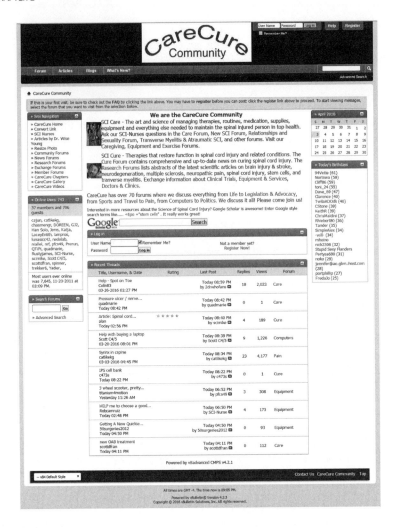

Figure 2.1. Screenshot of the CareCure Community homepage (http://sci.rutgers.edu/, accessed April 3, 2016).

Although the website is open to anyone in the world with an Internet connection, the dominant language is English and most participants hail from North America. Particular vernaculars continue to be key markers of difference and national identity dividing the World Wide Web into a patchwork of mutually unintelligible web pages. But determined participants can find socially or technologically enabled fixes to these linguistic challenges. On CareCure, for example, while the dominant language is English, multilingual participants often serve as the link between online communities that operate in different languages. CareCure members from non-English-speaking countries frequently translate important posts to online discussion forums in their own countries. BungeeEgg, for example, has translated information from CareCure into Chinese for members of the China Spinal Cord Injury Patient Forum (中国脊髓损伤者论坛 Zhōngguó jǐsuǐ sǔnshāng zhě lùntán). Free online language tools like the aptly named Babelfish website provide instant translations of entire web pages, converting between Italian and Chinese, Dutch and English, Spanish and Greek, and many other languages. I have used these automated translators to figure out the details of Dutch blog entries on stem cell research, for example. The results can often be quite comical: one online translator rendered the Dutch "stamcellen" into a puzzling "tribe warrants" rather than the more accurate "stem cells." However imperfect, these mediated approximations enable at least some Internet participants to share information across linguistic barriers.

The ways in which CareCure displays and organizes information also mediate users' experiences. Visitors to the website can browse nearly seventy public SCI Community Forums focusing on specific subtopics.[8] The signature Care and Cure forums create a crucial interface between treatment and research by bringing together information on "the art and science of managing therapies, routines, medication, supplies, equipment and everything else needed to maintain the spinal injured person in top health" with news on curing SCI (CareCure 2016). Dozens of other forums give members opportunities to discuss everything from politics and advocacy to recreation and sexuality. Moderators oversee specific forums, empowered with the ability to edit, delete, or move posts that they deem to be off-topic or offensive. They can also "stick" threads to the top of the list regardless of last posting date, indicating key priorities for members participating in the forum. In the Cure forum, for example, "sticky" threads included a "fundamentals crash course" on advocacy efforts to "speed up a cure," a description of current clinical trials for spinal cord injury, and a list of "ten frequently asked questions concerning cure of spinal cord injury."

This organizational structure creates localized groups of loyal participants attracted to specific topics. Rather than wading through hundreds of unrelated messages, members can jump directly into focused conversations of their choosing, thus fostering the creation of subgroups and subcultures. The topically stratified structure also helps incorporate new users into the community, who may be bewildered by the overwhelming volume of information on the forums. A New SCI forum welcomes people, families, and friends who have had a recent spinal cord injury, providing them with a separate space to ask urgent questions and receive immediate replies from experienced members. As neuroscientist and site administrator Wise Young writes to first-time visitors:

> The CareCure Community is uniquely equipped to provide information concerning acute spinal cord injury because over 70% of the members of this community have gone through the process, understand what is involved, and can offer in-depth advice and insights. (Wise Young 2003b)

From their first invitation, users are thus primed to think of CareCure as a community of like-minded (and bodied) people who share experiences and exchange information.

The sharing of information is the foundational mission of the CareCure platform, and this trumps even the protection of personal medical information and individual reputations. Although participants generally operate with the assumption that their screen names and contributions to thread discussions are matters under their own management, forum administrators ultimately retain control of members' information, from their individual posts to their membership accounts. Responding to member requests to delete posts or even their entire memberships, forum administrators dismissed this as

> frivolous because people have made indiscreet posts and have second thoughts about some information that have been posted or because they are upset or angry at people's responses to them. I therefore want to state the policy of the site concerning deletions of memberships, threads, or posts. Posts belong to the site. We reserve the right to keep, display, or delete posts for any reason. (Wise Young 2007)

Furthermore, CareCure administrators noted that they would not delete memberships of people who have already generated discussions with other members, because "this makes nonsense of other people's posts and the posts cannot be tracked by username" (Wise Young 2007).[9] In other words, the central purpose of the forum was to create an enduring record of information for a more broadly framed "community" that would endure over time beyond any individual member.

Several additional features of the electronic interface contribute to the development of a community consciousness among CareCure members. A special status box features members celebrating birthdays on each day, which encourages other members to post congratulatory messages on the forums. Another status box indicates the number of users currently online (including registered members and unregistered guests), and the website also lists how many people are currently viewing each forum. Registered members who are online at the same time can contact each other via a private messaging system. Members also know how many people are "lurking" on the site—viewing posts without officially registering. This list of fellow viewers heightens users' awareness of sharing a social space with others who are reading the same messages and learning about the same information. As one member commented soon after the feature was added, "It's great to see who is on the forum and to know you aren't out here alone" (mj 2002).

Within each of the SCI Community Forums, messages are grouped together in "threads"—series of replies stemming from an initial message. Members can choose to contribute to existing threads or post an independent message, which then becomes the start of a new thread to which others can reply. The forum software tracks and displays the number of replies and views[10] that each individual thread has received, which enables users to gauge the popularity of a particular discussion topic. The default display mode lists threads chronologically according to the date of the last post.[11] Visitors to a specific forum thus encounter the most recent activity first, which enables participants to find out immediately what is currently on the minds of other members. Not surprisingly, the threads at the very top of the webpage tend to attract the most number of replies as well as views, which creates a sense of momentum within the site as top-level threads take off and generate an increasing amount of interest.

LOGGING THE SPATIAL AND TEMPORAL DIMENSIONS OF CYBERSOCIALITY

The distinctive spatial and temporal dynamics of the CareCure forum play a key role in cultivating new social relations among people with spinal cord injuries. Tom Boellstorff (2008) has examined the dynamics of place and time in virtual worlds, focusing on an online graphical platform called Second Life developed by Linden Lab in 2003, which enabled users to create and interact with virtual representations of themselves and other people, objects, and places. Boellstorff has argued that placemaking is foundational to the experience of virtual worlds as "real" to their users—in other words, authentic, valued, and meaningful. This emphasis on place makes intuitive sense for the Second Life platform that Boellstorff studied, whose three-dimensional visuality enabled users to inhabit digital dwellings and create virtual landscapes that they experienced as homes and other places of significance. But what about a mostly text-based, two-dimensional platform such as CareCure?

I argue that the virtual "place" that CareCure establishes holds particular significance for people facing severe restrictions on their physical mobility. While some have been able to replace stairs with ramps, rewire their cars with hand controls, and install other assistive technology to extend their mobility, trying to get around poses significant challenges for many people relegated to a wheelchair-bound existence. The ongoing complications triggered by their injuries transform daily routines once taken for granted into protracted ordeals and pose significant challenges for venturing beyond their homes. CareCure's electronic forum system enables people based at different locations at different time periods to engage in ongoing conversations with each other. By collecting and displaying members' messages in a singular and publicly accessible location, the CareCure website creates an enduring record of ongoing conversations that creates a shared sense of community for its participants who might otherwise never have been able to meet given the restrictions on their physical mobility.

Furthermore, by archiving all messages, the CareCure forum enables users to retrieve and respond to messages posted from a minute to several years ago. Threads can stretch out over a period of days, months, or even years as members post new contributions and respond to earlier messages according to their own pace. This type of "asynchronic sociality" (Boellstorff 2008, 101), in which participants do not need to be present at the same time, plays a crucial role in community formation for participants living in geographically dispersed locales.[12] As the mother of a paraplegic son from Alabama wrote to a Hong Kong mother of a paraplegic son attending school in Vancouver, "There are no support groups around here so this site is wonderful. You all get me through the worst of days and nights" (bcmom 2003).

The spatial and temporal dynamics of CareCure thus enable a distinctive cybersociality among people with spinal cord injuries. By bringing together people who face similar challenges in a shared virtual space, CareCure provides a supportive environment for exchanging tips on self-care, commiserating about challenges, deriving comfort from others' encouragement, and countless other digital interactions that ultimately create a sense of a shared community among its users.

But as with most other groups both online and in the actual world, CareCure should not be romanticized as an idyllic community without conflict and disagreement. As users from the "Apparelyzed: Spinal Cord Injury Peer Support" online forum described their competitor's platform: "CareCure is an interesting place . . . sort of like a camping ground where gang wars are going on behind the scenes at certain sections" (WilliamCraig2007). Even CareCure's original founder and resident neuroscientist, Wise Young, bemoaned the frequent bickering and infighting that peppered the forum: "The first rule of the site is no attacks of other members. Unfortunately, many members break this rule all the time" (2010). Yet in spite of the eruption of personal attacks and even outright "gang wars," CareCure was still seen by insiders and outsiders alike as a distinct community. For the respondents from the Apparelyzed forum, this strong sense of shared communal identity at CareCure translated into a visceral feeling of exclusion for non-members:

> I certainly agree about the clicky [sic] type of feeling that I get when posting at CC [CareCure]. It seems to be a bit like Highschool—if your face fits then you are ok! lol, to be honest maybe it is because I am not a "gunho" cure-ite why I have trouble getting on there! Don't get me wrong, someone curing me would be fab, but I am not spending every waking minute and every breath obsessing about it. (kewlcatkez 2007)

Kewlcatkez's post suggests that CareCure's unique identity and the grounds for community membership revolved around a shared commitment to finding a cure for paralysis. Those who were not "gunho cure-ites" did not count as members of the CareCure community, even if they regularly browsed the forum and contributed posts. This impassioned belief in a cure constituted the most significant marker of community status for CareCure and was even embedded in the participatory forum's very name.

AN EXPERIMENT IN CURING

CareCure's founder, Wise Young, has played a crucial role in building the website as a community oriented around the search for a cure. He has single-handedly contributed nearly forty thousand articles and personal messages to the forums, devoting several hours each day to reading and responding to posts. Respected (and even beloved) by the CareCure community, the unpretentious founder posts on an affectionate first-name basis with members.[13] Wise is a fitting name for an eminent neuroscientist who was anointed by *TIME* magazine as "America's Best" in the field of spinal cord research (Kluger 2001) and chosen as one of the first inductees to the Spinal Cord Injury Hall of Fame (National Spinal Cord Injury Association 2005). Equipped with a medical degree from Stanford University, a doctorate from the University of Iowa, and clinical training in neurosurgery from New York's Bellevue Medical Center, Wise has conducted ground-breaking work in both the research and treatment of spinal cord injuries. He developed the first standardized rat SCI model that allowed researchers to compare results across different laboratories (Kwo, Young, and Decrescito 1989; Young 1993), helped discover and establish the drug methylprednisolone as the first effective clinical treatment for acute SCI (Bracken et al. 1990), and formed the first consortium funded by the National Institutes of Health (NIH) to test promising therapies for SCI. The director of neurosurgery research at New York University for thirteen years, he was recruited by Rutgers University in 1997 to serve as the founding director of the Keck Center for Collaborative Neuroscience in New Jersey.

Wise Young's commitment to both therapeutic help and scientific inquiry is reflected in the design of the CareCure website, whose two central forums, "Care" and "Cure," highlight the twin pillars of treatment and research in managing spinal cord injury. In particular, the Cure forum attracts the most attention from both registered community members and lurking visitors who scan the news. This signature forum consists of over 160,000 individual messages organized into more than 18,000 conversational threads. At any given moment, dozens to hundreds of people are viewing these Cure-related discussion threads. Members upload papers published in scientific journals such as *Nature* and *Spine*, discuss news reports on basic science discoveries in stem cell biology, and debate the significance these breakthroughs may hold for curing their paralysis. Some of the most popular discussion threads in the Cure forum compile lists of clinical trials happening around the world, providing members with opportunities to assess potential therapies, praise results deemed promising, or castigate the slow pace of research-oriented experiments.

Wise strengthens these online connections by hosting offline "open houses" at his neuroscience center at Rutgers. While these physical gatherings mostly serve those within driving range of New Jersey's flagship state university, some devoted CareCure members fly in from as far away as Chicago and California to attend. The Keck Center open houses enable members to meet each other in person and show off their talents, from modeling their latest creations in designer wheelchair fashion to sharing their triumphal stories of racing in ultramarathons across the Gobi Desert. ProfessirX, the Internet moniker of a spinal-cord-injured rapper, performs his tribute song "Bow 2 Wise" at the open houses on a regular basis, championing the achievements of his favorite researcher to the enthusiastic applause of the audience.[14]

Keck Center laboratory personnel provide tours of their wheelchair-accessible facilities and cutting-edge equipment, and doctors and scientists present talks on research results underscored by PowerPoint slides and testimonials from grateful patients. CareCure members who attend these open houses thus witness laboratory findings firsthand and discuss treatment strategies with leading experts in SCI research and treatment such as John McDonald, who accomplished what was widely believed to be impossible when he helped Christopher Reeve regain 20 percent of normal motor function and recover almost 70 percent of normal sensation seven years after an equestrian accident left Reeve entirely without motor or sensory function below the shoulders (McDonald et al. 2002). The question-and-answer sessions often extend far into the night. Those unable to attend in person can still participate vicariously, viewing digital photos and responding to detailed online updates from Wise and other CareCure members summarizing the open house events. As a visiting neuroscience nurse and clinical case manager from Virginia described:

> I have been in many research labs in my long life, and this is the most unique and special that I have ever been in. . . . The closest I can come to it, is the feeling I had when I was expecting babies . . . I am in this lab and I am always filled with the feeling that something very great will be achieved in this place . . . I keep meeting wonderful people there who are all tirelessly dedicated to resolving the problems that a spinal cord injury deliver to a person. When I am there, petty issues in my life melt off and away and I am constantly challenged and pressed by the need to continue my education and push my clinical experience in the right direction that would put me in the thick of the battle against this offensive injury. (Duramater 2002)

The pregnant expectations and hopes generated within the walls of the laboratory extend online through updates by members such as Duramater. The open houses thus facilitate community building both on- and offline while generating enthusiasm among CareCure members over the latest advances in spinal cord injury research.

Unlike earlier "patient education" initiatives such as St. Silicon's Hospital, the CareCure website is a participatory experiment in which neuroscientists and nurses are working alongside people living with spinal cord injuries in order to produce social and scientific change. As a senior CareCure member living with paraplegia in South Dakota speculated online:

> I believe Wise might be using these forums to conduct an experiment. The experiment is whether or not a group like SCI people can get together on a massive worldwide basis to learn about research, support research and raise money to promote research, and thus bring a cure faster. (bill j. 2002)

The active pursuit of and public commitment to finding a scientific cure are crucial features of CareCure that distinguish it from other patient support forums, medical organizations, and disability advocacy groups that help people living with spinal cord injury. Worried about giving patients "false hope," more conventional SCI researchers and physicians have tended to avoid using the word "cure." As Wise noted in a review of the scientific literature between 1950 through 2001 he posted for CareCure members, in over 23,000 articles on spinal cord injury, only 16 (less than 0.6 percent) referred to cure of the condition in the title or abstract (Wise Young 2001b). An editorial he wrote for the prestigious research journal *Science* addressed this fear of hope among his professional colleagues (Young 1997). Pointing out the long history of physicians who "have taken special pains to dash the hopes of people who have suffered spinal cord injury," he urged neuroscientists and doctors to adopt a more balanced attitude toward patients' potential for recovery. He countered his colleagues' overly pessimistic caution by citing basic and clinical studies that demonstrated the possibility of regeneration and functional improvement after spinal cord injury in both people and animals. As a researcher who maintained daily contact with people living with spinal cord injuries, Wise also gave them more credit and respect than did many other experts:

> People with disabilities are not so naive. Balancing hope and reality is a daily struggle for them. All people with disabilities have lived through surges of hope resulting from media reports of "cures." Many have adopted the philosophy of planning for the worst but hoping for the best. (Young 1997)

In contrast with the published scientific literature, a tetraplegic CareCure member from Australia vented his frustration with what he perceived to be the overuse of the term "cure" in popular discussions of new research advances:

> How many times have you heard of a cure, new cure, potential cure. may be, could result in or is a cure? How many potential cures have people seen in the last, say, 20 years? I am sick of all or any one "new" magic bullet [being] portrayed as a cure. All the fantastic hyped up discoveries like electric fields, 4-AP, magnets, schwann cells, stem cells, macrophages, exercise and lots more are not a cure on their own.

Therefore, I wish that doctors, scientists, organizations, media, etc stop using the word "cure" so liberally. I don't give a shit about your fund raising, science, research or membership numbers. Please stop giving me false hope and soliciting my money, support or whatever by using that word falsely. (Bruno S. 2002)

Bruno S. recognized the power of the term "cure" to generate interest, support, and ultimately dollars for researchers, clinicians, advocacy groups, and media outlets. His bone of contention was not with the pursuit of a cure but the indiscriminate use of the term as a form of false advertising. He felt it necessary to temper his critique with a public reaffirmation of his commitment to CareCure's foundational principle: "Before people call me anti cure or negative well I am 110% for cure. I still donate, support etc. It's just that I'd like some answers and hope people are realistic" (Bruno S. 2002).

Another CareCure member described his experiences grappling with the hopes and disappointments in spinal cord injury treatment advances as "the cure rollercoaster," noting that it "is not for the faint of heart":

One day up, the next day down. One day the cure looks like it will be here before we know it, the next day it looks like it will be twenty years. We all have to temper our expectations when reading any article. And the more we know the more we will ask the hard questions about any potential therapy. This is the only way to smooth out the ride. It's either that or get off. Some people choose to check in here only once a month. Others every few months. That way hopefully there will be something new to uplift them. Others choose to come here daily and just hang on and endure the peaks and valleys. We all have to do what's right for us. It's going to be a long haul. We need to buckle down for it. Some people adopt a twenty year time frame in their mind in order to keep from being anxious and disappointed all the time. We all cope in our own ways. Anyway, I feel the same pain as everyone else. We want it yesterday. (Jeff 2002, tetraplegic from New Jersey who moved to the Philippines)

Jeff's description of the "cure roller coaster" captures the affective state of people living with paralysis: immobilized by a sudden, life-altering injury and then confronted with the uncertain temporal horizons of a salvation that could be a few months or two decades or an entire lifetime away. CareCure helped mediate these emotions by enabling participants to express their anxieties, frustrations, and desires for a cure to their paralysis. Even more significant, CareCure members did not just think generically about the cure for paralysis, but they discussed, debated, and even tried specific candidates that had the potential of curing or at least bringing the community another concrete step closer to a solution. In the next section, I examine how CareCure mobilized users to evaluate and ultimately undergo an experimental fetal cell transplantation procedure in Beijing.

MEDIATING CHINA FEVER

China fever infiltrated the CareCure website at the end of 2002 with a report that Wise Young posted on an experimental fetal cell transplantation procedure developed by a military-trained neurosurgeon named Huang Hongyun based in Beijing (Wise Young 2002b).[15] Dr. Huang had conducted postdoctoral laboratory research at Rutgers' Keck Center a few years earlier, learning how to cultivate a special type of nerve support cell located in the nose. As one of only two areas of the central nervous system known to continually regenerate functional neurons in adults,[16] the olfactory bulb held particular promise for repairing damaged spinal cords. Scientists had discovered that olfactory ensheathing glial cells (figure 2.2), a type of support cell that wrapped around the olfactory nerve, attracted growing axons (Doucette 1984). They hypothesized that these olfactory cells (abbreviated in the literature as either OEC or OEG) played a key role in establishing a permissive pathway for the growth of olfactory nerve fibers (Doucette 1990; Raisman 1985; Ramon-Cueto and Avila 1998). Based on these properties, researchers speculated that OEG cells might also be able to create a bridge for damaged spinal cord neurons to regenerate across injury sites (Ramon-Cueto and Nieto-Sampedro 1994; Li, Field, and Raisman 1997; Raisman 2001; Fairless and Barnett 2005; Marshall et al. 2006; Ibrahim et al. 2006; Radtke et al. 2008). Huang pursued this tantalizing line of research in Wise's New Jersey laboratory, confirming that injecting OEG cells into the spinal cords of injured rats seemed to promote varying degrees of functional recovery (Huang et al. 2001).

Upon returning to the Naval General Hospital in Beijing in 2000, Huang worked on adapting the OEG cell transplantation procedure he had used in the laboratory on rats for a clinical study that would test the effectiveness of the intervention for human SCI patients. He performed his first clinical OEG procedure in November 2001, transplanting human fetal OEG cells into the injured spinal cord of a thirty-year-old Chinese woman.[17] Huang was the second clinician in the world to use olfactory ensheathing glial cells in clinical treatment. Just months earlier in Lisbon, a Portuguese neuropathologist had performed the world's first OEG transplantation procedure on a human patient (Lima et al. 2006).[18] But Huang outstripped his Portuguese counterpart in performing OEG transplantations since these initial clinical experiments. While the Lisbon neuropathologist conducted seven olfactory mucosa transplantations over the course of two years, Huang performed more than one hundred fifty fetal OEG cell transplantations in his first year (Huang et al. 2002; Huang et al. 2003). Wise spent five days at Naval General Hospital observing Huang's experimental neurosurgical procedure to investigate how research conducted on rats in the laboratory had been adapted for human clinical treatment. Wise reported to his CareCure audience that "most of the patients are getting some function back after the surgery," including increased feeling and a modest improvement in muscle movement (Wise Young 2002b).

As a research neuroscientist, Wise considered the underlying biological mechanisms that might explain Huang's clinical results. His speculations online to the CareCure community ranged from inducing placebo response and unmasking hidden functions to remyelinating[19] and even regenerating neurons—one of the long-cherished goals of the SCI cure movement (Wise Young 2002b). Since many patients regained function within just a few days after surgery, however, regeneration seemed an unlikely explanation for this immediate recovery. Much like hair, human axons grow approximately one millimeter each day, potentially requiring months to travel from the injury site back to the brain in order to bridge injured sections of spinal cord.

As a practicing neurosurgeon, Dr. Huang focused on generating clinical results. Although he had spent three years conducting laboratory research in the United States, his main focus upon returning to China now involved his clinical work as chairman of the Second Department of Neurosurgery at the Naval General Hospital, which had been established in recognition of his innovative procedures.[20] A surge of interest bombarded the hospital after a national broadcast by China Central Television featured his clinical successes (CCTV 2002), leaving Dr. Huang with a waiting list filled with thousands of domestic patients. His heavy operating schedule—which often included up to five open spine surgeries per day—left him with little time to devote to conducting painstaking laboratory work to confirm scientific explanations.

Wise described Huang's work to CareCure members as "a credible phase 1 trial"[21] that demonstrated the feasibility and safety of fetal OEG transplants and suggested some recovery of function (Wise Young 2002b). Despite these initial promising results, Wise cautioned that much follow-up work needed to be conducted in order to determine whether the functional recovery was maintained. Although OEG recipients might continue to experience long-term functional recovery as a result of regeneration, Dr. Huang lacked long-term data to determine this. This lack of follow-up data stemmed in part from the structure of the Chinese health care system. With the best hospitals historically concentrated in urban centers despite efforts during the socialist era to improve rural health care, China's afflicted developed a tradition of traveling for medical treatment. Chinese patients and their families often journeyed great distances and made significant sacrifices to seek therapy. As Dr. Huang's reputation grew, domestic patients came from farther and farther reaches of the country to seek his diagnostic skills and therapeutic help, returning home after exhausting their resources on the operation. Like many Beijing hospitals that treated patients from other provinces, Naval General had trouble staying in touch with these itinerant patients, making long-term follow-up a daunting task.[22]

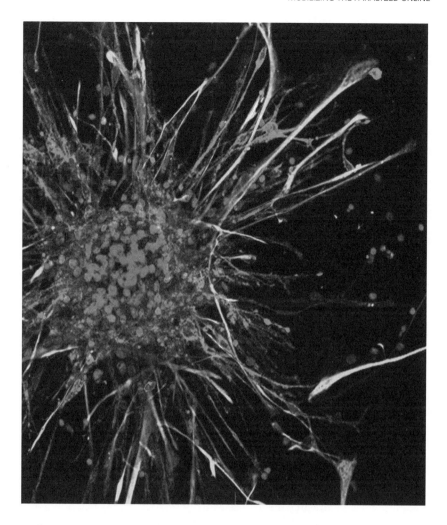

Figure 2.2. A human olfactory ensheathing glial (OEG) cell (Huang et al. 2009, 15).

SPATIALIZING HOPE ONLINE

Wise's December 2002 thread-starter describing Dr. Huang's clinical results attracted immediate attention from CareCure members, who responded with eager speculation over the possibility of a cure on the horizon in Beijing. While hope has most often been understood in temporal terms (e.g., as an orientation to the future, a state of not-yet, etc.), CareCure members also mapped out the spatial contours of hope in embracing China as a site of expanded possibilities.

Their online posts captured both their excitement over developments in China and the deep frustration many felt with the slow pace of clinical research in the United States:

> Seems that your China trip was very productive. Leave it to the Chinese to work out all the pitfalls. They have thousands of SCI patients to run experiments on without Gov't. regulations. They will have Phase 4 studies completed on OEG cell transplantation, before the US allows Phase 1. (giambjj 2002, applied science professor from Alabama with a tetraplegic son)

> When I was all about ready to forget about a cure, you showed the world it will be done. It seems your trip to [C]hina is proving more evidence that the human body wants to heal SCI easier than most think. . . . It seems these people can take leaps in progressing science compared to the US. (Felps 2002, paraplegic injured in 1992)

> I am just glad that they are doing what they are doing in China, they seem to be on the wild and wooly side when it comes to research/experimental therapies on people, and they don't have any religious nay-sayers badmouthing research either, which is great for us. With the safety conscious and generally restricted research in the Western world I suspect that China will be the first to come up with a cure if it is possible. Thumbs up for what they are doing there. (Andy 2003a, paraplegic from Chicago injured in 2002)

Contrasting China's "progressing" environment with the overly cautious mentality paralyzing American researchers, CareCure members such as giambjj, Felps, and Andy gave spatial form to their hope for a cure by leveraging the familiarity of biomedical science against a radical othering of China's "wild and wooly" regulatory environment.

This sense of hope became even more palpable on January 20, 2003, when Dr. Huang sent shock waves through the discussion thread by posting his willingness to take on foreign patients (hongyun 2003a). Dr. Huang had decided to leave the military medical system to work at Chaoyang Hospital, a major public hospital that served as the primary training ground for the Capital University of Medical Sciences. Located in the heart of Beijing's central business district near several foreign embassies as well as a McDonald's, Chaoyang Hospital provided a more accessible operating venue for both Chinese and potential foreign patients, as well as more flexibility for Dr. Huang himself to negotiate the terms of his employment.

The interest in Wise's China report had trickled to a halt just before Christmas, but Dr. Huang's post immediately hijacked the thread. The announcement set off a flurry of activity on the Cure forum, sparking eleven responses within ten hours that turned the abstract ruminations on research philosophy into concrete plans of action. A paraplegic engineer from Calgary proposed, "Now we need somebody to go give it a try and report back. I can offer a translator that lived in Hong Kong for 20 years if anyone needs it" (SCI PILOT 2003). There was no shortage of eager guinea pigs ready to take the risk on behalf of themselves and their fellow members:

> I am willing to take this chance and would document the entire procedure with regular Care Cure forum postings. Please e-mail me the translators name and contact info. (Schmeky 2003a, paraplegic engineer from Los Angeles injured in 2002)

> I would be willing to Volunteer and Document the procedure too. I am a t-4 Complete, 22 years post, in great physical condition. This is great news Dr. Huang. (Curt Leatherbee 2003a, forty-nine-year-old paraplegic from Rhode Island injured in 1981)

> C5/6 complete, 12yrs post from the UK also more than ready to volunteer and document. Just let us know how to apply and where to send MRI etc. (Andy C 2003, thirty-three-year-old British tetraplegic injured in 1990)

As CJO, who later became one of the first CareCure members to undergo OEG cell transplantation in Beijing, declared online to Dr. Huang: "I know that myself and others are very serious about having your treatment and you will find some good candidates here" (CJO 2003a). Some members even worried about the possibility of too many volunteers overwhelming Dr. Huang's precious time. Leo, the former South Dakota mayor turned cure crusader who had been injured for over a quarter of a century, chastised what he perceived as overeager upstarts cluttering the forum: "Ok you pups slow down! Hum, Seniority" (Leo 2003a). But he, too, succumbed to the euphoria a few days later, putting his name down on the growing list of volunteers (Leo 2003b).

Wise also tried unsuccessfully to urge restraint and encourage a more careful attitude: "There are indeed many questions that people need to be asking before volunteering for the procedure. Do people understand what the procedure is and what is involved?" (Wise Young 2003a). Although he listed a series of hard-hitting questions (involving complication rate, safety of transplanted cells, source of the aborted fetuses, nature of the rehabilitation program, best and worst results, and extent and duration of recovery), participants in the giddy discussion failed to pursue these pesky details with much interest. A few members did hesitate over the potential risks of undergoing the surgery, such as this forty-nine-year-old paraplegic from New Zealand injured in 1982: "I want to walk (and all other things) as much as anyone—I don't know if I could take the physical and financial risk of trying this procedure and I wondered if all you guys could" (Christopher Paddon 2003). Most of the posts from CareCure members, however, involved getting on Dr. Huang's waiting list or inquiring about practical details of accommodation rather than critical appraisals of the risks and scientific merits of the procedure.

Some years later, I asked Wise offline why he didn't more vigorously advise members to wait for validated results before risking their bodies, given his own critical stance toward unproven therapies and anger about "miracle cures" hyped by unscrupulous profiteers. He told me he constantly struggled with a delicate balance as the nominated champion for the scientific pursuit of a cure for SCI. As one of the founding members of CareCure, he had earned the trust and respect of the community built over years of research and tens of thousands of postings, and his opinions held much weight in the community. Yet members' ardent hopes for a cure and frustration about the slow progress of research easily turned against those scientists who were not being aggressive enough in pursuing potential solutions. CareCure members often branded many of Wise's colleagues as "lab rats" who did nothing for real suffering people, castigating "all the scams of false promises of rats" (Felps 2003). While longstanding CareCure members frequently defended him (e.g., "anybody who thinks the Wise-man is one of those lab rat types is mistaken" [Clay 2003]), Wise recognized that this support could dissolve in the volatile medium of an online forum, where any member could shoot off an angry response in seconds to complain about perceived injustices.

Voices of caution were submerged by a flood of posts from CareCure members expressing interest in being evaluated for the surgery after Dr. Huang posted his eligibility criteria for foreign patients to join his "clinical trial" (hongyun 2003b). Indeed, more critical posts were quickly challenged by those worried about offending Dr. Huang, as this exchange between two tetraplegic CareCure members demonstrated:

IP: What does three levels of recovery really mean? It would be great if the recovery moved in a clear, direct fashion down the spinal cord, so that use of triceps, and then hands would appear. But that is not the impression I'm getting. The impression I'm getting is somebody is able to jerk their leg, or now feels when their bowel is full. Why would anybody want that? So they can sit in pain for 12 hours until the personal assistant finally shows up? I personally would not want to feel that my bowel is full—at least not before i'm able to use my hands and do something about it. (2003a)

CJO: ip, Please don't show any negativity here. Dr. Huang has announced opening his trials up to foreign patients as a service to us. 3 levels would mean the world to some people, myself included. (2003c)

IP: I didn't mean my comment to be negative—just wanted to share how I critically think about whether I would go for this procedure or not. I am ecstatic that Dr. Hongyun is offering this procedure to foreigners. I am simply not brave enough to do it. (2003b)

With his "critical thinking" recast as "negativity," ip quickly retracted his cautionary attitude with an "ecstatic" endorsement, falling in line with the overwhelmingly upbeat tenor of the Cure thread. Few others ventured to raise substantive concerns.

The majority of posts came from members like Sfajt, a paraplegic from Houston, who declared, "Dr. Huang, I thank you so much for your willingness to help us. I am ready!" (Sfajt 2003). Between Wise's initial post in December 2002 and April 2003, thirty-five CareCure members publicly declared their interest in undergoing the surgery on the forum without any additional evidence for the treatment's therapeutic efficacy. Were all of these eager volunteers truly ready and willing to go to China, however? Schmeky, who was one of the very first to volunteer but ultimately never ended up going to China, explained his apparent lack of caution as a way to hedge his bets:

> My rational[e] is that if I (or anyone else) gets in line for this procedure, getting off a plane on Chinese soil is in all probability many months away. This may coincide with the one year follow up of those treated in the summer of 2002, at which point a more informed decision can take place. I envision that "if" results are positive, and you want to get this done in China, people from all over the world will stampede to Beijing. You probably would then be in for a long wait. This is why I am attempting to get my name in the hat. (2003b)

For CareCure members like Schmeky, this initial expression of interest was thus a maneuvering tactic for a better position in the impending stampede to Beijing, which was already beginning to occur even in the absence of more definitive evidence.

Indeed, others who were "100% serious" were already making concrete plans to go to Beijing (mk99 2003a, paraplegic CareCure moderator from Toronto who had undergone an experimental surgical procedure in Taiwan). The public Cure forum served as the primary method for interested members to establish initial contact with Dr. Huang, who was busy performing surgeries in China and only appeared online every few weeks. Further discussions with Dr. Huang occurred mostly along private channels such as email or PM (private message sent between forum members) as more committed members sent their MRIs and medical records to Beijing for evaluation and began making travel arrangements.

Although most public forum postings occurred asynchronously as members responded to messages according to their own schedules, clusters of related postings fed upon each other when members happened to be online at the same time. A determined CJO even tried using the thread itself to attract the neurosurgeon's attention: "Dr. Hongyun Huang, I notice you are online and I'm bumping this topic up in hopes that you'll contact me. Thanks" (CJO 2003b). Using the technique of "bumping," or posting to bring a particular discussion thread to the top of the list of active forums, CJO successfully caught the eye of the busy neurosurgeon and ultimately became one of the first three CareCure members to undergo the experimental procedure in Beijing.

CONCLUSION

Created from a neuroscientist's experiment in caring and curing, the CareCure website links the scientific pursuit of the cure with the construction of a community for those living on "Planet Paralyzed." By giving people with SCI and their families, clinicians, and researchers a virtual platform for discussing research innovations and building an extended community not limited by physical proximity, CareCure produces a new form of mobility that might otherwise be lost in the offline, visceral world of physical paralysis. I have examined how CareCure mobilizes users to challenge existing medical dogma and rally around new research advances by establishing a virtual space to engage collectively with these concerns. CareCure members' online discussion of Huang's OEG fetal cell therapy also illuminates how cultural difference becomes a resource in the process of pursuing hope. Contrasting China's experimental environment with the moribund state of American research on spinal cord injury, CareCure members concretized a sense of hope by leveraging the familiarity of biomedical science against a radical othering of China's differently situated regulatory regime. Spatializing difference becomes crucial to the formation of new experimental subjectivities in the unevenly globalized flows of capital, technoscience, and ethical norms. The opening up of virtual spaces for navigating those differences enables an explicit spatialization of hope predicated on the contrasts between different regimes of power and value.

This chapter has focused on the cybersociality and online mobilization of people grappling with spinal cord injuries. While CareCure serves as a rallying point for people living with chronic paralysis, those facing more acute diagnoses have turned to other forms of digital media. The following chapter takes a closer look at how the dynamics of illness and chronicity map onto different forms of mediation. I compare the CareCure SCI community with alternative digital platforms that people living with ALS have utilized to seek fetal cell transplantation at Huang's neurosurgery clinic. Paying close attention to the distinct timelines promised or threatened by various medical conditions, I demonstrate how different forms of mediation open up divergent horizons of hope for those living with dissimilar experiences of illness and paralysis.

CHAPTER 3

CYBERANATOMIES OF HOPE

In the next months we will see first hand accounts of [CareCure members undergoing OEG transplantation], and I will make my decision on whether to go or not then, but right now I kind of have the idea that I might be hopping a plane to China in my future. (Andy 2003c)

—Paraplegic CareCure member from Chicago injured in in 2002

It's precisely because the period of time available to us is so short that we are willing to undertake what we understand is an experimental procedure that may have no effect or only short-term effects. There is, after all, no alternative other than to do nothing at all. (Trophic 2004e)

—American expatriate blogger living in Moscow diagnosed with ALS in 2003

AS DIFFERENT BIOLOGICAL CONDITIONS BECOME increasingly mediated by digital modes of representation, these emergent forms of "biomediation" (Thacker 2004) catalyze new hopes and possibilities for those seeking to challenge orthodox prognoses and bodily limitations. In this chapter, I explore how the embodied dynamics of illness and chronicity shape online modes of health-seeking by comparing the experiences of people living with spinal cord injuries to those of people suffering from ALS. While the chronic nature of SCI enables the formation of robust and stable online communities such as Care-Cure, the cybersociality cultivated by people living with the immediate threat of ALS is much more contingent and ephemeral. The kinds of social connections forged online in turn shape the forms of mobilization and digital pathways to experimental medicine.

To illuminate how embodied experience, temporal dynamics, and mediated health-seeking are coming together in new ways, I will first take a closer look at CareCure members' online deliberations over the Beijing OEG cell transplantation procedure. As we will see, the eagerness or reluctance of different CareCure members to pursue experimental treatment must be contextualized in terms of the bodily reconfigurations and illness experiences delineated by each person's particular level of spinal cord injury—a phenomenon I characterize as "cyber-anatomies" of hope. I will then turn to an examination of how and why a very different group of patients have sought experimental fetal cell therapy in Beijing: people diagnosed with amyotrophic lateral sclerosis (PALS). Faced with a fore-shortened timeline of fatal neurodegeneration, PALS have employed alternative modes of digital health-seeking that involved poaching information from other websites, utilizing their own personal blogs to generate material support, and engaging in more private channels of communication. The distinctive ways in which people facing different illness experiences engage digital media technologies ultimately reveal the embodied dimensions of Internet-mediated quests for experimental therapy.

LIVING WITH CHRONIC PARALYSIS

The experience of spinal cord injury in the United States and other developed countries over the past several decades has shifted dramatically: from an acute cause of certain (if not immediate) death (Cushing 1927) to a chronic condition of paralysis for many (Bracken et al. 1997). As the U.S. National Institute of Neurological Disorders and Stroke describes in a fact sheet titled "Spinal Cord Injury: Hope through Research," this "revolution" in care has "greatly expanded life expectancy and required new strategies to maintain the health of people living with chronic paralysis" (NINDS 2013). This shift toward living with paralysis as a chronic condition has produced new temporal horizons for those living in the wake of SCI. While people who have suffered an SCI occasionally face acute complications that require immediate hospitalization, they more often deal with the everyday and ongoing challenges posed by chronic paralysis. Those who survive the initial catastrophic event face severe and often permanent disability. They must also adjust to a wide range of changes throughout their bodies as the original injury produces a cascade of changes in systemic physiology. Depending on the level of their injuries, many must learn to cope with ongoing bladder and bowel problems, sexual dysfunction, chronic pain, pressure sores, muscle spasticity causing uncontrolled jerking of their limbs, and/or autonomic dysfunction causing irregularities in blood pressure, heartbeat, and other involuntary reflexes. These bodily challenges are often exacerbated by dramatic reconfigurations in personal identity and social relationships.

The chronic nature of spinal cord injury meant that CareCure members needed to situate their considerations on whether to pursue experimental therapy in China along a much longer timeline. CareCure members each had their own complex calculus for deciding whether the potential benefits of the Chinese fetal cell transplantation would be worth the risks. Mk99 described making the choice "to go for it" as a matter of "reaching your tipping point" (mk99 2003c)—weighing the potential gains against the possible risks given one's particular physical, emotional, social, and financial situation. While best-selling author Malcolm Gladwell (2000) adopted this concept from epidemiologists to explain large-scale social phenomena in terms of "contagious" ideas and behaviors, mk99 used this term on a more intimate level to capture the decision-making process for individual CareCure members.

An online poll taken just before the first CareCure pioneers underwent their surgeries in Beijing illuminated members' thoughts on going to China for the procedure. Beaker,[1] a CareCure regular from Oregon who was following the pioneers' biomedical odysseys on the Cure forum with avid interest, set up the following hypothetical situation for members to vote on:

> If someone who was loaded offered to pay for you to go to China and have this surgery, would you:
>
> (a) GO!
> (b) No thanks, but I'd love the money to put a down payment on a house, make modifications to my current living conditions to make it more wheelchair friendly, purchase an iBOT, go on a fantastic vacation, go shopping, pay bills, or whatever you desire.
> (c) No thanks, but please give someone else the opportunity who does really want the surgery.
> (d) No thanks, but ask me again if/when the results improve and/or come to the United States.
> (e) None of the above. (Beaker 2003a)

Over the course of two days, a total of forty people voted before the poll was closed. Thirty percent chose an unqualified yes, although many more were interested: just over 42 percent chose to wait for further improvements before committing definitively.

CareCure's discussion-based format offers the anthropologist an unparalleled opportunity to examine how CareCure members negotiated high-stakes therapeutic choices. In addition to registering their votes, many members took the time to elaborate on their choices in the discussion thread linked to the poll. These attached discussions provide insight into the decision-making processes of members, revealing a depth of analytical sophistication that drew upon intimate knowledge of bodily processes, calculated evaluations of the available evidence, critiques of American politics under the George W. Bush administration, and even savvy predictions about medical innovations in the pipelines.

This particular poll focused on reasons why members might be hesitant about going to China, monetary issues aside. In other words, the poll assumed that wanting to go was the default choice that needed no qualification, while hesitation could potentially stem from many different sources. While these assumptions might seem skewed to the outsider, most voters shared the poll designer's point of view. CareCure members were part of a community devoted to finding a cure for SCI, and this placed them in a special ontological status compared with those who did not believe that a cure was possible. As one of the moderators noted, only 5 percent of CareCure voters chose to use the money for other purposes, and he speculated that this number would probably be higher among "non believers who just don't really seem to have much of an interest or motivation in Curative therapies" (Curt Leatherbee 2003e). As believers in the cure, the majority of CareCure members supported potential therapeutic advances in spinal cord treatment. For some, believing in a cure meant learning about and supporting research advances. For others such as Leo the cure crusader, it meant putting their own bodies to the test when a promising therapy became available:

> To me it was a no brainier decision, after years of shouting "oh to be a rat" someone said ok. Not long ago a SCI doctor said about one of our first guys "well he's just using them as guinea pigs" and at first I was pissed. Then I thought of the unknowledgeable doc who said it and thought yeah and a dam[n] good guinea pig, knowing [if] his kid [had] SCI they'd be off to China in a heartbeat. Also in July it will have been 28 years [since the injury] so it's time to rock. Time to start getting ready for that post SCI party since after this many years I'll have more work to do than most. (Leo 2004)

Tired of watching injured rats respond to experiments as they sat on the sidelines in their wheelchairs, activists like Leo were ready to board the plane to China. Indeed, some CareCure members had already tried other experimental treatments. As mk99, who underwent an experimental surgical procedure in Taiwan, explained two years earlier:

> I believe life is a balance between risk & reward and I am taking a calculated risk here with a potentially large reward. . . . I could not live with myself if I didn't try . . . sorry I just don't buy this bullshit that is fed to us here from the day you are injured. "go play wheelchair basketball", "get used to it", etc. You can't win if you don't play, simple as that. (mk99 2001)

Like Leo, mk99 also decided to pursue the experimental OEG transplantation in Beijing.

Other members were less sanguine about the Chinese procedure and engaged instead in meta-analysis of the poll's structure, commenting on the design of the questions or critiquing the proffered choices. While he praised "Beaker's well thought out choices," a self-declared "Monday morning poll designer" noted that the type of injury might impact members' decisions. With injuries to the upper spinal cord involving a greater degree of paralysis, this would-be pollster suggested adding the following option: "No, but if I had a cervical injury I'd be on the plane right now!" (Jeff 2003a). Another member noted that the options were not mutually exclusive—although the poll allowed him to select only one, he wanted to vote for all three "no" responses (Steven Edwards 2003a). Still others noted that the poll failed to distinguish between those who did not want the surgery and those who physically did not qualify for the surgery. One member observed that she was still experiencing return from her recent injury, disqualifying her since Dr. Huang treated only those who were neurologically stable (November 2003). Another just learned that he had a transected spinal cord, disqualifying him since Dr. Huang accepted only those whose spinal cords were at least partially intact anatomically on MRI examination. This latter member felt particularly despondent:

> I always thought my spinal cord was left partially intact but today I found out I'm one of the few with a completely transected cord. So right now I am left feeling like the light at the end of the tunnel just got turned off and I'm left here in the dark. So my answer is C) No thanks, but please give someone else the opportunity who does really *want* the surgery . . . but change the *want* to *can have* the surgery. Since I'm C6 complete, it might have made all the difference in the world to me.[2] (AO 2003)

LOCAL ANATOMIES OF SPINAL CORD INJURY

As both AO and the Monday morning poll designer's comments suggest, the type of spinal cord injury played a key role in members' deliberations. In order to understand why the OEG surgery "might have made all the difference in the world" for a "C6 complete" (a severe injury at the sixth cervical spinal cord segment), we need to understand how the anatomy of spinal cord injuries shapes sufferers' subjectivities, from their sense of self to their range of bodily experiences. This development of SCI subjectivity is an example of what anthropologists employing a biosocial approach have described as "local biologies"—the transformation of biological processes by social processes, and vice versa (Lock 1993; Ellison 1996, 1999; Kleinman 1999; Vitzthum 2008, 2009).[3]

People with SCI often categorize themselves based on the type of anatomical injury they sustained. Those injured in the cervical (neck) region generally refer to themselves as "quads"—shorthand for quadriplegia, denoting loss of movement in all four limbs. (The technical term used for injuries between the C1 and T1 segments of the spinal cord is "tetraplegia," which refers to damage in the upper neurons controlling sensory and motor function in the head, neck, shoulders, arms, and/or fingers.) Those injured lower down in the thoracic (chest), lumbar (lower back), and sacral (hip) regions of the spinal cord call themselves "paras," reflecting the technical classification of paraplegia for injuries between the T2 and S5 segments (which affect sensation and movement from mid-chest down to the toes).

People with SCI also describe themselves in finer-grained anatomical shorthand based on their precise neurological level of injury. These levels of injury are based on the lowest point on the spinal cord below which there is a decrease of feeling or movement, as determined by a neurological evaluation standardized by the American Spinal Injury Association (2015; Kirshblum et al. 2011b). Once the neurological level is determined, the injury is further categorized according to the extent of damage: those entirely without any sensation or motor function below the level of injury are considered "complete"; those with some movement or feeling are graded "incomplete."[4] This classification system (figure 3.1) has been adopted by most major SCI organizations around the world, resulting in more consistent terminology used to characterize injury types.

What do these anatomical classifications mean for the spinal-injured person? As an information sheet published by the Spinal Cord Injury Model System Information Network titled "Adjustment to Spinal Cord Injury" explains:

> You probably have a strong belief that your paralysis is only temporary, and you will soon return to your old, "normal" self. This hope is a common reaction after an injury. Unfortunately, it is far more likely for individuals to recover function based on their level and completeness of injury. . . . Almost all individuals with SCI continue to hope that they will walk again one day. However, a cure for paralysis may or may not come in your lifetime. A healthy approach to this reality is to move forward with your life after injury with the continued hope that advances in medicine will one day lead to a cure. In other words, do not wait on a cure to proceed with your life! (Rehabilitation Research and Training Center on Secondary Conditions of SCI 2004, 3)

This model rehabilitation center, based at the University of Alabama and funded by the National Institute of Disability and Rehabilitation Research, urged those with spinal cord injuries to focus on achievable goals within the context of their new lived reality. Oriented toward helping people adjust to their life after injury, the rehabilitation center emphasized that the specific neurological level of injury determined the realistic functional goals a person with SCI could expect to achieve (figure 3.2, figure 3.3).

Christopher Reeve, for example, became a "C2 complete" when he broke his neck in a horse-riding accident—a catastrophic injury that rendered the former Superman dependent on a ventilator and without any feeling or movement below his shoulders. Reeve explained the significance of these anatomical classifications in his biography, *Still Me*:

> A C2 incomplete means that the spinal cord is still intact, and one might have more recovery over time. Complete means there will be no further recovery because the spinal cord has been transected or so badly damaged that there is no hope for repair. At C2 you can move your head and you can talk; at C3 you can breathe a little bit; at C4 you can breathe normally; at C5 you gain some use of your arms; at C6 you might begin to get use of your hands. So when someone injures their spinal cord, the first question is: What level? Because this will give you an idea what their future is. (Reeve 1999, 40)

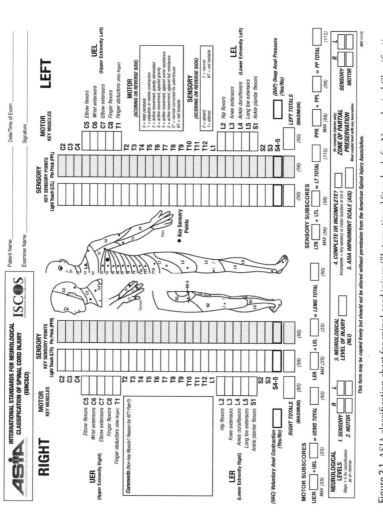

Figure 3.1. ASIA classification chart for spinal cord injury ("International Standards for Neurological Classification of Spinal Cord Injury" reprinted with permission from the American Spinal Injury Association, Atlanta, revised 2011, updated 2015).

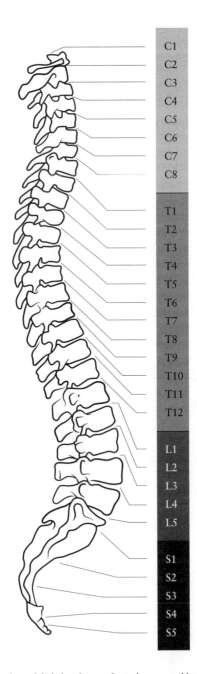

Figure 3.2. Human spinal column labeled with neurological segmental levels (illustration designed by Oikeat Lam).

Level	Functional Abilities	Prospects and Goals
C1–C3	Limited if any movement of head & neck	Dependent on ventilator to breathe; talking may be impaired; 24-hour care & assistance required with nearly all activities
C4	Some head & neck control	May be able to breathe without ventilator; assistance required with most activities
C5	Full head & neck movement; good shoulder control; can raise arms & bend elbows	Some independence in feeding and personal hygiene with equipment; can operate power wheelchair and car with hand controls
C6	Full head, neck & shoulder movement; can move arms & wrists	More independence in eating, drinking, personal hygiene, housekeeping tasks with special equipment
C7	Has added ability to straighten elbows	Need fewer adaptive aids in independent living; daily use of manual wheelchair
C8–T1	Has added strength and precision of fingers resulting in more hand function	May live independently without assistive devices; can transfer independently from wheelchair to bed or car
T2–T6	Has full motor function in head, neck, shoulders, arms, hands & fingers; more trunk control	May be totally independent with all activities of daily living
T7–T12	Has added motor function from increased abdominal control	Able to perform unsupported seated activities
L1–L5	Has additional return of movement in hips & knees	Walking may be possible with help of specialized leg & ankle braces
S1–S5	Various degrees of return in bladder, bowel, sexual functions	Increased ability to walk with fewer or no supportive devices

Figure 3.3. Functional abilities and goals correlating to specific levels of complete spinal cord injury (chart designed by Oikeat Lam). Information compiled from Rehabilitation Research and Training Center on Secondary Conditions of SCI (2000).

Formerly considered a permanent life (or death) sentence for people with SCI, this injury level-constrained future was now in flux as CareCure members embraced the possibility of a cure in China. Initial evidence (based on Wise's anecdotal observations during the December 2002 trip and a presentation Dr. Huang gave at the Keck Center in September 2003) suggested that many of the OEG surgery recipients experienced sensory gains of four to five dermatomes (key sensory points used to assess the level of feeling) and motor recovery of one to two levels. The significance of this potential recovery depended largely upon the anatomy of their injury, however, so it was not just a simple matter of how much but what kind of improvement it would entail. Wise hypothesized:

> Let us assume optimistically that the long-term results will show that 80% of the patients regained an average of four sensory dermatomes and partial recovery of two motor levels below their preoperative level. Let us further assume that partial motor recovery means getting 2 motor points per muscle. In other words, a person who has weak wrist extensors (C6) with a muscle score of 1 (flicker) gets slightly stronger with a score of 3 (anti-gravity), i.e. a score gain of 2. Let us further say that the person gets movement of triceps (from zero to a score of 2) and that pinprick sensation improves from C8 to T4. Would people consider this degree of recovery sufficiently worthwhile to warrant the cost and risk of surgery? Some might, others may not. (Wise Young 2003c)

As this hypothetical analysis suggests, a general statement about OEG surgery's potential to improve sensory and motor function was meaningless without being evaluated in light of the particular anatomical considerations of a given person's specific injury. Members needed to assess the significance of these few levels of improvement in the embodied context of their own injury levels—a matter of interpreting "local neuroanatomies," one could say.

In deciding whether to travel to China for the OEG surgery, CareCure members thus based their evaluation on a close interpretation of what the purported gains meant for their particular levels and types of injury. For tetraplegics with higher levels of injury such as Christopher Reeve, a motor recovery of a single level could mean the difference between being ventilator dependent or not. Recognizing the potential of the treatment to transform his local anatomy, Reeve attended a presentation Dr. Huang gave in September 2003 for a Keck Center open house (figure 3.4).[5]

Those with lower cervical injuries could also benefit significantly with even a small neurological improvement. A "C8/T1 complete" noted that "gaining at least one level of function will mean having full hand function"—the difference between pinching instead of grabbing, or the difference between typing freely on a computer keyboard instead of jabbing awkwardly at the letters while gripping a typing stick (jimnms 2003). Not surprisingly, the first CareCure pioneers to China all had cervical injuries.

Those with paraplegia had a more equivocal time deciding whether the gains would be worthwhile. Several discussion threads sprouted up to discuss whether "paras" should undergo the OEG transplants: some who posted were adamant that Dr. Huang had already demonstrated that many Chinese paraplegics had benefited from his procedure (Jeff 2003c) while others remained less certain that there would be any meaningful gains. A Hong Kong–based mother of a teenager who had been injured in a skiing accident even traveled twice to Beijing in order to interview paraplegic OEG recipients. She concluded that "my observation is T12 paras do not recover as significantly as those with higher levels of injuries" (poonsuzanne 2003), and her son decided to wait for future improvements. Some paraplegics even gave up altogether on changing their local anatomy. As one member with a mid-thoracic injury declared:

> As a T4–6 complete, I've made my peace with living this lifestyle. The person it's helped me become I wouldn't trade and would rather see some of the people I've met here on CC gain what benefits there may actually be and what may come down the road from this. (Anonymous 2003)

Those who were reconciled with their post-injury lifestyle formed a distinct minority within the CareCure community, particularly among those who frequented the Cure forum. Notably, the few voices who seemed content with their current status did not choose to identify themselves even with a screen name, preferring to post anonymously. The most active participants in the Cure forum were those in search of potential therapies to alter their local anatomies. The question for them was whether the particular therapy in question promised enough transformation to warrant the risks of undergoing an experimental operation.

Beaker, who had started the China poll, reflected a more common attitude among paraplegics on CareCure:

> For me, I'm not interested in this surgery (at least right now). I'm pain free, and as a para, independent. I don't think going from T4/5 to maybe T6/7 and incomplete would really benefit me much. . . . If I had less function, I think I would be much more interested in having this surgery for myself. (Beaker 2003a)

According to Beaker's calculus, while an improvement in one or two motor levels would potentially entail increased use of her rib and chest muscles, this would not translate into meaningful improvements in her functional abilities. As her rationale suggests, the matter of independence was a significant factor for those living with SCI. As one tetraplegic CareCure member from Texas responded:

> I would definitely go. I am a C6 with strong arms and some movement of my fingers but no function. I have a small amount of return in my abdominals. A couple of levels of return would probably mean a huge difference in my independence. (rapid524 2003)

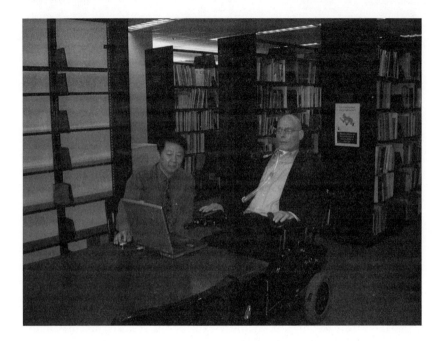

Figure 3.4. Chinese neurosurgeon Huang Hongyun with Christopher Reeve at the W. M. Keck Center for Collaborative Neuroscience in New Jersey, September 2003 (photograph courtesy of Huang Hongyun).

Thoracic-level paraplegics, on the other hand, were already able to perform many daily activities on their own. Many of them thus dreamed of a more radical possibility: walking out of their wheelchairs. To be able to walk, however, paraplegics needed to experience functional descent to at least L1 in order to move their hips. Dr. Huang's surgery, which suggested motor improvements of only one to two levels, was still a far cry from walking for "complete" paraplegics with upper thoracic injuries.

Mk99, who shared the same neurological injury level as Beaker, had a different take on his condition and the possibility of improvement: "I am also a T4 like Beaker and agree that becoming a T6 will not change my life too much. And yet I am scheduled to go to Beijing in January. Why? Because I would love to be incomplete vs. complete" (mk99 2003c). For mk99, the shift to being "incomplete" represented a categorical break in experience that made the crucial difference for him—his tipping point for taking on the risks of experimental surgery. If he were to become an "incomplete," he speculated that the possibilities could be endless for him: "Because then I have a CHANCE to get out of the chair. Because there is a possibility that suspended treadmill training, FES & intense physio will actually bring an incomplete some functional recovery. And because there is also a chance to recover some B&B&S [bladder, bowel, sexual] function" (mk99 2003c). Whereas a "complete" had no realistic basis to hope for neurological repair, an "incomplete" might dare to dream of recovering lost function.

Mk99's reasoning tempted other paraplegics like Andy, who wavered on the brink of tipping:

> I'm in the same boat as the other T-levels as well. Will a couple levels help me being a T6 complete? Probably not much with the exception of having a better cough (I smoke, yeah, I know) and maybe a little better push while taking a dump than just my diaphragm. It sure won't help with trunk control as I have rods to T12 and that is too far away. BUT, the chance of being incomplete is a really interesting prospect for me. I would love to have some feeling below what I have now, even some motor control for that matter, no matter how "nonfunctional". BBS possibilities too? Sign me up! Yep, this procedure is a godsend for a C level injury and they benefit most from it, but I want more than I have now also. (Andy 2003c)

Indeed, the possibility of regaining bladder, bowel, and sexual function even made thirty-three-year-old Beaker reconsider her position: "It would be awesome to get some B&B control. And considering I was injured when I was 8, I might get to feel some things that I've never felt before. That'd be cool!" (Beaker 2003b). Despite these tempting possibilities, however, Beaker still faced one frightening consequence that outweighed any potential gains for her: the specter of pain:

> I guess the biggest thing for me is the fear that it would result in having to deal with pain for the rest of my life. I'm thinking that if I am complete now but moved to incomplete, I might be able to feel some pain that I'm not feeling now because I'm complete? Maybe I'm wrong about that. (Beaker 2003b)

Others like Mike C agreed with Beaker, having witnessed the agony of those on CareCure unfortunate enough to be afflicted: "Yeah Beaker, for me it's the pain issue as well. After reading all about the horror stories of neuropathic pain over the years, I can understand your position. And I share it" (Mike C 2003).

Mk99 was undeterred, however, arguing that for him the risks did not outweigh the potential benefits. Indeed, he believed that he couldn't get any worse than he already was, as a "T4 complete" without any sensation or motor function below his injury level. As he explained in an earlier posting, "I am now approx 15 months post injury (T4 complete) and have gotten NOTHING back in that time. I can't see how I can become more "complete" than "complete". It's like comparing degrees of death . . . can one person be more dead than another?" (mk99 2001). Confronted by the possibility of neuropathic pain, he replied that his existential pain was worse: "I'll deal with the risk of great pain. There's nothing more painful than sitting in a wheelchair watching time pass you by while you can't do anything that used to mean everything to you" (mk99 2003c). As a former motorcycle joy rider and now the father of two rambunctious children, he was determined to give himself a shot at escaping his bodily constraints:

> My new babies bring me lots of joy and happiness each day and provide a strong
> reason to "soldier on."... A cure (even a partial one) will make everything so
> much better... including parenting. I want to teach them to ride a bike and not
> how to insert a catheter or magic bullet.[6] (mk99 2003d)

Members such as mk99 assessed the significance of potential improvement in
the embodied context of their own injury levels. Rather than universalizing
knowledge about morphology and bodily structures, these CareCure participants drew on scientific discourse about their specific injuries to localize anatomical knowledge to their specific lived experiences.

As these examples demonstrate, personal exegesis of local anatomies shaped
each member's deliberations, rendering generic conclusions about the therapeutic decision-making processes of "paras" versus "quads" ineffectual. Whereas a
paraplegic like mk99 might defy expectations by choosing to go, some tetraplegics who might have much to gain from the slightest descent in neurological
levels might not be so quick to get on the airplane to Beijing. For example, a
"C3 complete" dependent on ventilator assistance at night surprised his fellow
CareCure members by voting a definitive "no" on Beijing:

> JEFF: Steven—I was shocked to see your response. At your level, you potentially
> have a lot to gain... I was surprised in part due to the amount of time you spend
> reading and participating in the Cure Forum. And even doing so much research
> on your own. Can you elaborate at all as to why you categorically would not go?
> (2003b)

> STEVEN EDWARDS: I potentially have a lot to gain, but at the same time I poten-
> tially have a lot to... well, "gain." As a C3, I use my neck to do pretty much every-
> thing I can, like using the computer. What if I have the surgery, gain to a mid-level
> C4 functionality and lose the full ROM [range of motion] in my neck I currently
> have? That would suck for me.... Having an injury this high up sucks as it is, but
> what if I had pain added to it? That would totally make it suck. (2003b)

Although Steven acknowledged the benefits he stood to gain, a careful consideration of his precarious local anatomy made him realize that he had perhaps
more to lose than others given his already limited functionality. As he pointed
out, people with high cervical injuries relied almost entirely on the movement
of their necks to substitute for their motionless arms and hands. They typed by
using mouth-sticks or voice-recognition software, and those like Steven who
continued to adhere to conventional norms of punctuation, capitalization, and
typo editing in their online postings demonstrated truly impressive willpower.
More typically, people with limited or no hand mobility tended to forego these
niceties in the interests of time and energy.[7] As a C4 tetraplegic patient of Dr.
Huang's informed me in an email: "Hi Kid, No disrespect ment, I type with
a mouth stick and short cuts are nice. Also my gramer is not so hot so try to

read what i'm saying not how i say it" (personal email to the author, April 30, 2005). In addition to typing emails, those with high cervical injuries also used mouth-sticks to turn pages, dial telephones, push buttons, turn knobs, toast bagels, write longhand (by attaching a pen at the other end of the stick), and even draw and paint. Thus, for a C3 like Steven, the neck was sacrosanct territory. Although descending to C4 level functionality might give him some degree of shoulder control, for Steven the danger of disrupting the hard-won movements he had trained his neck to perform outweighed this potential gain.

The effects of local anatomy extended far beyond an individual's injured spinal cord to the collectively shared "local moral world" (Kleinman 1999) in which he or she was immersed. For some tetraplegics dependent on caregivers for everything from bathing to scratching an itchy nose, an improvement that allowed even limited use of their arms would be a huge improvement in the quality of life for not only themselves but also their families. As CJO, the twenty-five-year-old "C5 complete" tetraplegic who underwent the OEG transplant in September 2003 explained:

> The one thing I hate the most is my dependence on others. I can't get out of bed without help. I can't get something to eat or drink without help. I'm always at the mercy of others, mostly my angelic mother who has dedicated her life to caring for me and constantly tells me she wishes she could trade places with me. (That's just crazy talk; I don't wish this life on anybody.) My six year old niece has a more independent life than I do. I would literally die if left alone for a few days. That's not hyperbole; that's a fact. Like prison, quadriplegia consists of routine, and then more routine. Getting ready for the day used to take me mere minutes. Getting out of bed, showering, going to the bathroom, dressing, etc. now takes hours. There is no break; I must do this every day. Paralysis is an all day, every day condition. They don't tell you that when you sign up. Read the fine print, people. Feeling like a burden to others has been a constant for me. My mother selflessly gives of her time, but I feel like a hindrance on her life and those of others who lend a hand. I always have to ask for help from others. I bet I say "please" and "thank you" more than most anybody, but that doesn't make me feel less bothersome. (CJO 2007)

Facing the ongoing, relentless experience of quadriplegia that transformed quick habits into arduous processes, CJO felt the terrible burden of chronic paralysis weighing down an entire lifetime not just for himself but also for his uncomplaining mother and family. As these online deliberations reveal, the eagerness or reluctance of different CareCure members to pursue experimental treatment must be contextualized in terms of the bodily reconfigurations and local moral worlds induced by each person's particular level of spinal cord injury. The embodied dynamics of chronic paralysis play a crucial role in mobilizing CareCure members' quests for a cure through this online discussion forum and beyond to China.

ALS: FORESHORTENED TIMELINES OF NEURODEGENERATION

The temporal horizons for those diagnosed with amyotrophic lateral sclerosis are very different from those of people living with chronic paralysis. While people with SCI contended with an ongoing but generally stable condition, PALS such as Colorado firefighter Jeff, Yankee baseball star Lou Gehrig, and reportedly China's Chairman Mao grappled with an inexorable downward decline. ALS is a lethal motor neuron disease that acts quickly and spares few. Most patients die within three to five years of the onset of symptoms. There is no cure, and doctors do not know the root cause of the disease. Although the etiology is unknown, the so-called progression of the disease is clear: ALS attacks the nerve cells that control the voluntary muscles of the body. These motor neurons play a crucial role in transmitting messages from the brain through the spinal cord to the muscles. As these neurons degenerate and die, the muscles are no longer able to function and begin to atrophy. Affected individuals eventually lose their ability to move their limbs and other parts of their bodies. When the muscles of the chest wall and diaphragm begin to fail, PALS can no longer breathe on their own. With no cure or even effective treatment for the degeneration of motor neurons in ALS, patients have very little recourse beyond waiting for the inevitable wasting away of their muscles even as their intellect and higher cognitive functioning remain intact.

How have the temporal dynamics of ALS affected the digitally mediated health-seeking of those living with this incurable neurodegenerative disease? In an open letter to his American neurologists that he posted on his public blog, Trophic explains the foreshortened timeline he faced as an ALS patient as the driving force for his decision to pursue experimental treatment in Beijing:

> The advice given by Dr. Wise Young, director of the Keck Center, who was Dr. Huang's supervisor during Huang's residency at Rutgers and who is following the procedure closely, is that SCI patients should wait. Since their condition is stable and the procedure continues to be perfected, there is no reason for them not to see how things develop and perhaps improve further. . . . As concerns ALS patients, my perception of the time frame available to us suggest[s] little opportunity for waiting. Generally, our condition is not stable and the disease can change from a slow advance to one that's disconcertingly rapid. In my case, I seem to be entering one of those disconcertingly rapid phases. Almost every couple of days I notice some slight diminution in function. A month and a half ago, before I saw you in the US, I could walk unaided or, at worst, with the aid of a cane. I am now totally dependent on crutches. And so with numerous other small things. In any case, I don't have the time to wait to see what the future brings. At very worst, the procedure can't have consequences worse than those I'll face anyway. At better, it may help stabilize things until something better comes along. At best, it may encourage some improvement. The risk-benefit ratio is all in favor of benefit. (Trophic 2004c)

For someone afflicted by the rapid degeneration of their motor neurons, the "risk-benefit ratio" that Trophic invokes seems clear: he faces certain death if he does nothing. Recounting his response to his neurologist's warning against trying the experimental Chinese therapy, another ALS patient from Texas asked: "What do you want me to do? Buy a coffin and make myself comfortable in it?" The Texan chose instead to fly to Beijing and underwent the OEG fetal cell transplantation in May 2005.

POACHING ON CARECURE

Although CareCure was an online platform devoted to spinal cord injury, it became a key pathway for people with ALS to obtain OEG fetal cell therapy in Beijing. Their use of the CareCure forum to obtain contact with Dr. Huang could be characterized as "poaching." As outsiders and newbies to the online world of spinal cord injury treatment and research, people with ALS generally made very few contributions to the SCI community (as measured by number of public posts). Most instead pursued a utilitarian focus on mining the website for any useful leads to treat their rapidly progressing neurodegenerative disease. Longstanding CareCure members generally tolerated this type of "poaching" from ALS patients, recognizing the severity of these interlopers' disease and the dearth of viable online communities for neurodegenerative disease elsewhere in cyberspace. A few of the ALS "poachers"—almost always caregivers rather than ALS patients themselves—did try to offer a more substantive contribution to the spinal cord injury community in grateful recognition of the assistance that other CareCure members offered in the form of therapy suggestions and general emotional support.

Of the people with ALS whom I met in Beijing or encountered online, many of them connected to Dr. Huang through the CareCure thread "Beijing—Wish to contact Dr. Huang? Please post here!" This thread had been set up in September 2003 by CareCure moderators, who admonished OEG therapy seekers to "please use this thread to keep the other ones from getting swamped. I will attempt to move all previous posts from other threads into this thread. I'd like to try to keep this as organized as possible! Thank you!" (mk99 2003b). This thread generated 524 inquiries and over 119,560 unique views in the following decade, making it one of the ten most popular threads in the Cure subforum.

While several of the initial thread contributors were regular "members" or "senior members" living with spinal cord injury who had posted dozens or even hundreds of contributions to the CareCure forums, the vast majority of participants in this thread were "junior members" who set up an account on the CareCure forum for the express purpose of contacting Dr. Huang. These participants generally made a single public post consisting of their basic demographics (level of injury or disease status) and email information. They then continued their correspondence with Dr. Huang and his staff through private email, never making another public contribution to the CareCure forum.

This type of targeted, online health-seeking was particularly common among patients and families facing ALS. A typical inquiry looked like this one from jshoham, a junior member who created a CareCure account in March 2004 to initiate Post #254 on the Huang contact thread:

> Hello Dr. Huang, I would like to see if my father who has Bulbar ALS can undergo your olfactory ensheathing cell transplantation. He would be a very good candidate. He was diagnosed on 3-26-04. If you do not have time to do this procedure could you refer me to another chinese doctor that could? If you could or an assistant of yours email me contact information that would be great as well. I will be traveling to China in June on business and would like to set up a time where I could meet with you or another DR that you recommend for this procedure. (jshoham 2004)

Jshoham appended his email address at the end of his post and never made another contribution to the CareCure forum, although the website enabled him to make successful contact with Dr. Huang.[8] His father became the fourth foreign ALS patient (and thirty-third ALS patient overall including Chinese recipients) to receive the experimental OEG fetal cell transplantation in Beijing at the end of April 2004—a mere three weeks after his initial diagnosis of ALS in the United States.[9]

Although jshoham made only one public post on the CareCure forum, his wife created her own CareCure account in April 2004 with the username iublondie25 to report on the results of her father-in-law's experimental surgery. As she explained in opening her thread titled "I have just returned from Beijing . . .":

> I know this forum is mostly for spinal injuries but I wanted to let people know that I was there and I have perspective on the whole "Beijing Experience". There really isn't an "ALS" forum anywhere that I have found . . . and the procedure is similar so I decided to post here. LOL. I also met the infamous Leo and Jeanie. I know Leo is on his way home and I hope he has a safe flight. But if anyone has any questions please let me know. You can post here or e-mail me . . . I will answer anything to the best of my ability. (iublondie25 2004a)

She was inspired to contribute to the online spinal cord injury forum precisely because of the face-to-face connections she made with other CareCure members undergoing the experimental procedure during her trip to Beijing. But after just three months of posting updates on the CareCure forum, she publicly announced that she could no longer handle the onslaught of queries regarding Huang's procedure:

> Hello all. I am afraid that I can no longer accept e-mails from people asking about Dr. Huang. I have gotten overwhelmed. I suggest you follow this thread along with others like it. Dr. Wise is more of an expert than I am. I am so sorry but it has

become very time consuming and I frankly do not have the time or energy to answer personal emails anymore. With running our company, taking care of my family, taking care of my health and pregnancy I just cannot do it all anymore. Please keep having faith. I will continue to post updates on this board and braintalk. But please do not contact me via e-mail anymore. I am sorry. (iublondie25 2004b)

As iublondie25's post suggests, people living with ALS and their loved ones face the ever shrinking temporal horizon of inevitable degeneration, placing increasing burdens on their caregivers as their muscles continue to atrophy and they become increasingly unable to function independently. These individual and family demands often leave little time for contributing to a broader community beyond immediate social circles either on- or offline.

Even CareCure members who were not personally grappling with the neurodegenerative disease found it challenging to manage the onslaught of inquiries from PALS seeking Dr. Huang's experimental fetal cell therapy. Inundated by private requests for more information, CareCure moderator Wise Young started a public thread on the spinal cord injury Cure forum devoted to "OEG Treatment of ALS" in June 2004. He featured this thread as a "sticky" at the very top of the Cure forum to enable ALS visitors to find the information more easily. The intense interest from people and families with ALS even led CareCure administrators to consider setting up a separate forum on ALS, although Wise worried that this might "compete or take away from the discussions of other sites" (Wise Young 2004). The brother-in-law of an ALS patient from Brooklyn, New York, responded:

> I feel that any contribution to the ALS community by the members of this forum could only be considered a helpful addition. Although I am also relatively new to the communities being provided, such as that at "braintalk" I find myself frequenting this forum regularly as it is. Furthermore, given the recent exposure that you have had on national television specific to ALS, and the interest by individuals visiting and calling your place of research, I believe that people will naturally be visiting here in search for more information. This should stand in stark contrast to any thought that you may be "taking away" from the other ALS community boards. (golanbenoni 2004)

Like golanbenoni, most of the people searching online for information about ALS were "newbies" to the digital world of patient advocacy websites who generally stumbled onto the CareCure forum.

Diagnosed with ALS twenty months prior to his first post on CareCure, Trophic, the American expatriate lawyer living in Moscow, could be considered an old hand in the online quest for information about possible treatments for ALS. Although he maintained his own personal blog and regularly scoured the Internet for potential leads, Trophic emphatically declared his preference for the CareCure spinal cord injury forum as his central source of information:

I've found more useful information relative to my specific needs regarding als (dx Jn'03) here than virtually anywhere else. And, like most of us, I've looked everywhere. The contributions made here, and specifically those of its extraordinary moderator, add a great deal to what can be found elsewhere and detract from absolutely no one else's work. (Trophic 2004b)

For Trophic, the careful scientific evaluations and responsiveness of CareCure's founder, Wise Young, trumped any disease-specific modes of organization. According to Trophic's reasoning, a forum on spinal cord injury research and treatment could prove more useful than a different forum devoted to ALS, depending on the experience and expertise of the participants.

BLOGGING FOR LOCAL AWARENESS AND SUPPORT

Many ALS patients who pursued experimental therapy in Beijing chose to maintain public blogs about their experiences before, during, and after the procedure.[10] Prior to their transnational journeys, these blogs functioned as a mechanism to raise awareness about their plight and generate material and emotional support. Jeff, the Colorado firefighter fighting ALS, was a case in point. His blog was hosted by his fire department's main professional website and served as a way to publicize the chili suppers, Harley-Davidson motorcycle raffle contest, and other fund-raising efforts that his fellow firefighters, paramedics, EMTs, engineers, and lieutenants organized to support their comrade. After the successful fund-raising that enabled Jeff to make his journey to China in November 2004, the blog continued to function during his transnational quest as his primary means for staying in touch with his friends and family members.

American PALS were not the only OEG fetal cell recipients to utilize blogs as a mechanism to stay in touch with far-flung family and friends. The hired British "carer" for an irascible former lawyer rendered speechless by ALS initiated a joint blog in order to keep family, friends, and colleagues appraised of their journey to Beijing:

I'm writing this first post sitting in the departure lounge at Heathrow—with just 90 minutes to go before our flight to Beijing is due to depart. . . . [T]he overnight in the hotel was "interesting". Within 5 minutes of entering the room [Duncan] had managed to fall "base over apex" and land unceremoniously on the floor between the bed and the wall. Although he might only look skin and bones—I can tell you that [he's] quite a "lump" to pick-up. I've told him that if he performs any more antics like that I'm not going!! We're now both sampling the complimentary booze—there's no food of course because of the strike by Gate Gourmet. Hopefully my next post will be tomorrow—once we've settled in our new (but temporary) home. . . . Cheers for now from us both." (Sweet N Sour 2005b)

Both Brits enjoyed a "wicked" sense of humor, with Duncan often interspersing his carer's garrulous blog posts with cutting commentary rendered in all capital letters:

> ALMOST 24 HOURS SINCE I WAS BEING BORED RIGID AND SO FAR NO OBVIOUS DIFFERENCES HAVE MANIFESTED THEMSELVES. I AM TAKING PATCHES TO KEEP MY MOUTH DRY BUT ON THE OPERATING TABLE I WAS AS DRY AS A BONE—FEAR FEATURED HEAVILY WHEN THEY STARTED TO MEASURE ME UP FOR THAT NEVER TO BE REPEATED "BLACK AND DECKER" MOMENT. I'M NOT SURE WHAT THEY DISCOVERED WHEN STICKING COTTON BUDS INTO EACH EAR—MAYBE TO SEE IF THEY COULD SPOT ANYTHING IN THE MIDDLE. [GERALD] ASSURES ME THAT ONLY TWO HOLES WERE BORED BUT IT CERTAINLY FELT LIKE 4 TO ME—AND I OBVIOUSLY HAVE A THICK SKULL JUDGING BY THE PRESSURE APPLIED AND MY HEAD SINKING INTO THE PILLOW. (Sweet N Sour 2005c)

As Gerald and Duncan's joint blog illustrates, these personal websites enabled the personalities of the online contributors to shine through, providing more options for control and customization than online discussion forums such as CareCure.

The blog format also enabled PALS to engage in long digressions on their personal webspaces. Trophic, the American expatriate lawyer, subtitled his blog as follows:

> Random and not random materials on ALS / amyotrophic lateral sclerosis / боковой амиотрофический склероз / motor [neuron] disease / maladie de Charcot / αμυοτροφική πλευρική σκλήρυνση / 馬達神經元疾病 / Lou [Gehrig's] / Steven Hawking's Disease / Dr. Huang Hongyun's OEC/OEGC transplants / rehab options / and other matters related and unrelated, not excluding political irritations, commentary on the exceptional, interesting, awful, and unspeakable, and other matters as they arise. (Trophic 2004a)

Ruminating about how he found himself awaiting an injection of fetal cells into his brain, Trophic indulged in a long rant about what he viewed as the hypocrisy in U.S. politics:

> But why, I wonder, are we Americans, citizens of what we like to think of as the most advanced and certainly the richest country in the world, here in China? Well, a great deal of it has to do with U.S. politics. We may be advanced, but the question is, in what? Increasingly it looks like our advancement is not only in the voodoo economics of the Republican[s]' "supply side" nonsense and the Democrats' "strategic trade" nonsense, but voodoo medicine as well. . . . It's because of the advanced state of our science that the FDA acted quickly to prevent any intellectual conflict of interest in its consideration of dangers in arthritis medications

in addition to Vioxx by banning one of the scientists who knows most about the issue. I kid you not, that's the phrase their spokesman used "intellectual conflict of interest." A government that invites logging companies to write forest regulations, drug companies to write drug rules, oil companies to write environmental standards, and sees nothing wrong in a system where the regulators and regulatees routinely change places (and salaries) may genuinely believe that disagreement constitutes something called "intellectual conflict of interest". That would go a long way to explain why reality has such a difficult time intruding on these people's perceptions. "Intellectual conflict of interest," you understand, is a no-no; financial conflict of interest, on the other hand, is a yes-yes, is highly recommended, and often appears to be obligatory. (Trophic 2004d)

These personal rants contrasted sharply with Trophic's shorter, more succinct posts on the CareCure forum, which he utilized for informational purposes only regarding possible therapies for ALS.

The personal blog format was particularly popular with people from the Netherlands living with ALS.[11] Ardi Bouter was the first Dutch patient to receive the OEG fetal cell transplantation procedure in September 2004 (Boer 2005). Like many other family members facing ALS who ultimately ended up traveling to China for the experimental neurosurgical procedure, Ardi's son had first discovered and made contact with Dr. Huang through the CareCure forum:

Hi Dr. Huang, I am writing this message on behalf of my father who is suffering from ALS. I have searched over the world to find something else than Rilutec to help him. My father would really like to be treated as soon as possible no matter what the costs are. Could you please let me know anything about the procedure and timings? Thanks in advance, Eric Bouter (son of Ardi Bouter) (ericbastiaan 2004)

Fluent in English, the Dutch son was able to establish a connection with the Chinese doctor on this American spinal cord injury website in their shared second language, securing a surgical appointment in Beijing for his father two months after his initial inquiry.

Fielding a constant stream of requests for more information about his China surgical experiences from his compatriots, Bouter became Huang's semiofficial patient coordinator for Dutch-speaking patients over the next six months. Less comfortable with writing in English than was his son, Bouter chose instead to create his own personal website titled "Voor en Door ALS patienten" (For and by ALS patients) in Dutch and "Fight against ALS Together" in English. Bouter's website included detailed information in Dutch about Huang's experimental therapy, an interactive "guest book" where family, friends, supporters, and other PALS could leave personal messages, and a general "message forum" where online visitors could exchange and discuss information related to ALS. As he described on his website's homepage in a mix of mostly Dutch with some English included as a recognition of the interest from PALS around the world:

Deze site is een interactieve gemeenschap van ALS patienten. Op deze site kan informatie worden gevonden over het leven met ALS, de laatste ontwikkelingen van behandelmethoden en hulpmiddelen. Please sign the guest book and be part of the ALS community. [This site is an interactive community of ALS patients. On this site you can find information about living with ALS, the latest developments in treatment methods and tools. Please sign the guest book and be part of the ALS community.] (Bouter 2004)

More accessible for Dutch ALS patients and their families than the English-language dominated CareCure website, Bouter's website played an important role in establishing an online community for Dutch ALS patients and families who sought experimental therapy in Beijing.

I tracked the experiences of twenty PALS from the Netherlands who underwent OEG fetal cell transplantation after Bouter at Huang's neurosurgery clinic during 2005, and nearly all of them either posted updates on Bouter's guest book or linked their own personal blogs to his central clearinghouse. For example, Loes Claerhoudt, the third Dutch ALS patient to undergo Huang's procedure in January 2005, launched her personal blog in conjunction with her quest for fetal cell therapy in Beijing. Diagnosed with ALS in 1999, she already wrote a regular column about her experiences living with ALS for the Utrecht-based newspaper *AD Utrechts Nieuwsblad*. Her newly created blog served as a way to keep family, friends, and interested observers more immediately apprised of her experiences. As she declared in her inaugural post from Beijing:

We zijn er! Na een prima vlucht bevonden we ons opeens in een andere wereld. China! Inmiddels zijn we in het ziekenhuis van dokter Huang . . . Ik houd jullie op de hoogte! [We are here! After a good flight we found ourselves suddenly in another world. China! We are now in the hospital of Dr. Huang . . . I'll keep you up-to-date!] (Loes Claerhoudt 2005a)

True to her word, Claerhoudt continued to post multiple times a day during her nearly monthlong treatment in Beijing. These posts attracted dozens of replies from supportive family and friends back home in the Netherlands. Following her return to Utrecht, she continued to post regularly on her personal blog in addition to writing about her experiences in more conventional formats such as her newspaper column. The newspaper also bundled some of her columns into a book titled *Loes* in 2006, and she subsequently published a second book in 2009 titled *En dan is er altijd nog de hoop* . . . (And then there's always hope . . .).

CONCLUSION

This chapter has examined how the embodied dynamics of illness and chronicity shape online modes of health-seeking. By comparing the varied experiences of people living with chronic paralysis to those of people suffering from ALS, I have identified distinctive "cyberanatomies" of hope that illuminate how embodied illness experiences enable or foreclose particular forms of mobilization and digital pathways to experimental medicine. While the chronic nature of SCI has enabled CareCure members to engage in reasoned debate over the benefits and risks of experimental therapy within the context of a robust and stable online community, the acute threat of ALS has produced much more contingent and ephemeral engagements with digital modes of health-seeking.

The ALS blog launched by Loes Claerhoudt was still active over a decade later, in no small part because of the unusually slow progression of her disease. But nearly all of the other blogs authored by the Dutch ALS patients I started following in 2005 have long since disappeared from cyberspace. Ardi Bouter's once-vibrant website suffered the all too common fate of personal websites whose webmasters are no longer able or willing to maintain them. A few months after Bouter's death in May 2005, his website and message forum were converted to "read only" status by his son. Languishing online with no new contributions, Bouter's website was ultimately taken down by his Internet hosting provider after his domain name expired in 2006.

As I discussed earlier in the book while analyzing the demise of the CareCure precursor website CanDo.com, broken links and ephemeral information pose significant challenges to community building and group mobilization. The contingent nature of personal websites is particularly problematic for people diagnosed with ALS, as patients succumb to the ravages of the terminal neurodegenerative disease and are no longer willing or able to update their websites.[12] Over the course of my research, I tracked dozens of blogs as well as patient information websites curated by PALS around the world (many of which I read with the help of online translation tools). Only a handful of these websites are still accessible—and even fewer of the PALS whom I met in Beijing are still alive. As information disappears with their creators, new PALS must constantly reinvent the wheel and repeat the same questions as they confront the untimely dictates of their disease, often without the hard-earned knowledge that previous PALS accumulated, distributed, and evaluated.

WHERE THE VIRTUAL
BECOMES VISCERAL

THE PRECEDING CHAPTERS HAVE EXAMINED the online deliberations of people living with paralysis and neurodegenerative conditions as they considered whether to pursue experimental therapy in China, mapping the hyperlinked pathways they've traveled along their biomedical odysseys. This chapter follows these experimental pioneers onto Chinese operating tables to undergo fetal cell transplantation. What happens when the hope they construct online runs headlong into the visceral discomforts and moral challenges of undergoing an experimental therapy that requires cells from aborted fetuses? I provide ethnographic insight on how these fetal cell recipients from around the world have operationalized hope in Beijing hospital wards, immersing themselves in the practical details of navigating an unfamiliar medical system while circumventing existential debates over the moral status of aborted fetuses.

I begin by analyzing the online surgical report threads of the first three foreigners to receive Dr. Huang's fetal cell transplantation.[1] All three were men from the United States who had suffered cervical-level spinal cord injuries. As we will see, CareCure played a key role in mediating their transnational encounters, offering a digital "umbilical cord to hope" as they made sense of a radically different world. I then incorporate the experiences of a wide range of other fetal cell recipients in order to address the key points of disjuncture that Dr. Huang's foreign patients had to negotiate during their cross-cultural encounters in Beijing: conflicting expectations about caregiving, moral qualms about the use of fetal cells, and the embodied vicissitudes of experimental surgery.

THE CARECURE PIONEERS

Tim C. became paralyzed from the chest down in 2002 at the age forty-two, when a collision with a tree during his first ride in an all-terrain vehicle injured the cervical vertebrae of his spinal column. His doctors told him that he would never regain functional control of his hands, legs, bowel, or bladder. Refusing to accept a life sentence of complete tetraplegia, Tim C. turned to the Internet to search for alternatives. Like Leo, Beaker, mk99, and many others, he discovered the CareCure website. Through the online Cure forum, Tim C. learned that Chinese SCI patients had experienced some recovery of motor function and sensation after undergoing Huang's fetal cell transplantation procedure.

After making contact with Huang through the CareCure forum, Tim C. became the first American to undergo the experimental OEG surgery in September 2003 at Chaoyang Hospital, one of the busiest public hospitals in Beijing with over 1,900 patient beds and 2.8 million surgeries performed yearly.[2] He was followed in quick succession by his fellow CareCure compatriots: Handibob (a forty-six-year-old "C5–6 incomplete" from Michigan) and CJO (the twenty-five-year-old "C5 complete" from South Dakota we met in the previous chapters). These three men were no longer simply contemplating but actually experiencing the quest for the cure in China, and they embodied the hopes of the cure movement for their comrades back in cyberspace. As Tim C. declared, "i'm a rip-roaring C4/5, asia A, complete. fix me and you'll fix most" (Tim C. 2003f). The three pioneers remained in constant communication with the CareCure community throughout their trip (even sometimes from their hospital beds while hooked up to IVs), each starting their own dedicated "Beijing OEG Surgery Report" threads to help other CareCure members follow their progress. The live updates they posted on the Cure forum about their experiences garnered a cult following that hung onto every byte of information coming from Beijing.[3]

As the first foreign patients treated by Huang and his staff, the three CareCure pioneers bore the brunt of the cross-cultural miscommunications and conflicting expectations about caregiving, as well as more mundane annoyances such as voltage incompatibilities. They provided frequent updates of their experiences at Chaoyang Hospital for their fellow CareCure members, describing everything from minor frustrations and bodily symptoms to encounters with hospital personnel and surgical procedures. Their online postings detailed grimy hospital conditions that "would not win any awards for cleanliness by our standards" (Tim C. 2003a), outdated equipment such as hand-crank operated hospital beds and old transformers that "appeared u-boat vintage" (Tim C. 2003b), and the difficulties they faced in trying to fit their bulky power wheelchairs through narrow bathroom door frames. As Tim C. lamented to his online audience:

> Needless to say my power chair drew attention to people in the street as if the martians had landed. clearly, we're not dealing with the most advanced technology, yet just think how much more advanced would the OEG therapies be if it was allowed to exist in places such as the U.S.? how unfortunate is it that many people in foreign, less technologically developed countries, come to the U.S. to take advantage of our medical technology, when because of the few "righteous" decision makers

in our government, i must travel around the world for what could be so much more in terms of advancing treatment for sci. (Tim C. 2003a)

Despite the difficulties of navigating the foreign Chinese hospital environment, sympathetic CareCure members saw this as a better alternative than what was on offer in the United States. As Schmeky from California wrote: "Currently, NOTHING is actively taking place for SCI victims in the US (other than research). How incredibly heartbreaking. Tim C., you're making history" (Schmeky 2003c).

CareCure members heralded the voyage as a momentous occasion: "I've been having the sensation that I'm watching this huge event unfold, like developing the a-bomb without a bad side. And the rest of the world doesn't know it's going on! . . . I am so excited and scared for our SCI astronauts" (betheny 2003). Others echoed the otherworldly reference, underscoring the significance of the voyage for those fervently hoping to leave behind their wheelchairs:

> I wish you all the best guys your our ambassadors now there in China, and I feel that your mission is better & worth something more than that of Armstrong when he landed on the [moon]. I hope you will be able to say with proud "One small step for man, One giant leap for mankind"! (drnader 2003)

CareCure members were rooting for their own astronauts' history-making quest for the cure, filled with anticipation that the three men would soon be taking their first post-SCI steps.

From "SCI astronauts" to "heroes," warriors," "pilgrims," and even "our American martyrs," CareCure members repeatedly championed the bravery of Tim C., Handibob, and CJO in undergoing a risky operation on the other side of the world (which seemed as far away as the moon for many American CareCure members immobilized by their paralysis). The three China travelers were most frequently anointed "pioneers."[4] A modest CJO, arriving in China a week after Tim C. and Handibob, called his predecessors "the true pioneers" who "have paved the way and given great comfort to me and those that will be accompanying me overseas." As for himself: "I'm not a pioneer and I'm not brave for doing this; I'm just like many of you who are striving for increased functionality to alleviate the obstacles that our spinal cord injuries have presented us with" (CJO 2003d). Rallying around the importance of the first journeys to China for the entire community, CareCure members were quick to disagree with CJO's self-assessment:

> You really are a pioneer for us, one of the first to have this done that actually can give us first hand accounts of their experiences with this, you have my respect for doing this. (Andy 2003b)

> CJO, Tim and Bob—you are all pioneers. You are all heros to all of us. You are all so very brave. Just imagine the hope that fills the hearts of all of us. Please take that

hope with you as a gift for your continued bravery! As other types of procedures become available, we will need more like you. (Chim-Chim 2003)

Indeed, not all CareCure members who rushed to sign up were willing to follow through with the risky foreign procedure. As Curt Leatherbee admitted, "I should be going there too, but I chickened out" (2003d).

While established CareCure members avidly awaited news from China, new members began swamping the forums with requests to sign up for the procedure even before the three pioneers had received the transplanted cells. In an attempt to manage the requests overwhelming various Cure forum topics, CareCure moderators started a new discussion thread devoted specifically to those wishing to contact Dr. Huang (mk99 2003b).[5] Writing from Chaoyang Hospital a few days before his surgery, Tim C. called this thread the "Soon-to-Be Infamous Huang List." He registered his shock over fellow members' overeager behavior in capital letters:

AS AN SCI PATIENT SCHEDULED FOR HUANG'S PROCEDURE NEXT WEEK, I AM WITNESSING AN INCREDIBLE EVENT ON CARECURE. CARECURE MEMBERS ARE SIGNING UP BY THE DROVES EVEN BEFORE THEY HAVE THE BENEFIT OF LEARNING THE OUTCOME OF THE FIRST THREE U.S. PATIENT SURGERIES. WILL WE EXPERIENCE SOME DEGREE OF RETURN AS THE RESULT OF THE PROCEDURE? OR WILL WE FALL VICTIM TO THE "P.T. BARNUM EFFECT." (Tim C. 2003e)

Despite his capitalized harangue, Tim C. himself had admitted that "the 'duped probability' was quite low" on his own surgery report thread after seeing the dramatic results of two post-operative Chinese patients (Tim C. 2003c). With three trusted representatives on the ground in China, the tantalizing possibility of a "China cure" was enough to assuage CareCure members' fears over being duped and stoke their "medical imaginary." As Mary-Jo DelVecchio Good has noted in her analysis of cancer patients who embrace experimental treatments, "enthusiasm for medicine's possibilities arises not necessarily from material products with therapeutic efficacy but through the production of ideas" (2001, 397). The buzz generated by the pioneers' touchdown in Beijing was enough to convince some CareCure members that the surgery was legitimate and persuade them to place their own bodies under the knife—or at least get on the growing list of eager candidates.

THE UMBILICAL CORD TO HOPE

CareCure members celebrated every minute detail they gleaned from Beijing. Their burgeoning hope was a collectively produced phenomenon linking together the SCI astronauts with their virtual community. The CareCure pioneers recognized the importance of sharing their experiences with their fellow community members back on "planet paralyzed" (Morgan 2003c). As Tim C. told devotees of his postings: "CareCure is the umbilical cord to hope and recovery. Status of my progress, for better or worse, as the result of my OEG transplant belongs to the CareCure community" (Tim C. 2003j).

Members checked for new posts repeatedly every few hours, disappointed if they came away with no new updates from Beijing. Indeed, many community members tried to follow the China activities down to the minute. As an eager caregiver from Texas wrote to Tim C. and Handibob: "The chatroom experts have determined that your surgeries will be at 7:00 PM tomorrow Central time. We have been glued to this site for days now, but look forward to the post that you are once again comfortable in your rooms" (The mom 2003a). She reported to CJO that the first question her teenaged son asked after he came home from his high school homecoming dance—the same day as CJO's surgery—was whether there was any news from China (The mom 2003b).

Many readers of the CareCure surgery reports were people living with spinal cord injuries, trying to decide for themselves whether they wanted to make the trip to China. As Rustyreeves told the pioneers, "thank you for wandering into this 'Indiana Jones' like world looking for the Grail we all seek. You are our eyes and ears on this journey and our prayers, thoughts and futures accompany you every step of the way" (Rustyreeves 2003a). As Red_1 Canada told his buddy CJO:

> I am so thankful to all of you guys for doing this. You guys to me are people we can all trust. It means alot to have "close friends", if by nothing else the # of times we log-in, actually going over there and basically testing this whole OEG thing out for us . . . I just wish there was more we could do for you and the others . . . GOOD Luck to the three of you and those who are soon to follow . . . possibly me?? (Red_1 Canada 2003, T12 paraplegic from Canada injured in 2002)

These injured CareCure members held onto the pioneers as their primary hope for a better future. In more practical terms, Tim C., Handibob, and CJO were "test subjects" who could generate reliable evidence for whether the experimental Chinese operation worked:

> Thanks god everything goes well in your surgery. In Turkey doctors still say that they do not believe in this kind of surgeries. You are my only evidence. Do not let us to broke our hopes. We will always watch you please do not forget to updating us. (mka 2003, brother of a thirty-four-year-old C6–5 incomplete tetraplegic from Turkey)

Other anxiety-ridden posts came from friends and family members of the pioneers, desperate to hear news of their loved ones. As the sister-in-law of Handibob's wife exclaimed after not receiving any news for two days after the surgery:

I know things must be busy there and all right now but, waking and finding NO post or No e-mail from you is just plain right awful and makes us worry here a bit. Whats going on there? You know I am the patient one and your brother has none what so ever and thats why I am having to write this. He calls me every morning from work to find out anything and looks for the mail and then again at night when he comes home from work and there hasn't been anything I can tell him or he can see from you. Write us and let us know whats going on there will ya please. (llarose2 2003)

If too much time passed between China updates, a vigilant member would usually pipe up: "[CJO], If no news soon i'm having the governor call up the national guard, lets not make an international issue out of this" (Leo 2003c). Ironically, Leo himself was the cause of anxiety several months later when he failed to post his own China surgery results as often as members wanted. As larwatson, a C5–6 tetraplegic lawyer injured in 1982, urged:

Leo, I want to know everything. I want to know every new sensation, movement, etc. . . . imagined or not . . . because its your experience. I admit that I am greedy. But the paucity of information is killing us. The great thing about yourself, CJO, Tim C. is that we know you guys. You're like family. Brothers in arms. Your successes, failures and inbetweens are more than understood. We need to hear your guys' experiences. The good, the bad, and the ugly. In fact if you guys posted a weekly diary of your experiences I would be eternally grateful. (larwatson 2004)

Although most CareCure members had never met each other in person, many used familial metaphors such as "umbilical cord" and "brothers in arms" to invoke the close relationships they had built up together online over the course of commiserating over their everyday challenges, sharing their excitements, and comforting each other about disappointments.

The "big extended family" demonstrated their support in material ways as well. When Tim C. posted about his inability to find a commode in Beijing, members immediately responded. As Tim C. bemoaned his toileting situation from Beijing ("i can't imagine reverting back to bed baths for the duration" [Tim C. 2003b]), CareCure members organized a fund-raiser in cyberspace that illustrated the power of virtually mediated "real-time" mobilization efforts. The appeal began with Rustyreeves, who started a separate thread in the Cure forum devoted to the "Tim C shower chair fund" (2003b). Within thirty minutes ip offered to donate one of his extra commodes (ip 2003c). Sympathetic members eager to show their support for the CareCure pioneers posted additional contribution offers and logistical suggestions: "If it were me waiting to take a shower, I'd be in a bit of a hurry. Can ip or anyone else be ready to ship by tomorrow?" (dahliasinbloom 2003). CareCure cheerleaders praised their fellow members as more people continued to join the effort: "That's the spirit! Fantastic! . . . Let's get this shitter in the air" (Rustyreeves 2003c).

Federal Express gave the Shower Chair Fund contributors an incredible case of "sticker shock" when they discovered that the heavy, bulky chair would cost nearly five hundred dollars to ship using FedEx Economy service or a whopping $950.21 with FedEx Priority (ip 2003d)—twenty times more than the cost of the commode itself! Undeterred by the setback, CareCure members redoubled their efforts to raise more money: "I'm in, $25. Come on people, this won't be hard to do. I can't imagine being w/o my shower chair to deal w/ my morning routines" (jmublueduck 2003a). In less than twenty-four hours, the CareCure supporters exceeded the target. As Rustyreeves announced to Tim C:

> IP has donated a shower/commode chair and everyone is chipping in to have it FedEx'd to you by the 23rd/24th. Shipping is only a paltry [$468.86]—Let's pray it fits the door jam. If not, at least you can do the BM [bowel movement] sitting up. Best of luck my friend. You have an army of well wishers back here hanging on your every action. (Rustyreeves 2003d)

The chair arrived in Beijing three days after Tim C. and Handibob underwent the OEG surgery. As Tim C. reported on his OEG surgery report thread, "I awoke this morning to the chatter of several doctors and nurses gawking at the newly arrived shower chair from the US. i suppose on behalf of the PRC [People's Republic of China], thank you. they appeared to want to configure a bathroom for patients to be able to use it" (Tim C. 2003h). He thanked his fellow members, underscoring his gratitude in capitalized letters: "CARECURE IS EVERYTHING ANYBODY COULD HOPE FOR. WE FEEL VERY FORTUNATE TO HAVE THE SUPPORT OF EVERYONE BACK HOME" (Tim C. 2003i).

As Shower Chair Fund contributor jmublueduck replied, "it's great to hear FedEx pulled through. very cool! anyway, just know we're here for you guys. the shower chair was just a tangible way we could express our care" (jmublueduck 2003b). Through these expressions of care—invoked by shower chairs, intimations of anxiety, and kinship metaphors displayed online—CareCure members participated vicariously in the quest for the cure undertaken by their SCI pioneers.

AROUND-THE-CLOCK CAREGIVING

Back on the ground in Beijing, flesh-and-blood family members played a vital role in facilitating and managing these biomedical odysseys. This stemmed in part from the nature of the neurological conditions with which they were grappling. Attending to the needs of someone living with a neurological injury or degenerative disorder was a grueling endeavor. As CJO described in the previous chapter, those living with high cervical spinal injuries depended on others for even the smallest tasks of daily life, from getting out of bed in the morning to getting something to drink and taking a bath. Only his "angelic mother" was capable of and willing to fulfill these relentless needs.

The context of the experimental treatment also elevated the role of family participants. Undergoing hospitalization and surgery in Beijing heightened both the practical and moral demands on family caregivers to attend to the needs of their OEC pioneers. In China, as with many other developing countries, the work of providing care for hospital patients falls largely to family members. The hospital staff focuses on medical treatment, while family members are held responsible for all other needs of the patient. This contrasted sharply with contemporary American expectations about medical care. In his social history of American medicine from 1850 to 1920, historian Charles Rosenberg (1987) has documented the transfer of health care from the family to formalized institutions in which strangers render care to strangers. This reorganization of American health care established the now taken-for-granted assumption that hospitals are responsible for the complete care of patients. In this context, which has been reinforced by American hospital practices such as limited visiting hours, family involvement takes a largely peripheral role.

But hospital care has been organized differently in China (Henderson and Cohen 1984). Family members serve as the main caregivers for patients during hospitalization (Schneider 1993). Their intensive participation is necessary to ensuring patients' well-being, including attending to personal hygiene and nutritional needs, as well as making advance payments for all medical services. Nurses, who typically bear much of the burden of care in American hospitals from feeding patients to changing bed pans, play a more technical role in Chinese hospitals. Their focus is on assisting physicians in delivering specialized medical treatments and managing the administrative tasks of keeping the hospital ward running smoothly. Both the structure of health care delivery and the cultural logic of filial piety in China have reinforced family involvement as a key component of patients' treatment process during hospitalization and beyond.

Huang's American patients and their family members thus entered into a very different cultural milieu upon landing in China. Huang explicitly required all of his foreign patients to come with at least one caregiver. Thus CareCure pioneers Tim C. and Handibob came to Chaoyang Hospital with their wives (Mrs. Handibob was a registered nurse with twenty-three years of professional experience) while CJO brought his mother along. As tetraplegics with cervical-level injuries, the pioneers were all to some extent dependent upon their caregivers to help them get through their daily routines and survive their extraordinary adventures. Their familial caregivers sometimes even took over the work of posting updates on behalf of the busy pioneers, who were often preoccupied with an endless battery of tests. As they assured anxious CareCure members looking for updates:

> Right now the most important thing is for the three of us to have the surgery and to hopefully have the results to be able to prove that it works. So everyone just take a deep breath quit worrying about all of the maybe issues the three of us will

keep you posted in our progress hopefully on a daily basis. If not us as we will be a little incapacitated, our Beautiful caregivers will take over. P.S. my beautiful wife is typing this message (Hahahahaha) Talk to you all soon. (Handibob 2003b)

From companions and cheerleaders to laundry maids and ad hoc typists, family members (most often women) played a crucial role in managing the cross-cultural experiences of undergoing experimental treatment in a foreign country. When Huang moved his operations to New Century Hospital at the end of 2004, one of his key upgrades was to provide private rooms for each patient with an additional hospital bed so caregivers could stay with their loved ones around the clock. The caregiver's lodging and meal costs were factored in the $20,000 price tag for the OEG procedure and monthlong hospital stay.

ALTERNATIVE ARRANGEMENTS

While the majority of Huang's foreign patients came to China with at least one family member, a small number were unable to find a blood relative or close friend to accompany them. These patients thus turned to hired aides to assist them during their monthlong treatment in Beijing. The anomalous experiences of these solo patients and their alternative caregivers reveal much about the interpersonal relationships and expectations shaping the cross-cultural encounters between the Chinese medical staff and their foreign patients.

Frau K. was an imperious seventy-five-year-old Swiss woman who landed in Beijing in October 2005 without an appointment for the OEG surgery. She suffered from tethered cord syndrome, which created excess tension in her spinal cord and had led to urinary incontinence and progressive neurological deterioration. Frau K. was one of the only OEG surgery seekers who did not find out about Huang from Internet sources. The septuagenarian didn't even own a computer. Instead, she had seen a German TV report on Huang's procedure and managed to track down the physical address of New Century Hospital after a series of phone calls. Dr. Huang took pity on her and agreed to treat her, even though by then he had a waiting list of hundreds of other patients seeking to undergo OEC transplantation.

Frau K. was accompanied by a Russian woman named Yana who spoke five different languages, including Chinese and German. Yana worked as an independent tour guide and had lived in China for several years. After meeting Frau K. she volunteered her services to her new "friend," sensing an excellent business opportunity. While most of the New Century staff members viewed Yana as an opportunist who barely disguised her desire to make a profit from the clinic, Dr. Huang seized upon the potential of Yana's linguistic abilities for serving his increasingly diverse patient population. Proclaiming that "we can no longer just use English" since the patients now came from countries all over the world, Huang invited Yana to give a talk on cross-cultural communication issues at the weekly staff meeting. Yana turned the opportunity into a platform for flagrant self-promotion. Criticizing the gathered staff for not doing an adequate job communicating with their foreign patients, Yana declared that hospital needed to hire someone like her who could speak multiple languages and, more important, who could understand what foreign patients wanted. But Yana's vision of herself as Frau K's translator and companion clashed with the Chinese staff's expectations about how best to meet the needs of a foreign patient. Bird, one of the clinic's patient coordinators, faulted Yana for not being willing to carry out most of the physical tasks of caregiving, including bathing and turning Frau K. over in bed to avoid pressure sores. Yana's lack of care manifested in a festering bedsore that Frau K. developed during her second week at New Century Hospital.

Frau K. was an impetuous, demanding patient who caused endless trouble for the New Century nurses and physicians. Dr. Brian, a young Chinese neurosurgeon assigned as her attending physician, took the brunt of Frau K's frustrations. He had adopted the English name "Brian" because it sounded like "brain," an apt moniker for an aspiring neurosurgeon.[6] After enduring yet another tirade, Dr. Brian theorized that since Frau K. had never been married before and lived on her own, she did not know how to interact socially with others. Frau K. had an inflated sense of her own importance. One afternoon, she beckoned me into her room and announced that the "King of Kuwait" was being treated in Room 18 and he had kissed her hand twice.[7] Smiling, she told me that his son promised to bring flowers for her. She speculated that if she were twenty years younger, he would have fallen in love with her. Gesturing at her own face, she told me that "they really like blue eyes."

Frau K's infatuation with neighboring royalty contrasted sharply with her disregard for the Chinese staff. I found Dr. Brian slumped at his desk in our shared office one afternoon, his head cradled in his hands. Dr. Huang had chastised him for "not taking better care of the old Swiss lady." Frau K. had to be given intravenous fluids to replenish her nutrients, and Dr. Huang blamed Brian for not doing a better job encouraging her to eat her meals. But from what I could see, Brian was trying his best to deal with his challenging patient. I watched Frau K. fling her cup to the ground on numerous occasions and order Dr. Brian to bring her a new one filled with colder water. Dr. Brian lamented in Chinese, "I've never even treated my own mother this well! I spent this entire day sitting by her side, getting her water, peeling apples for her." He had even skipped the clinic's anniversary banquet celebration in order to sit with Frau K. But she did not appreciate his efforts, pushing him away when he approached too closely. Pointing at her mouth and puffing, she muttered, "Chinese men not good. Chinese men smell bad here."

Without an attentive family caregiver by her side, Frau K. required an inordinate amount of resources and attention from the Chinese clinic staff. The nurses would often find her stark naked with all of the covers thrown off her bed, and she constantly berated them for not meeting her needs. She made several nurses cry, and a few of them refused to go into her room after being physically slapped by her. During an emergency staff meeting convened to discuss her situation, Dr. Huang's second-in-command, neurosurgeon Dr. Liang, tried to assuage the nurses' complaints by placing Frau K.'s pitiable situation in context: "She's all alone, an old woman, it's not easy for her to come here to us for treatment." Dr. Liang assigned four neurosurgical trainee residents to her room, ordering them to take turns accompanying the old woman at all times. The four residents looked dismayed at their unfortunate luck as the others snickered. Sophie, the head Chinese nurse, exclaimed: "Hang in there everyone, let's keep it up!" Meanwhile, I could hear Frau K.'s screams emanating from the end of the hallway: "I have never been sicker in my life! Chinese people are DUM DUM DUM!" Throughout the entire meeting, the indicator light for Room 1 flashed continuously as Frau K. pressed her call button repeatedly.

Frau K.'s case was an extreme outlier and it was easy for everyone to criticize her "friend" Yana's failings. But even in cases where hired caregivers acted with impeccable professionalism and selfless devotion, the Chinese staff at New Century did not see these individuals as adequate replacements for a close family member. Gerald, the British carer we encountered in chapter 3, was a case in point. A semiretired solicitor from a village in central England, Gerald had come to Beijing as a substitute "carer" for his former boss, Duncan, who had sought Dr. Huang's surgery in a desperate attempt to stave off the ALS that had already claimed his abilities to walk and talk. Duncan, a divorced father of two grown children, did not have any family members able to accompany him to Beijing so he had turned to Gerald for help. Both approaching their sixties, the two British men shared a "wicked" sense of humor that they displayed prominently on their online chronicle of their China experiences. Their blog, titled "Sweet N Sour" to reflect Gerald's view of their contrasting personalities, began with a gruesome photo of a samurai with a hatchet through his skull and adorned with the caption: "In the beginning, Dr Huang's early attempts at the procedure were less sophisticated!" (Sweet N Sour 2005a).

The two men had been only casual acquaintances before embarking on their "Beijing adventure" together, although Gerald claimed that this made him a more effective caregiver for his wheelchair-confined employer. Unlike family members enduring the agonizing wait outside the operating room with tears streaming down their faces, Gerald explained that he provided "compassion without the excess emotion." He could thus focus more effectively on the practical details of ensuring his cantankerous charge's comfort, carrying out tasks ranging from the entertaining (shopping for beer and "ice lollies" to satisfy Duncan's discerning palate) to the distasteful (cutting Duncan's overgrown toenails). The irascible patient presented a less rosy picture of his designated caregiver's qualities, however. As Duncan declared in capital letters on their blog: "GERALD WAS AN INSPIRED CHOICE OF COMPANION AND HIS INSISTENCE ON GOING TO THE HOTEL EVERY NIGHT REALLY GETS

UP THE NOSE OF THE HEAD NURSE" (Sweet N Sour 2005c). Duncan was one of the only patients at New Century Hospital's Neurosurgery Ward for Foreigners whose caregiver did not stay overnight in the extra hospital bed that the clinic placed in each room. Instead, Gerald slept on a custom-designed pillow-top mattress at the five-star Shangri-La Hotel in a different district of the city. What Gerald rationalized as fair recompense for his volunteered services most of the nurses perceived as a moral failing in an otherwise likable foreigner who entertained them with free English lessons.

These everyday interactions and misunderstandings on the hospital ward caused both consternation and amusement among patients, their caregivers, and the Chinese medical staff. But all of these details were overshadowed by the main purpose of these foreigners' visit to China: to undergo a potentially life-altering fetal cell transplantation operation.

THE UNNAMED FETUS IN THE OPERATING ROOM

Huang's experimental protocol required extracting olfactory ensheathing glial (OEG) cells from the olfactory bulb of fetuses aborted during the second trimester of pregnancy. Although olfactory receptors begin to form early in the embryonic period, the olfactory bulb does not mature until mid-gestation. Huang thus needed second-trimester fetuses in order to produce enough of the right kind of cells for his procedure. This posed both practical and moral quandaries for patients and families seeking OEG fetal cell transplantation.

Huang's domestic Chinese patients and families were responsible for procuring the aborted fetuses—an arrangement that he had established during his tenure at the Naval General Hospital and continued to maintain during his stint at Chaoyang Hospital and more recently at New Century Hospital. How did this work in practice? The head nurse of the neurosurgery ward would provide would-be Chinese patients with the phone number of an abortion clinic. These patients (or more often their family members) would have to contact a nurse or physician at the abortion clinic, obtain referrals for pregnant women seeking second-trimester abortions, and then negotiate payments for the donor and the associated abortion clinic staff in order to obtain access to the fetal remains following the abortion procedure. Only after the payment and agreements were secured would the Chinese patient be able to arrange an appointment with Huang's staff for the OEG fetal cell transplantation. While Huang had decided to focus primarily on foreign patients by the time I started my fieldwork at New Century Hospital, I had the opportunity to interview some of his Chinese patients who returned for follow-up examinations. Brother Lu, an SCI patient from Zhejiang province who had undergone the OEG fetal cell transplantation in Huang's early days at the Naval General Hospital, described the arduous fetal procurement process for me. As someone who had traveled over 1,500 kilometers from home to seek Huang's experimental treatment, Lu faced particular difficulties locating pregnant women in Beijing who were willing to have late-term abortions. After finding willing donors, he had to pay for the cost of the abortions and nutritional and recovery fees for the women, as well as offer *hóng-bāo* (红包) (monetary gifts enclosed in red envelopes) to the various medical personnel involved.

When Huang began accepting foreign patients such as Tim C., Handibob, and CJO, this procurement process quickly became untenable. While he might reasonably expect his Chinese-speaking patients from Taiwan and Hong Kong to obtain their own fetal tissue, his patients from the United States and Europe did not have the linguistic capacity or cultural knowledge to approach pregnant Chinese women or their Chinese obstetricians to negotiate an arrangement. Huang's clinical staff thus began to obtain the fetal tissue on behalf of the foreign patients, as part of the $20,000 price tag of the surgery and monthlong hospital stay.[8]

Beginning in 2005, Huang executed a formal "Scientific Research Cooperation Agreement" (科研合作协议书 *kēyán hézuò xiéyì shū*) with a hospital located five hundred kilometers away in Shandong province. This agreement specified the "Cell Research Center's Fetal Sample Derivation Requirements" (细胞研究中心胚胎标本取材要求 *xìbāo yánjiū zhōngxīn pēitāi biāoběn qǔcái yāoqiú*); namely that the Shandong hospital would provide Huang's laboratory with a supply of aborted fetuses (流产胚胎 *liúchǎn pēitāi*) of gestational age sixteen weeks or older, as well as certification that the fetuses did not have any brain malformations and the pregnant women did not have HIV, Hepatitis B, or Hepatitis C. If a pregnant woman refused to submit to testing for these infectious diseases (which she would need to pay for out of pocket), then the research collaborators were instructed to conduct the tests on a sample of maternal blood instead. The "cooperation agreement" also specified the optimum abortion procedure: induction of abortion by water balloon (水囊引产 *shuǐ náng yǐnchǎn*). A commonly used procedure in China for inducing abortion during the second trimester of pregnancy, this method involves inserting an artificial bladder (often constructed of a doubled condom attached to a rubber catheter) between the uterine wall and fetal membrane. Sterile saline would then be injected into the artificial bladder to increase intrauterine pressure and provide mechanical stimulation of the cervical canal, ultimately inducing uterine contractions and prompting the expulsion of the fetus and placenta. The entire induced abortion process generally took approximately seventy-two hours, giving the research collaborators plenty of time to prepare for the retrieval of the aborted fetus and the subsequent cultivation of the olfactory bulb cells. Recognizing the critical importance of documenting informed consent for a potentially controversial step in his experimental procedure, Huang's "cooperation agreement" also mandated an "Authorization for the Disposal of Induced/Aborted Remains" (引产物 / 流产物处置授权书 *yǐnchǎnwù/liúchǎnwù chǔzhì shòuquán shū*) to be signed by the pregnant woman.[9]

As an American coming from a sociopolitical context where abortion providers were harassed and even killed for performing late-term abortions, I was surprised that Dr. Huang and the Chinese hospital staff members I interviewed were unperturbed by the use of second-trimester fetuses for their experimental procedure. For these Chinese health care workers, abortion was a standard medical procedure routinized by nearly three decades of state-mandated birth-planning policies that limited most urban families to a single child. Huang explained his decision to outsource the fetal cell procurement to a hospital in another province as both a practical matter and a public relations move. In cosmopolitan Beijing, female urbanites who wanted abortions generally obtained them early in the pregnancy. During my fieldwork, one of the New Century nurses got pregnant after having sex with her fiancé for the first time. Prepared neither emotionally nor financially to give birth to a child, the nurse terminated her unwanted pregnancy as soon as she could (in her case, forty-four days after the first time she had sexual intercourse). Outside the main metropolitan centers, rural women tended to have less access to medical facilities, often resulting in abortions performed later in the pregnancy process.

Although his Chinese patients and staff members seemed unbothered by the ethics of abortion, Huang was sensitive to Western media portrayals of his experimental therapy. He wanted journalists to focus on his potentially paradigm-changing medical achievements rather than getting bogged down with what he considered to be unimportant distractions. By executing this fetal procurement agreement in a different province, Huang physically removed inquiring journalists and foreign patients (as well as curious anthropologists) from encounters with pregnant women who underwent childbirth-like processes to abort late-term fetuses on the brink of viability. In their analysis of emerging tissue bioeconomies, Catherine Waldby and Melinda Cooper observe that while women play an essential role as the primary tissue donors in the new stem cell industries, these feminized forms of "regenerative labor" remain largely unacknowledged (2010, 3). Adapting a Marxist theory of alienation to show how women participating in the tissue bioeconomy become alienated from the products of their regenerative labor, Waldby and Cooper argue that "formally 'reproductive tissue' enters into another epistemological space where the potentiality of the germ cell is defined in radically different ways" (2010, 14–15). Although Huang utilized olfactory bulb cells rather than oocytes or embryos, these aborted fetal cells underwent a similar epistemological transformation as they moved to a different institutional, legal, and scientific context.

This epistemological transformation enabled many of the foreign patients to avoid dwelling on the morally and viscerally repugnant aspect of their otherwise exalted quests for a cure. Not surprisingly, the words "abortion" and "fetus" did not appear at all in the surgical report threads of the CareCure pioneers who underwent Huang's procedure in Beijing. The only public acknowledgment of the source of the cells made by the first three American OEG recipients was the following CareCure update from Tim C. a few days after he arrived in Beijing: "[Huang's] staff doctor repo[r]ted that my blood test results were fine and confirmed my blood type. He would now obtain the fetal tissue" (Tim C. 2003b). In Tim's rendering, the unmentioned aborted fetus has already been transformed into "fetal tissue," conveniently procured and matched by an anonymous staff doctor.

Excited about the possibility of a cure within reach, CareCure members were particularly circumspect about the moral quandaries posed by a procedure that required aborted fetuses and even engaged in self-censorship online to avoid emphasizing the fetal origins of the OEG cells and attracting unwanted attention to their discussion forum. When junior member and family friend PaulaMc enthusiastically announced that she had informed *Dateline MSNBC* about Tim C.'s journey to Beijing, a senior CareCure member quickly warned her about jeopardizing Huang's operation:

> PaulaMc, i would urge you to consider the possible consequences of media publicity at this stage . . . the pro lifers may have a "welcome home celebration" waiting for these people on their return to the US. i am guessing this, but it may have implications for Dr Huang to Publish in Scientific Journals. it would not be difficult for the Brownback Bill[10] to be modified to include a clause that US citizens who receive therapies involving fetal cells be arrested and charged on their return to the states. if you do get media attention for this procedure, i would suggest that you ask other patients permission before mentioning their names, and i would implore you not to mention this [CareCure] site." (dogger 2003)

Recognizing the delicacy of the situation surrounding Huang's experimental fetal cell procedure, PaulaMc immediately responded: "Dogger, You're probably right, it could result in bad consequences. I'll just keep my mouth shut should I hear back from them" (PaulaMc 2003).

Despite being protected from many of the moral quandaries and questionable black market exchanges posed by obtaining fetuses from late-stage abortions, foreign patients were still subject to the practical constraints of a cell-based therapy. Obtaining an adequate supply of fetal olfactory cells was the key rate-limiting step of the experimental procedure. Aside from the practical challenges of obtaining aborted fetuses, the subsequent preparation of OEG cells was itself a tedious and labor-intensive process. Although immortalized OEG cell lines had been produced from rat olfactory bulbs (Moreno-Flores et al. 2006), this laboratory achievement had yet to be duplicated for human OEG cells when Huang initiated his clinical treatments. Furthermore, since creating immortal cell lines required transforming the original cells with viruses, this could potentially affect the cells' regenerative properties or pose a safety risk for use in human patients. Thus scientists and clinicians seeking to utilize these cells needed to continuously establish primary cultures from a fresh source material such as fetal olfactory bulbs or adult nasal mucosa.

For Huang's staff, this meant that OEG cells had to be cultured on the spot for each surgical recipient. As they described in a paper for the research journal *Anatomical Record* (Liu et al. 2010), the intact olfactory bulb was extracted from the aborted fetal remains, washed in an ice-cold saline solution, and diced into small fragments. This mix was then digested with trypsin, a reagent commonly used in cell cultures to dissociate tissue into individual cells. These olfactory bulb cells were then seeded onto petri dishes. After culturing and propagating the olfactory cells for two to three weeks, Huang's laboratory staff was able to obtain approximately one million cells from each fetal olfactory bulb. They ensured that the propagated cells were the desired type through visual inspection (OEG cells had a distinct morphology consisting of small nuclei, thin cytoplasm, and fine processes) and immunostaining with the p75 antibody (a neurotrophin receptor specific for OEG cells). The laboratory staff also performed human leukocyte antigen (HLA) typing to ensure histocompatibility between the donor fetuses and the surgical recipients. Depending on the available supply of aborted fetuses, they used one to two fetal olfactory bulbs to obtain enough OEG cells for use in the transplantation procedure.

Although foreign patients were shielded from the nitty-gritty of procuring and preparing the fetal cells, they still felt the ramifications of any complications in this process. The availability of the cells affected the timing of the surgical procedure for patients. Particularly when an influx of new patients arrived in quick succession to Beijing, Huang's clinical and laboratory staff members often had difficulty preparing enough cells to meet the demand for the transplantation procedure.

Dutch columnist Loes Claerhoudt arrived in Beijing at the beginning of January 2005. Her sons had accompanied her to Beijing during their Christmas holiday, expecting to provide help and support during her surgical operation. They had hoped to witness their mother's first improvements following the surgery and "the beginning of a new life" ("begin van een nieuw leven" [Claerhoudt 2005b]). But they ran headlong into the challenges of supply and demand, with sixteen patients from Belgium, Croatia, Greece, Holland, Hong Kong, the U.K., the United States, and Yemen arriving within days of each other after the new year. As Loes explained in her blog for anxious family and friends back home awaiting news:

> Wat betreft de cellen: het is in de eerste plaats moeilijk om er aan te komen. Als de cellen er dan eenmaal zijn, moeten ze nog in het laboratorium verder worden gekweekt. Dit proces is kennelijk niet helemaal te beinvloeden. [With respect to the cells: it is first of all difficult to get them. Once the cells are there, they still have to be grown in the laboratory. Apparently it is very difficult to influence this process entirely.] (Claerhoudt 2005a)

As the days dragged on without any available cells for transplantation, her sons finally had to return home to Utrecht in mid-January, leaving their mother's care to their father alone. Loes finally underwent the experimental surgery sixteen days after she first arrived in Beijing, troubled no longer by the lagging status of the cells in question. Her immediate focus, as evidenced on her public blog, was recovering from the operation and striving for a reversal in neurodegenerative processes that had taken away many of her functional abilities. Like Loes, many of Huang's foreign patients avoided grappling with the morality of abortion or chose instead to emphasize more personally pressing concerns about surgical recovery and functional gain.

REDEEMING THE FETUS

There were, however, some OEG surgery patients who struggled with the morality of abortion. I was surprised to meet a significant number of pro-life Southern Baptists undergoing fetal cell transplantation in Beijing. The Southern Baptist Convention has long opposed the use of human stem cells and fetal tissue in research or treatment. An early resolution in 1992 challenged "the unethical practice of using fetal tissue from induced abortions in experimental research, whether privately or publicly funded," noting that it would allow "electively aborted babies to be exploited for scientific and commercial purposes" (Southern Baptist Convention 1992). A 1999 resolution vigorously opposed human embryonic and stem cell research, noting that "some forms of human stem cell research require the destruction of human embryos in order to obtain the cells for such research and Southern Baptists are on record for their decades-long opposition to abortion except to save the physical life of the mother and their opposition to destructive human embryo research" (Southern Baptist Convention 1999). A resolution issued the following year on "human fetal tissue trafficking" continued to condemn "elective abortion [as] an act of violence against unborn human beings, and the sale of their tissues is an assault on the biblical truth that all human beings are created in the image of God" (Southern Baptist Convention 2000).

Given these unequivocal condemnations of abortion and the use of human fetal tissue, how could a Southern Baptist pursue Huang's treatment in good conscience? I discovered that even those with strong religious views condemning abortion usually found a way to justify the procedure when they or their loved ones were faced with the choice.

A couple I met from Kentucky actively drew on their faith as Southern Baptists to reconcile their church's stance against abortion with their choice to pursue a procedure that utilized cells from aborted fetuses. Describing their trip to China as part of "God's plan for us," Roberta, whose husband, Sam, suffered from ALS, recounted the story of how they had discovered Huang's experimental therapy. Their pastor had come across a story in the *Baptist Standard* about a paper mill worker in Alabama who had undergone the OEG fetal cell transplantation procedure in Beijing. This Alabaman was no ordinary ALS patient:

he came from a staunchly religious family with a father-in-law who was a Baptist pastor. As reporter Karen Tolkkinen described in the news story that convinced the Kentucky couple to go to China:

> Lyles' father-in-law, Pastor Benny Harrison of Christian Fellowship Baptist Church in Thomasville, Ala., was lying awake in bed one night, seeking an answer from God as he was torn between his son-in-law's terrible future and the dilemma over the aborted babies in China. An Old Testament passage came to him—the story about how Joseph's brothers sold him into slavery in Egypt. The story begins with a terrible act—the sale of their brother. But it ends with redemption, when Joseph, who has risen to a position of power in Pharaoh's palace, saves his family from famine.
>
> "They meant for bad," Harrison said. "God meant for good."
>
> It's like that with the babies, he said. Abortions are wrong. But maybe the babies can help his son-in-law and others.
>
> [Lyles's wife] also found comfort in those words.
>
> "Something good can come out of something bad," she said. "They will continue the abortions anyway. They're throwing these cells away every day." (Tolkkinen 2004)

Faced with a horrifying terminal illness, the Alabama and Kentucky families, together with their pastors, believed that the potential positives outweighed or even justified the use of the fetal cells, given that these babies were already going to be aborted under the Chinese government's policy of one child per family.

Like the Lyles family, Sam and Roberta obtained the spiritual and financial support of their congregation back home—including daily prayers and $30,000 in donations—and traveled to Beijing in the hopes of halting the rapid deterioration of his motor neurons. By the time Sam arrived in Beijing, he had already lost control of his lower facial muscles and even his wife had difficulty understanding his garbled speech. Trying to talk with Sam reminded me of labored conversations with my husband's aunt, who had died the previous year of complications from multiple sclerosis (MS), another neurodegenerative disease that also affects a person's ability to talk. Difficulty in communicating is probably the most disheartening aspect of neurodegenerative diseases such as ALS and MS. I remember sitting in the nursing home with my husband's aunt with a strained smile on my face, desperately grasping for the barest thread of conversational continuity. As Sam struggled to participate in our conversation that April afternoon as a sandstorm darkened the windows of his hospital room, I had that same awful feeling as I made every effort to decipher what he had to say. In the end, Roberta and I had to nod cheerfully and pretend we understood him as he tried to control the excessive saliva pooling in his mouth with a small suction machine. Less sure of herself now, Roberta told me, "If it doesn't work, that means it just wasn't God's plan and we'll just take each day as we have been and keep praying."

Glancing furtively at the door, she pulled her suitcase out from under her husband's bed and showed me a beautifully embroidered cloth. "It's a prayer blanket," she told me. "The congregation back home gave us a few to take with us. . . . I don't know if it's okay to take them out here." I nodded as she caressed the corner of the prayer cloth and explained their decision to undergo the fetal cell transplantation surgery as a way of redeeming the immoral practice of abortion in China. "My husband and I don't believe in abortion. But China does it for other reasons besides research. . . . It's like making lemonade out of lemons. We feel like this is a way God has of taking something bad and making something good out of it." Roberta resolved their uneasiness about benefiting from abortion by placing the exchange firmly within a Christian narrative of sacrifice. Her husband's use of the cells ensured that the death of the fetus was not in vain, effectively transforming an otherwise unholy act into a meaningful sacrifice.

This logic of retroactive redemption effectively enables the cells of the donor (i.e., the aborted fetus) to be framed as a sacrifice whether they were gifted, sold, or even stolen. This has important implications for the anthropological literature on organ transplantation and more broadly the economy of bodily transactions. Writing about living donor kidney transactions in India, Lawrence Cohen (2001) observed that patients in need of kidneys often preferred to purchase them through illegal brokers rather than to take them from family members.[11] The family member's life was granted a social and political value that allowed a loss of life or health to be identified as sacrifice, while the anonymous seller's life was framed as "bare life" (Agamben 1998)—a life unworthy of being lived, one that can be allowed to die within the regime of biopolitics, and ultimately a life whose loss can therefore never be considered a sacrifice. Cohen notes that this distinction results in the selective suppression of "difference" essential to the politics of transnational organ sales. According to this selective logic, the tissues are equivalent enough to be exchanged, but the value of the lives is different enough to enable the trade. It is ironic to draw on Agamben to think through how Southern Baptists with ALS justify the use of aborted fetuses, given that both figures fall under his definition of "bare life."[12] Returning to the logic of sacrifice invoked by Huang's Southern Baptist patients, lives which had been written off as "devoid of value" (whether the incurable patient or the aborted fetus) were ultimately rescued and redeemed by the experimental fetal cell transplantation procedure.

THE "BLACK AND DECKER" MOMENT

Once the OEG fetal cells were procured and cultured, how did the experimental surgical procedure unfold? Huang's OEG fetal cell transplantation protocol for patients with spinal cord injury was based on well-established surgical procedures.[13] After putting the patient under general anesthesia, the next step involved performing a laminectomy, a common surgical procedure used to remove a portion of the vertebral bone.[14] Huang and his neurosurgical team then opened up the dura mater membrane in order to expose the spinal cord. After removing visible adhesions (scar tissue), the neurosurgeons injected approximately two million cultured olfactory ensheathing glial cells above and below the injury site. They then sutured up the dura and sewed the bony lamina back in place.

While Huang and his neurosurgical team initially applied the same procedure to all of their patients, they modified their protocol for patients with ALS and other neurodegenerative diseases. The compromised respiratory function of ALS patients made general anesthesia a risky proposition. The Chinese neurosurgeons thus decided to forgo the spinal cord injection and inject the cells directly into the brain, which would enable them to perform the intracranial transplantation procedure using local anesthesia only. Huang's analysis of ALS patients' MRI scans indicated abnormally high signaling along the pathway of the corticospinal tract, a key area of the brain implicated in motor function. He thus decided to perform the intracranial transplant in this region, targeting the bilateral corona radiata of the brain's frontal lobes (Victor, Ropper, and Adams 2000; Chen et al. 2007; Huang et al. 2008).[15] While the precise etiology and mechanisms of motor neuron degeneration in ALS have yet to be determined, the prevailing consensus suggested multiple pathogenic processes including genetic alterations, oxidative stress, glutamate toxicity, protein aggregation, and other environmental factors (Bruijn, Miller, and Cleveland 2004; Shaw 2005). By injecting OEG cells into the corona radiata, Huang attempted to alter the neurochemical environment in this critical region in the hopes of staving off motor neuron death. His neurosurgical team located this "key point for neural network restoration" (Chen et al. 2010) using a combination of neuroimaging scans and stereotactic techniques (a method of locating targets of surgical interest within the brain relative to an external frame of reference). They then drilled two small burr holes into the skull at the identified key points, injected a suspension of approximately one million cells into each hole, and then sutured the scalp to close the incision.

Why did the divergence in clinical procedures matter for how patients experienced the fetal cell transplantation? Since SCI patients underwent the experimental procedure under general anesthesia, none of them consciously experienced the operation itself. They only had memories of entering the operating room, being transferred to the operating table, and then waking up afterward back in their private hospital room. Not surprisingly, most of Huang's SCI patients had little to say about the actual surgical experience. Their discussions, on- and offline, focused on the battery of tests they underwent before the procedure and their recovery afterward.

ALS patients, on the other hand, had a completely different relationship to the surgical procedure. Unlike their fellow SCI patients, the majority of ALS patients who underwent the fetal cell transplantation received local anesthesia and were thus conscious throughout the entire operation. The experience of what British patient Duncan described as "THAT NEVER TO BE REPEATED BLACK AND DECKER[16] MOMENT" was disconcerting for many of the ALS patients, to say the least (figure 4.1). While I had ample opportunities to scrub into the surgeries and observe the operations, witnessing the procedure as a bystander was a completely different experience than actually lying down on the steel surgical table and getting fetal cells drilled into your head.

To illuminate the material and affective dimensions of this experience from the perspective of an experimental pioneer, I turn to Jeff Dunn's online account of undergoing the OEG cell transplantation procedure in November 2004 at New Century Hospital. As a former firefighter and paramedic before ALS struck him down, Jeff was used to rushing head-on into raging flames in the line of duty. Despite facing risks and dangers on a daily basis, even he found the experience of getting fetal cells injected into his head nerve-wracking. Jeff described his surgery day on his public blog hosted on the Castle Rock Professional Fire Fighters and Paramedics Local 4116 website:

> Limbo is the best description for the hours pre-surgery. There were three of us scheduled, another ALS and a SCI, but no one knows the schedule. So, we wait. Around 2:00 PM, without any notice, the nurses showed up and said it is time. Wow, talk about surprised, I mean, I like to psych myself up for these kinds of things. They asked if I wanted a wheel chair to which I said hell no, I'm walking in and walking out. Admittedly my legs did get a little stiff the closer I got to the surgery rooms. [My wife] Cyrilla gave me a kiss as I passed through the doors and told me she would be waiting.
>
> The following is hopefully an honest depiction of the procedure as best as I can describe using facts and emotions simultaneously. I walk into the first room on the right, which is approximately 10 x 15 feet and nothing like the surgery suites I have so often found myself in through the years. The paint is old and the light is an older type two tube florescent. I spend as much energy as possible checking out the equipment and am pleased. They have state of the art cardiac, SpO2 (oxygen monitoring), respiration monitoring and oxygen delivery equipment. I am asked to lay down on the table, which is a typical hard table with removable armrests, and all the equipment is on my left. Behind me and to the left is a lighted x-ray panel where I can see my MRI films. A nurse initiates an IV in my right hand, small gauge butterfly, with a 250cc bag of a clear solution but

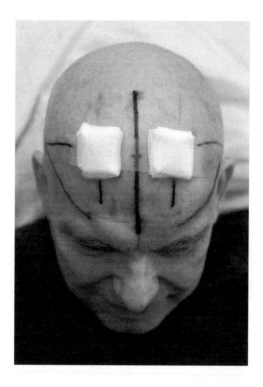

Figure 4.1. That "Black and Decker" moment (photograph by Doug Kanter). Gauze pads and lines drawn on his skull mark the site of fetal cell transplantation surgery on an American ALS patient at New Century Hospital.

the label is in Chinese so I have no idea what it is. All the equipment is applied expertly except they have to change electrode patches twice because they weren't reading—probably dry. Hate to think what kind of shape their defibrillation pads are in, if they use them.

As I lay there I can feel my anxiety level rising and I wonder why. I mean, I've had surgeries, I have ALS and nothing should scare me. It is the language barrier, I cannot understand anything happening or what everyone is talking about and this is a very scary thing. I think back to all the patients I have seen on 911 calls who could not understand anything I was saying. This is a surgery where I have interacted with these doctors for 8 days, imagine experiencing a heart attack, calling 911 and having 5 or 6 guys walk through the door with equipment and begin working on you without any understanding of what is happening. It is an enlightening experience.

The doctors, three plus Dr. Huang, begin marking lines on my head repeatedly referring to the MRI films and then continuing. This takes about fifteen minutes followed by some reassuring pats on my shoulder and then my face is draped and I am blind. The next noise I hear, other than Chinese, is a drill getting fired up. Man, I jumped about a foot off that table when they did that and almost bolted for the door. It sounds like a DeWalt 18v and I wonder if they use a hammer drill.

Haven't they ever heard of Valium? I mean I'm tough, or so I thought, but I am getting pretty wigged out. Next comes the local anesthetic, without warning, and soon I can't feel my head or at least the important areas. Another pat on the shoulder and here comes the drill. Nothing in life can prepare you for the sensation of a drill being pressed to your head and someone drilling. Scenes from every horror movie, those that involve someone meeting an untimely death by drill bit are racing through my mind and I silently repeat, don't slip, do a good job! Along with that are about 50 Hail Mary's and 20 Our Fathers. The pressure they are applying is significant, enough to move my whole body down on the table. Half way through the first [hole] there is a pause; a lot of Chinese and I can hear them changing bits. I always knew I had a hard head but this is surprising, must be cheap bits. As drilling resumes, so do my Hail Mary's, and the other thoughts mentioned above. Breakthrough! What an odd sensation and sound, a hissing sound. Okay, bring on the airhead jokes and your welcome for the easy setup. Everything is the same on the second hole with the exception of changing drill bits and upon breakthrough the same hissing noise, which would mean that the air bags are compartmentalized. . . .

If you are wondering about pain, all I will say is it beats going to the dentist. I wait for what seems like a long time with nothing happening and lots of Chinese conversation. I am beginning to wonder if something is wrong but cannot ask. Eventually I feel someone touching my head and then searching for the hole. Once Dr. Huang finds it there is a squishing noise as the cells are injected. He has to dig quite a bit longer on the left side and I start to consider the possibility that a second hole will have to be drilled. The Hail Mary's come back into my head immediately and soon, success, marked by the squishing noise. There are some more reassuring pats on the shoulder and I hear the word, successful, spoken by someone. Music to my ears. There is a sharp sting, again without warning, as someone pulls a suturing needle through my skin, but I am worry free by this time. Moments later the drapes are removed from my face and all I see is a janitor . . . just kidding, I see four smiling doctors and a nurse who again repeat, "successful." I am helped to a seated position and the only pain I feel is in my lower back from being on a flat surface without anything under my knees. I immediately realize that I am not walking anywhere because my legs are like stone. Evidently I had kept every available muscle tensed up for the entire procedure and I have turned into Medusa. Oh well, time to swallow pride and I climb into a wheelchair.

The first thing I see as they open the doors is my wife and I get another kiss. I also note the Rosary in her hand and know that she has been stressed also. Back to our room, there are no recovery rooms I guess. The oxygen, IV, and monitors remain in place and we are checked by two nurses every 5 minutes and a doctor every 10 or 15 minutes. I feel pretty good, maybe a little shaky, but immediately feel the urge to get up and be free of these machines. The entire procedure lasted 50 minutes start to finish. I am finally freed 3 and a half hours later and ravenously dig into dinner. I find that I am not tired and wish to begin therapy immediately to tell the new cells where I need them. I finally give in around eleven and drift off thinking of new cells swimming around my head. Hope I don't sneeze! I miss everyone, especially my children.[17]

Jeff's blog was a testament to his enduring wit, fortitude, and humanity in the face of a devastating disease. Titled "The Dunns go to China: Why is it that someone has to travel halfway around the world to get ALS treatment?" the blog was witness to the dramatic lengths Jeff had to undertake to seek medical care. It was also material evidence of the devotion of hundreds of people who supported his biomedical odyssey: his beloved wife, Cyrilla, who found herself transformed from life partner to full-time caregiver; his colleague Oren Bersagel-Briese, who maintained the fire department's website and facilitated Jeff's online posts; his fellow firefighters in the Castle Rock Local 4116 who took turns working Jeff's shifts so that their stricken colleague could continue to receive his paycheck and medical benefits; and the hundreds of other firefighters and their families, friends, and community members who followed his Internet-mediated quest, sent encouraging emails, participated in fund-raisers, and helped raise awareness for his fight against ALS.

CONCLUSION

This chapter has examined the diverse hospital experiences of several experimental pioneers who underwent olfactory ensheathing glial cell transplantation in Beijing. Although these foreign patients were physically engaged in the quest for a cure rather than just debating about it online, Internet communication technologies continued to play a key role in mediating their cross-cultural encounters in Beijing. Online communities such as CareCure offered a digital "umbilical cord to hope" as these experimental pioneers made sense of a radically different world. I analyzed the key points of disjuncture that these fetal cell recipients had to surmount during their hospital stays in Beijing, providing ethnographic insight into how various individuals and their families dealt with the visceral discomforts of negotiating an unfamiliar medical system and the moral challenges of undergoing an experimental therapy that required cells from aborted fetuses.

Adriana Petryna has demonstrated how "practical issues have overwhelmed ethics" in the globalized pharmaceutical trial industry (2005, 183), with bioethicists and contract researchers focusing on procedural questions of recruitment rather than broader concerns about inequality and exploitation. For many of the foreign patients who went to Huang's neurosurgery clinic seeking an experimental cure, a similar turn to the pragmatic helped foreclose troubling concerns about the ethics of the fetal cell procedure. While most chose to focus on mundane practical concerns, a small subset of Southern Baptist patients "theologized" their moral qualms by invoking a Christian narrative of sacrifice to grant moral value to the fetal cells potentially saving their lives. Caught up in the immediacy of undergoing an experimental surgery in an unfamiliar environment, others like Duncan and Jeff chose self-deprecating humor to mediate the overwhelming viscerality of their "Black and Decker" brain-drilling experience.

The preceding three chapters have examined how the dynamics of illness and chronicity map onto distinctive digital pathways to experimental medicine. I have tracked the mediated experiences of foreign patients seeking olfactory ensheathing glial cell transplantation in Beijing, exploring how they mobilized and operationalized hope in different ways throughout their biomedical odysseys. Part 2 of this book will shift perspective to consider these transnational encounters from the perspective of the Chinese clinicians performing the experimental therapies.

PART II

CHINESE EXPERIMENTS

ODE TO OLFACTORY ENSHEATHING CELLS

A WITNESS TO HISTORY: MEDICINE'S SPLENDOR
NEUROLOGICAL DISORDERS CENTER ANNIVERSARY SONG

历史的见证：医学的灿烂

神经疾病中心一周年之歌

BY WANG FENGMING (王凤鸣) (known to his foreign patients as Dr. Pain for his vigorous *tuīná* [推拿 Chinese massage techniques])

当阳光拨开云雾	When sunlight pushes aside the clouds and mist,
大地一片生机盎然之时	When Mother Earth overflows with life,
当世界令人信服地证明	When the world offers convincing proof of
嗅鞘细胞的神奇	The miracle of olfactory ensheathing cells!
神经疾病中心迎来了	The Neurological Disorders Center welcomes the first
她诞生一周年	anniversary of her birth.
翻开历史	Opening up history,
我们惊人地发现	We discovered to our surprise,
嗅鞘细胞对神经疾病的	The application and treatment of olfactory
应用和治疗	ensheathing cells for neurological diseases.
竟是世界医学史上	Never before had the world opened up this door of
没有敲开的门典	knowledge in the history of medicine;
竟是先人从未涉足的领域	Never before had our ancestors set foot in this
	uncharted territory;
竟是人类没有解决的病难	Never before had humanity solved these catastrophic
	illnesses;
竟是被宣判了这些人	Never before had these people escaped from the
死亡的断言	verdict of death.

于是在这个盲区	Whereupon in this land of blindness,
这些患者	These patients
失去了掌握自己命运的权力	Lost their power to control their own destiny,
失去了改善自我功能的机缘	Lost their opportunity to improve their functioning,
失去了家人亲友的爱恋	Lost their family and friends' affection and love.
有的萌生退意, 每况愈下	Some wished to withdraw, worsening evermore
对生活失去了信心	No longer any confidence in life,
对美好世界失去了向往	No longer any desire for the beautiful world.
有的则用扭曲了的灵魂	Some used their twisted souls
去看绚丽多彩的人生	To look upon the glory and color of life,
更有患者想去自我了断	Some wished even more to cut themselves off
结束自己宝贵的生命	And end their precious lives.
啊!	Ah!
多么残酷的现状	How cruel the status quo!
多么悲惨的病患	How tragic the patients!
多么让人痛心, 可叹	How distressing to see!
然而, 历史并非无情	But history is not merciless.
并非忘记那些受煎熬的人群	She did not forget the tormented.
并非忘记让他们享受人间的 欢乐	She did not forget to give them earthly happiness.
如果说天到酬群	If we say Heaven rewards the people,
那么更应酬报研究出治疗 这种病的人	Then she should provide even more reward to those who find a way to treat these patients.
他就是走在世界医学顶端的	He is the one who has reached the pinnacle of world medicine:
黄红云教授	Professor Huang Hongyun.
他夜以继日, 废寝忘食, 不顾一切	He works from night until day, forgetting food and sleep, heedless of everything else.
千百次的试验, 希望和着汗水	Hundreds of thousands of experiments, hope driving him to sweat harder,
终于成功了	At last achieving success.
他用嗅鞘细胞打开了 患者的天门	He used olfactory ensheathing cells to open up the heavenly gates for patients;
他用嗅鞘细胞注入了 患者的体内	He used olfactory ensheathing cells to infuse the bodies of patients;
他用沸腾的热血溶进了 他们的心田	He used his hot boiling blood to flow into their hearts;
奇迹出现了	Producing a miracle.

有的人站起来了	Some people stood up.
有的人能走路了	Some people began to walk.
有的人能开口说话了	Some people opened their mouths and talked.
绝大部分的患者改善了 　　自己的功能	The vast majority of patients improved their function.
他们激动不已	In endless excitement they
伸开双臂	Reached out their arms,
热烈拥抱着黄教授	Warmly embracing Professor Huang,
幸福的泪水沾湿了衣衫	Their happy tears staining his clothes.
如果说, 他们要说一句 　　感谢的话	If they wanted to say words of appreciation;
那么, 不同国家, 不同肤色 　　用了同一种语言	Then, different countries, different skin colors, 　　　all used the same language:
Thank you very much	Thank you very much
道出了他们发自内心的呼唤	Reveals the essence of their heartfelt call.
他们用重新燃起的希望	They used rekindled hopes
恢复了做人的尊严	To restore the dignity of being human.
啊!	Ah!
这是多么精彩的世界	What a splendid world!
这是多么高尚的医患	What a noble relationship between a doctor and a 　　patient!
不是吗?	Aren't they?
在这里充满着爱, 　　和家人一样的爱	Here we are filled with love, a love like a family's.
在这里充满着责任, 　　一丝不苟的责任	Here we are filled with duty, a duty in which not even 　　one thread is loose.
在这里充满着温暖, 　　春天般的温暖	Here we are filled with warmth, a warmth like that of 　　a spring day.
还有护士小姐	And there are the lady nurses,
她们以白衣天使的人道	Using the humanity of their angelic white dresses
热情的服务	To provide passionate service
到位的护理	To offer authentic care
给神经疾病中心平添了一道	Adding to the Neurosurgical Disorders Center
可爱亮丽的风景线	Lovely and beautiful scenic landscape.
虽然只有短短的一年	Although this has only been one short year,
医疗条件又很有限	And our treatment conditions have been very limited,
又存在着这样那样的困难	And we have faced many other difficulties,
却治疗了 300 多来自世界 　　各国的患者	Yet we treated over 300 patients coming from 　　　countries around the world.

还有大批国外患者的治疗	And large numbers of foreign patients seeking treatment
被排到两年以后的时间	Are on a waiting list two years long.
许多国家的媒体、电视台、网站	The media, television, and websites of many countries
专派记者前来采访、报导	Have sent dedicated reporters to cover the news
还特邀教授去做学术报告	And have specially invited the Professor to give academic reports.
这本身就是医学史上的一个奇观	This in itself is a miracle in the history of medicine.
一年来的成就和花环	The achievements and garlands of the past year
成为他们动力和源泉	Become their momentum and headspring.
他们没有停止前进的步伐	They never stop their forward march,
反而更加坚定了信念	But remain all the more steadfast in their faith.
这里聚集着一批精英、专家	Gathered here in the company of elites and experts,
他们将去研究解决一个个专题	They will study and solve one problem after another,
以深邃的理论和实践	With profound theory and practice
去攀登世界医学的峰巅	They will ascend the pinnacle of world medicine.
尽管前进路上还有很多问题	Even though the road ahead has many questions
甚至还有意想不到的难关	And even unimaginable difficulties
但终究会被他的执著	But in the end through his perseverance,
会被他的无言的事实	Through his unspoken facts,
会被他的利剑所击穿	Through his sharp sword these will be pierced.
风雨过后	After the storm
必定是晴朗的天空	Clear sky appears without fail.
他们必定会为中国、世界医学	On behalf of China and the world of medicine they will without fail
创造出更大的辉煌和灿烂	Create even more glory and splendor.
2005. 10. 28 夜	The night of October 28, 2005

(Translated from the Chinese by Priscilla Song)

MEDICAL ENTREPRENEURS

WHILE THE PRECEDING CHAPTERS HAVE detailed how and why Americans and Europeans living with neurological disorders have pursued fetal cell transplantation in Beijing, I now shift optics to examine these transnational encounters from the perspective of the Chinese clinicians performing the experimental procedures. The following chapters reveal the effects of state-led capitalism and globalization on the experiences of biomedical practitioners immersed in a changing health care system. Since the founding of the People's Republic, ideological mandates have shifted from Mao Zedong's call in the 1950s to "serve the people" (为人民服务 *wèi rénmín fúwù*), Deng Xiaoping's economic reforms in the 1980s to "let some get rich first" (让一部分人先富起来 *ràng yībùfèn rén xiān fù qǐlái*), Hu Jintao's efforts in the 2000s to "build a socialist harmonious society" (构建社会主义和谐社会 *gòujiàn shèhuì zhǔyì héxié shèhuì*), and more recently Xi Jinping's "Chinese dream" targeting the "great renewal of the Chinese nation" (实现中华民族伟大复兴的中国梦 *shíxiàn Zhōnghuá mínzú wěidà fùxīng de Zhōngguó mèng*). As the former emphasis on state-funded preventive care has yielded to a market-driven pursuit of high-tech interventions and subsequent efforts to redress growing health inequalities, Chinese clinicians have faced increasing threats to their professional identities and their very livelihoods as they negotiate the tensions between individual interest and collective good. Yet these politico-economic changes have also enabled novel experiments in profit-making and professional success for an emerging class of medical entrepreneurs.

This chapter explores the ethnographic contours of medical entrepreneurialism in contemporary China. Entrepreneurs are conventionally understood as self-employed individuals who develop and operate independent business ventures, including taking responsibility for the associated risks and profiting from the rewards. Inspired by a Foucauldian approach to power and subjectivity, social theorists have reclaimed the term from economics departments and business schools to explore the broader ways in which entrepreneurialism offers a template for remaking the self that is becoming increasingly aligned with neoliberal projects. In describing the emergence of a transformed *homo economicus* (economic man) under a new neoliberal regime, Foucault argued that this figure is no longer a "partner of exchange" in the classical economic sense based on a rational calculation of utility but is rather "an entrepreneur of himself, being for himself his own capital, being for himself his own producer, being for himself the source of [his] earnings" (Foucault 2008, 225–26). For Foucault, this is the quintessential figure linking together the cultivation of the self and the practice of governance.

Nikolas Rose (1992) builds on these insights to articulate a new regime of political subjectivity based on the "enterprising self" that emphasizes personal fulfillment, individual choice, and self-governance. Like Foucault's, Rose's insights are largely based on examples from Western liberal democracies; ethnographers have subsequently sought to pinpoint the ethnographic specificities, deceptive similarities, and pivotal differences in entrepreneurial self-making in other contexts. Most notably, Carla Freeman's (2014) analysis of the rise of an entrepreneurial middle class in Barbados theorizes the cultural specificity of postcolonial neoliberalism in the Caribbean by teasing out the analytical tensions between competing regional idioms of reputation and respectability. By highlighting the affective dimensions of entrepreneurial narratives in Barbados, Freeman demonstrates how entrepreneurialism is not just a mode of self-employment but also must be understood as an emergent way of life.

Anthropologists studying contemporary China have seized upon these Foucauldian approaches to understand how market reforms have transformed Chinese citizens into active agents seeking to maximize their own human capital while simultaneously aligning themselves with a multilayered state's political objectives in a variety of different domains (e.g., Hanser 2002; Zhang and Ong 2008; Hoffman 2010; Yan 2010; Kleinman et al. 2011). While this analysis may seem similar to other narratives of entrepreneurial self-making around the world, Chinese accounts of entrepreneurialism must be grounded in the fraught history and politics of entrepreneurship in the People's Republic. Formerly vilified during the collectivist era, which centralized economic production and abolished private property, the status of entrepreneurs in China began to revive in the 1980s in the wake of economic reforms that enabled individuals to pursue alternative work opportunities outside the state-controlled economic sector. No longer stigmatized as "capitalist roaders" (走资派 *zǒu zī pài*), new entrepreneurs in the post-Mao era were reframed as hardworking proprietors helping to set the country on a course of national prosperity. Anthropologist Judith Farquhar has drawn attention to the specific Chinese term for entrepreneurs invoked in post-Mao official discourse: *gètǐhù* (个体户), which literally means "one-body-household" (1996, 242–43). Farquhar highlighted the embodied and personal nature of these individual and family-run enterprises, contrasting them to the Maoist era's emphasis on the collectivized work unit (单位 *dānwèi*). Farquhar has traced the implications of this embodied entrepreneurial logic in the context of a rural county town in north China during the early 1990s. Her research in Shandong province examined how traditional Chinese medical practitioners transformed themselves into *gètǐhù* doctors: self-employed, fee-for-service petty proprietors operating small-scale storefront clinics that capitalized on the unmet needs of localized clientele.

Unlike the *gètǐhù* doctors studied by Farquhar in the 1990s, urban clinicians working within state-owned hospitals in the new millennium have contended with a different set of institutional logics generated by successive rounds of hospital reform. These urban medical entrepreneurs have experimented with rapidly changing regulations to capitalize on new services and identify new (and potentially more lucrative) patient-consumers. For these enterprising urban clinicians, the revival of the individual pursuit of profit in contemporary China must be understood in the context of state efforts to shape the economic prospects of the country. These interests converge most dramatically in the pursuit of advanced technology, which is not just a money-making scheme for individuals but also a broader state strategy for national development. This chapter situates the role of urban medical entrepreneurs in promoting a technology-intensive tertiary health care sector within an older history of geopolitical humiliation and more recent experiences of sweeping politico-economic changes in the People's Republic. I argue that Chinese medical entrepreneurialism is not simply an economic mechanism for generating income; it must also be understood as a cultural phenomenon enabled by technonationalism. Scholarship on Chinese technonationalism has addressed the development of "strategic" technologies underlying national security and economic competitiveness, focusing on the establishment of the Chinese nuclear weapons program (Lewis and Xue 1988; Feigenbaum 2003).[1] An ethnographic exploration of why Chinese doctors pursue advanced biomedical technologies presents a very different perspective on technonationalism, however. As an "applied" scientific discipline engaged with promoting well-being and alleviating suffering on the intimate level of human bodies, biomedicine offers an on-the-ground view of human experience that elite policy analyses of weapons of mass destruction often overlook. Anthropologists have drawn attention to the ways in which state promotion of biotechnology reconfigure notions about the ethics of belonging and the collective fates of populations in a variety of Asian contexts (Ong and Chen 2010). In a global era of proliferating risks to health and wealth, various Asian governments have come to understand biotech enterprises as key to both economic development and national security.

I build on this project by exploring how state entrepreneurialism converges with the experimental activities of urban Chinese clinicians. Drawing on a series of extended interviews I conducted between 2005 and 2015 with neurosurgeon Huang Hongyun (figure 5.1), I examine how an exceptional Chinese medical entrepreneur has leveraged the hope and hype of experimental fetal cell medicine to attract a global clientele of patients and build a profitable business venture. Huang's neurosurgery career provides a fascinating lens for understanding the emerging culture of Chinese medical entrepreneurship in the new millennium. In the ode to Huang and the "miracle of olfactory ensheathing cells" penned by a traditional Chinese medical practitioner working at New Century Hospital, the admiring author concludes that "they will without fail create even more glory and splendor" for "China and the world of medicine." This ode invites us to consider Huang's neurosurgical enterprise not in terms of its lucrative potential but rather in terms of its role in glorifying the Chinese nation. As we will see, Huang draws upon the narrative trope of technonationalism in projecting his autobiography to deflect critics' accusations of profiteering and reframe medical entrepreneurialism as a moral duty.

The transnational marketing of medicine in service of the nation is not a new phenomenon in China. As historian Sherman Cochran (2006) has documented, "Chinese medicine men" acted as "agents of consumer culture" during both war and peace in late imperial and Republican China, utilizing diverse print media to market Western-style drugs across national boundaries and political barriers. Highly trained urban physicians in the post-Deng era such as Huang are deploying new forms of digital media to extend their reach even farther. Their ambitions span the globe as they pursue advanced biomedical training abroad, introduce new technologies and fields of study to China, and bask in national and even international media attention as they treat both Chinese and foreign patients. As a successful medical entrepreneur in the new millennium, Huang has created a transnational and transcultural enterprise that has attracted thousands of patients from over eighty countries around the world.

In order to understand how this has happened, I will first present a broad overview of how changes in the political economy of the Chinese health care system have encouraged hospitals and doctors to provide advanced medical technologies to foreign patients. The second half of the chapter provides ethnographic insight into these processes by exploring how Huang, a consummate medical entrepreneur, has drawn upon the trope of technonationalism to catapult his experimental therapy to international prominence.

HEALTH CARE UNDER "SOCIALISM WITH CHINESE CHARACTERISTICS"

When Mao Zedong and the Chinese Communist Party established the People's Republic of China in 1949, they rebuilt the war-ravaged country through a series of national campaigns based on class struggle and centralized bureaucratic control. The new socialist planned economy eliminated private ownership, collectivized agriculture, and nationalized manufacturing and commercial enterprises. In the medical sector, the socialist reorganization of health care placed urban medical facilities under state ownership and management while health care in the countryside came under the jurisdiction of rural cooperatives. Urban hospital workers became state employees whose training opportunities, wages, and job assignments would be dictated by the fledgling country's needs rather

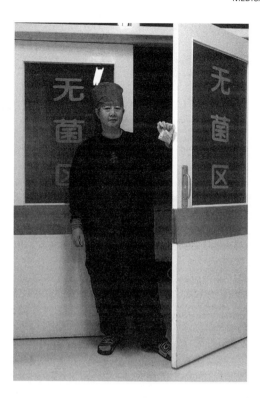

Figure 5.1. Chinese neurosurgeon Huang Hongyun stands outside the surgical operating theater at New Century Hospital (photograph by Doug Kanter).

than by individual incentives. Rural medical practitioners likewise had their schedules and earnings controlled by collective rural production brigades. The first National Health Congress in 1950 established the guiding principles of the new socialist health care system: (1) to serve workers, peasants, and soldiers; (2) to prioritize preventive care over expensive curative treatment; and (3) to unite Chinese and Western medicine (Chen 1989, 80). These new objectives were often carried out through massive public health campaigns that swept the entire country, from patriotic crusades to "eliminate the four pests"[2] to coordinated immunization efforts and sanitation crusades to eradicate schistosomiasis and sexually transmitted diseases (Hesketh and Zhu 1997a).

Despite the ideological orientation toward basic preventive care for the masses, systemic health inequalities persisted during the collectivist era. The limited budget of the national Ministry of Health, coupled with the practical challenges of escalating medical costs, resulted in significant burdens on lower levels of administration to come up with strategies to extract more central subsidies, control the provision of services, and generate local sources of revenue by levying mandatory "self-help" contributions and use fees (Lampton 1977). These localized financing methods exacerbated the gap in medical care between urban and rural areas. The rural majority relied on increasingly insolvent cooperative medical stations staffed by local "barefoot doctors" trained in rudimentary primary care, while urban workers and government cadres enjoyed subsidized and even free access to advanced medical services provided by college-educated physicians working in large hospitals (Davis and Chapman 2002). The persistent inequalities of the two-tiered health care system prompted a scathing critique from Mao in 1965, who castigated the Ministry of Health for failing to serve China's rural population: "The vast majority of peasants are not able to obtain health care. First, there are no doctors. Second, there are no medicines." He proposed renaming the ineffective agency the "Urban Lords and Masters' Ministry of Health" (城市老爷卫生部 *chéngshì lǎoyé wèishēng bù*) (Mao 1965).[3]

Mao's intensified attacks on urban privilege and professional power sparked a decade of political struggle targeting perceived traitors in the party establishment, from counterrevolutionaries to intellectuals. Medical schools and universities stopped admitting students at the outset of the Cultural Revolution as a mass movement of young Red Guards shut down classes and engaged in revolutionary attacks to rout out the "Four Olds" (四旧 *sì jiù*): old ideas, old culture, old customs, old habits. When schools reopened in 1970, entrance examinations were abolished and training was reduced to abbreviated programs emphasizing practice over theory (Pang, Wong, and Ho 2002). The Cultural Revolution channeled health care workers to underserved rural areas through a concerted national campaign that compelled urban medical students and subspecialists alike to work in the countryside.

Deng Xiaoping, who eventually emerged as China's paramount leader in the political reshuffling following Mao's death in 1976, set the country on a radically different path of "socialism with Chinese characteristics" (有中国特色的社会主义 *yǒu zhòng guó tèsè de shèhuì zhǔyì*) with his policies of "reform and opening up" (改革开放 *gǎigé kāifàng*). The targeted market-driven reforms and open-door policies officially announced by Deng in December 1978[4] launched the fastest pace of sustained economic growth in world history (Economist 2007).

Following policies of decentralization and privatization that proved phenomenally successful in increasing the profitability and efficiency of agricultural, industrial, and commercial sectors, the central government significantly reduced its role in health provision and financing. As early as 1979, then minister of health Qian Xinzhong suggested "using economic means to manage health care" (Cao and Fu 2005). Although budgetary spending on health continued to rise during Deng's Reform and Opening Up period, the Chinese state's share of the country's total spending on health declined from 36 percent in 1980 to 15 percent in 2002—placing China in the bottom 10 percent of the world's countries in terms of government share of health spending (Duckett 2011, 4). In addition to its decreasing fiscal commitment to health provision, the central government's "retreat from health" also entailed cutting back on health risk protection for both rural and urban residents and transferring responsibility for financing medical services to lower-level authorities (Duckett 2011).

In rural areas, the dismantling of the commune system led to the demise of the cooperative medical system that had compensated practitioners for providing health services to villagers. A 1980 Ministry of Health report noted that many former commune doctors were informally practicing medicine by "hanging up signs to advertise their services or seeing patients within pharmacies," "operating individual household clinics overseen by street committees," or even "setting up medical stalls at markets and peddling itinerant medical services" (People's Republic of China Ministry of Health 1980, 515). This Ministry of Health report, which was subsequently adopted by the State Council as national policy, recommended granting formal legal status to these private practitioners in order to resolve their employment problems, fulfill the medical needs of patients, and strengthen oversight of these medical practitioners (ibid.). Thus many rural doctors became legal fee-for-service private practitioners who relied predominantly on drug sales to make a living.[5]

Although the 1980 directive specifically prohibited medical workers in state- and collectively owned medical institutions from engaging in private practice,[6] a new round of medical reforms authorized a "reward and punishment" (奖惩 *jiǎngchéng*) system for hospital employees based on performance in order to encourage economic development in the health sector. The 1985 reform initiative identified the "slow development of health enterprises" as the major problem causing "incompatibilities between China's economic construction and its people's medical needs" (People's Republic of China Ministry of Health 1985, 378). The report blamed the egalitarian mantra of "eating from the big pot [吃大锅饭 *chī dàguōfàn*] as a serious problem impeding the active mobilization of all aspects of the medical sector" (ibid.). In order to "speed up the development of health enterprises," the Ministry of Health recommended increasing the "autonomy" (自主权 *zìzhǔ quán*) of hospitals through the "necessary implementation of reform, loosening policies to allow greater freedom, streamlining administration and instituting decentralization, utilizing multiple methods of financing, broadening the path of development for health enterprises, and enlivening medical work" (ibid.).

Domestic critics have noted that the central government's health reforms during the 1980s amounted to "giving policies but not money" (Cao and Fu 2005). The state's reduced share in funding the health care sector created mounting pressure for hospitals to maintain their own operational costs, pay for staff salaries, and purchase equipment. Even as the government reduced its fiscal responsibilities toward hospitals, however, it continued to regulate medical prices in the urban health sector. Although the 1985 directive recognized that these "standardized medical fees were too low" (医疗收费标准过低 *yīliáo shōufèi biāozhǔn guò dī*) and needed to be "gradually reformed" in order to encourage the "development of health enterprises" and "improve the quality of medical service," the Ministry of Health noted that the "adjustment of standard medical fees was too difficult to overhaul in the first year of health reforms" (People's Republic of China Ministry of Health 1985, 380–81). Seeking to ensure access to basic health care, the Ministry of Health thus continued to enforce below-cost charges on a wide range of routine medical services. Over two decades later, essential services such as outpatient consultations and per diem inpatient hospitalization charges continue to be priced below the actual costs of treatment. As an internist at an elite Beijing hospital complained to me during an interview in 2004, an outpatient appointment with him cost the same as using a public toilet.

These features of Chinese health care policy reflected the peculiar political economy of what Mao's political successor Deng Xiaoping branded "socialism with Chinese characteristics": a volatile combination of decentralization coupled with continued state control over strategic sectors.[7] While these shifts threatened hospitals' financial viability and doctors' livelihoods as exploding health care costs have far outpaced government financing, they simultaneously enabled novel opportunities for a new class of medical entrepreneurs to pursue more lucrative forms of health service provision.

In particular, developing advanced medical services became a crucial strategy for generating revenues at public hospitals. Whereas the Ministry of Health declined to adjust basic prices of established health services, the 1985 directive provided a key loophole that enabled hospitals to set higher charges for new instruments, new equipment, and newly developed medical treatment services (People's Republic of China Ministry of Health 1985, 381). Indeed, this strategy aligned well with national priorities. Of the "Four Modernizations" (四个现代化 *sì gè xiàndàihuà*)[8] embraced by the Communist Party leadership, Deng declared in the inaugural address of the 1978 National Science Congress that the modernization of science and technology should be the country's top priority (Chen 1989, 148). Deng's Marxist-inspired slogan that "science and technology are the primary forces of productivity" (科学技术是第一生产力 *kēxué jìshù shì dì yī shēngchǎnlì*) became the central government's battle plan for the country's rapid development.

Following the national emphasis on scientific and technological development, Chinese government agencies through the 1980s and 1990s provided hospitals with incentives for developing new medical technologies. In 1988, for example, the Ministry of Health, Ministry of Finance, Ministry of Personnel, National Bureau on Commodity Pricing, and National Taxation Bureau joined forces to actively encourage the expansion of health services. In this jointly issued recommendation subsequently adopted as national policy by the State Council, the multiagency effort legitimized differential pricing in the health sector based on the level of technological advancement: "Health service fees should be spread out according to the condition of the facilities and the level of the medical technologies." Once hospitals fulfilled their obligation to provide essential health care services, the government agencies encouraged them to branch out into more lucrative directions:

> After completing routine health care duties [正常医疗任务 *zhèngcháng yīliáo rènwù*] and ensuring their quality and quantity, a portion of major urban hospitals are allowed to establish special examination rooms [特诊室 *tèzhěn shì*] staffed by high-level health care workers [高水平医护人员 *gāo shuǐpíng yīhù rényuán*] for the purpose of providing high quality services [高质量服务 *gāo zhìliàng fúwù*]. They can implement high fees [高收费 *gāo shōufèi*] (not reimbursable by public and labor medical insurance plans) in order to open up new services for society and meet different levels of health service needs. (People's Republic of China State Council 1989)

Although the guidelines admonished hospitals that the "use of new technologies and equipment should be offered to patients at a reasonable cost after factoring in wages," the overall tenor of the policy urged hospitals to embrace new technologies and offer higher-quality services through the incentive of charging higher fees. Not surprisingly, many hospitals responded by creating elite wards offering a range of high-tech services catering to wealthy consumers.[9] Encouraged by material incentives and an ideological shift to pro-market policies as the best way to improve the quality and efficiency of health care, health service providers blazed the way for the commercialization of China's health system along a distinctive path.

By the early 1990s, the development of high-tech medicine as a key method for revenue generation was in full swing. In a national policy recommendation on "deepening the health reforms" (深化卫生改革 *shēnhuà wèishēng gǎigé*), the Ministry of Health exhorted every level of government as well as medical and public health work units across the country to "accelerate the transformation of research results into the practical forces of production [现实生产力转化 *xiànshí shēngchǎnlì*] [and] promote the commercialization [商品化 *shāngpǐnhuà*] of research results" (People's Republic of China Ministry of Health 1992). To accomplish this transformation, the ministry recommended "actively advancing the alliance between scientific institutions and business enterprises" and suggested that "work units and individuals who manufacture, develop, and popularize new advanced technologies with significant results should be amply rewarded" (ibid.). The 1992 directive articulated the philosophy driving Chinese health reform during this era: "以工助医, 以副补主" (*yǐ gōng zhù yī, yǐ fù bǔ zhǔ*), which exhorted industry to subsidize the development of health services while also encouraging hospitals to engage in sideline enterprises to support their own operating costs.

Enshrined as a national agenda and reinforced through subsequent adjustments in health pricing policies, the pursuit of advanced medical technologies thus became a foundational revenue-generating strategy deployed by entrepreneurial hospital administrators and clinicians in urban centers throughout the 1990s and into the new millennium. In their overview of Chinese health care reform published in the influential newspaper *Southern Weekend* (南方周末 *Nánfāng Zhōumò*), Cao and Fu (2005) characterized the entire decade of the 1990s as dominated by "the voice of marketization" (市场化的声音 *shìchǎnghuà de shēngyīn*). This period marked the most drastic stages of China's health care stratification, with legal reforms authorizing the increasing marketization and privatization of health services. A 1997 national directive urged party and government leaders to "further strengthen and deepen health reforms" by implementing differential pricing for different types of medical services. While the central government continued to promote universal access to health care as a key goal of "socialist modernization" (社会主义现代化 *shèhuì zhǔyì xiàndàihuà*) by controlling the prices for "basic medical services" (基本医疗服务 *jīběn yīliáo fúwù*), this directive explicitly allowed the "liberalization of prices for voluntarily chosen special needs services" (自愿选择的特需服务价格放宽 *zìyuàn xuǎnzé de tèxū fúwù jiàgé fàngkuān*) in order to "guide the rational separation of the flow of patients" (引导患者合理分流 *yǐndǎo huànzhě hélǐ fēnliú*) (People's Republic of China Community Party Central Committee and State Council 1997). While anthropologists and public health analysts have critiqued the role of these health policies in deepening socioeconomic inequalities in both rural and urban China,[10] I follow a different line of analysis in this chapter by tracking how the technological imperative in Chinese health care has shaped the cultural logics underpinning medical entrepreneurialism with "Chinese characteristics."

CURING THE SICK MAN OF EAST ASIA

The pursuit of advanced technology is not just a money-making scheme but also a specific cultural strategy for national salvation. While the recent changes in the financing and organization of health care sparked by China's transition to market socialism have enabled and encouraged entrepreneurial doctors to develop advanced therapeutic interventions, these high-tech desires must be situated in a broader Chinese program of scientific and technological modernization (科学技术现代化 *kēxué jìshù xiàndàihuà*).[11] Social historian David Rothman (1997) has traced the technological imperative in American health care, tying the pursuit of advanced medical technologies to a history of American exceptionalism rooted in middle-class priorities. The Chinese passion for science and technology arises from a very different cultural sensibility: a history of geopolitical humiliation framed in terms of medical pathology. Branded the "sick man of East Asia" (东亚病夫 *Dōngyà bìngfū*), late imperial China suffered crushing setbacks from technologically superior Western nations. "Learning from the barbarians"[12] became a key strategy for modernizing China and catching up with the West.

Increasing numbers of Chinese students began studying abroad, sparking successive waves of social and political transformations throughout the twentieth century. The knowledge and values they brought back home played a crucial role in shaping the development of modern China. As Shu Xincheng argued in his history of the Chinese study-abroad movement first published in 1927: "No foreign-educated students, no Chinese new culture" (C. Li 2005b, 69). Even a cursory review of Chinese history since the Qing dynasty reveals the dramatic influence of foreign-educated Chinese students. Sun Yatsen, who studied medicine in Hong Kong and lived in exile in Hawaii, Japan, Southeast Asia, and Europe, played a key role in the overthrow of China's imperial system in 1911 and became the first provisional president of the new Republic of China. Chinese intellectuals who studied in the United States and Britain under the Boxer Rebellion indemnity funds spearheaded the May Fourth Movement of 1919, which rejected Confucian principles in favor of science and democracy. Chinese students who studied Marxist theory in France and the Soviet Union helped establish the Chinese Community Party in 1921. Prior to Mao's split with Khrushchev in the early 1960s, thousands of "Soviet experts" (苏联专家 Sūlián zhuānjiā) provided technical aid in China while thousands of Chinese students studied at Soviet institutes of higher education (McGuire 2010).

Deng Xiaoping's efforts to accelerate China's scientific and technological modernization after the disruption of the Cultural Revolution paved the way for the "largest study-abroad movement in Chinese history" (C. Li 2005b, 69–70). Normalizing relations with foreign countries and signing bilateral agreements on scientific and cultural exchanges, Deng began sending large numbers of students and scholars for advanced training overseas in 1978 as a cornerstone of his "Open Door" policy. The American Committee on Scholarly Communication with the People's Republic of China noted that the "overwhelming majority" of Chinese students and scholars returned home during the early years of the Open Door exchanges (Lampton 1986). These early students and scholars tended to be older, married, and more established; their personal, familial, and structural ties to their homeland brought them back to China.[13]

By the late 1980s, Chinese government officials began worrying about the loss of scientists and engineers to other countries (Zinberg 1988; Orleans 1988) even as American congressional reports noted a "tremendous 'brain-gain' in favor of the United States" as a substantial number of Chinese citizens remained in the United States following their studies (U.S. Bureau of Oceans and International Environmental and Scientific Affairs 2005, 74). The Chinese government's suppression of Beijing students protesting in Tiananmen Square on June 4, 1989, intensified the exodus as sympathetic governments around the world responded by providing Chinese students studying abroad with favorable immigration policies. In the United States, for example, former president George H. W. Bush signed a temporary executive order in 1990 allowing Chinese citizens in the United States to extend their stay. The subsequent Chinese Student Protection Act of 1992 made over seventy thousand Chinese students and scholars automatically eligible for lawful permanent residency status (Brooks 1992). A 1993 survey of Chinese students and scholars residing in the United States noted that respondents cited "political instability" as the most common reason for not returning to China (Chen, Rosen, and Zweig 1995, 3).

In her ethnographic study of multiple passport-holding Hong Kong executives and their "computer widows" and "parachute kids" during the 1990s, Aihwa Ong emphasized the racialized constraints these "flexible citizens" experienced in their adopted European and American homes. Despite their economic success and educational credentials, these elite members of the Chinese diaspora faced "structural limits to the accumulation of cultural capital" as they "[ran] up against regimes of racial difference and hierarchy" (Ong 1999, 91, 93). When leveraged back home, however, these foreign connections became "transnational capital" that provided returnees with increased rewards, recognition, and power (Rosen and Zweig 2005). More recently, Vanessa Fong (2011) has examined how China's first generation of singletons, which has come of age under the one-child policy, has pursued study abroad as a method of achieving social and cultural (if not legal) citizenship in the developed world.

As memories of Tiananmen recede to the background, a new generation of returnees have chosen to develop their careers in China rather than hitting a discriminatory "glass ceiling" abroad. Following the meteoric rise of the Chinese economy, this "tidal wave of returnees" is reversing the former brain drain as they pursue lucrative opportunities back home (C. Li 2005a, 2). In a study comparing returnees and locals at seven universities in China, Rosen and Zweig noted that returnees made more significant contributions to their universities and received preferential treatment, from increased administrative responsibilities to higher success rates in receiving national and provincial-level awards. While resentful locals who had never gone overseas cited preferential treatment and failure to succeed overseas as the dominant forces bringing returnees back, the new generation of returnees focused on favorable domestic factors as their reasons for returning to China, including the ability to "do their own thing" and higher social status (Rosen and Zweig 2005, 125).

Unlike the overseas Chinese (华侨 *huáqiáo*) of the 1990s described by Ong, who emigrated to foreign lands in search of better opportunities in newly adopted homelands, China's new mobile elite are called *hǎiguī* (海归)—literally "return from the sea," a colorful homonym for "sea turtle."[14] For these foreign-educated Chinese who have come back home to pursue professional careers in the new millennium, return plays a fundamental role in their identities and strategies for success. They view their time abroad as a temporary stint for learning new skills and acquiring new technologies rather than as a permanent relocation and realignment of national loyalties. Capitalizing on their foreign-acquired knowledge, these sea turtles pursue professional careers in the twin service of national development and personal profit. In a feature story on this new breed of Chinese returnees, the *Economist* (2003) explicitly described them as "Chinese entrepreneurs on their way back . . . [to] a land of boundless opportunity."

Studying abroad has become an increasingly important rite of passage for medical professionals interested in advancing their careers.[15] In a study of emergency medicine physicians employed at eight public teaching hospitals in Beijing, 17 percent (25 out of 143 respondents) went abroad to engage in short-term study, obtain an academic degree, or attend a foreign conference (Gupta and Walline 2008). Respondents reported that studying abroad increased their familiarity with a broader range of advanced procedures and enabled them to access more opportunities for professional advancement. For these state-employed physicians, foreign educational opportunities contributed to their perceived medical expertise and workplace status.

The prestige of studying abroad plays an even larger role in securing the credentials of private medical entrepreneurs offering experimental stem and fetal cell therapies. Shenzhen Beike Biotechnology Company, dubbed "China's most prominent stem-cell therapy company" by the prestigious scientific journal *Nature* (Cyranoski 2005), is a case in point. According to company literature, Beike's chief executive officer and founder, Sean Hu, obtained his doctorate in biochemistry from Gothenburg University in Sweden and conducted postdoctoral research at the University of British Columbia before returning to China. The chief scientific officer, Susan Jiang, conducted postdoctoral research at the University of Arkansas and Stanford University after receiving her doctorate in clinical medicine in China. The company's website prominently featured Hu's and Jiang's foreign academic pedigrees, utilizing them for marketing purposes to drum up business from foreign patients interested in obtaining the company's experimental stem cell therapies.[16]

In the following section, I take a closer look at the career trajectory of Chinese neurosurgeon Huang Hongyun, who has leveraged his studies abroad to develop a "cutting edge" experimental procedure that has attracted the attention of patients and doctors from around the world. Huang's neurosurgery career provides a fascinating lens for understanding the ethnographic contours of medical entrepreneurialism in contemporary China.

A SEA TURTLE'S NAVAL CAREER

An exemplar of China's mobile professional elite, Huang Hongyun was born in eastern Shandong province in 1955. His penchant for traveling received an early start when he moved across the country as a teenager to Urumqi, the Chinese government's administrative seat for the Xinjiang Uyghur Autonomous Region in northwestern China. Unlike many who were sent to remote areas during the radical reeducation campaigns of the Cultural Revolution, Huang's family moved out West by choice in order to pursue better work opportunities. These pioneering families from Shandong were on the leading edge of the Chinese state's efforts to bring the predominantly minority-inhabited area into the national fold by sending growing numbers of Han Chinese to work in the fertile, resource-rich, and politically strategic border region.

Huang received his medical degree[17] in 1982 from Xinjiang Medical School (新疆医学院 Xīnjiāng Yīxué Yuàn), marrying the daughter of two faculty members soon afterward. Like Huang, his wife's parents had come to Xinjiang from Shandong province. The circumstances of their cross-country migration were very different, however. Formerly staff members of Shandong Medical School, they had been forced to move to Xinjiang during the 1950s in a patriotic mission to help establish the region's first medical institution. The building of Xinjiang Medical School—designated as one of the key national projects in China's First Five-Year Plan—involved the conscription of hundreds of experts from eastern China's established medical schools (L. Wang 2006).[18]

As a medical graduate in Deng Xiaoping's era of Reform and Opening Up, Huang had more flexibility and freedom in his career options than did the doctors of his in-laws' generation. He initially began working in the neurosurgery department of Xinjiang Medical School's affiliated hospital, but he subsequently enlisted in the People's Liberation Army (PLA, 中国人民解放军 Zhōngguó Rénmín Jiěfàng Jūn) for the opportunity to pursue graduate training in neurosurgery. Huang moved back across the country to study at the Military Academy for Advanced Medical Studies (军医进修学院 Jūnyī Jìnxiū Xuéyuàn) in Beijing, receiving his M.S. in 1988 and his Ph.D. in 1991. He joined the staff of the Naval General Hospital (海军总医院 Hǎijūn Zǒng Yīyuàn) in Beijing, whose prestigious neurosurgery department received the distinction of serving as the entire military's key neurosurgery center in 1992. An ambitious Huang quickly worked his way up the military medical ranks at Naval General, rising to director-level neurosurgeon in the course of six years.[19]

Huang joined the military medical system during a period of aggressive expansion that capitalized on new market-driven possibilities enabled by Deng's politico-economic transformations. The Chinese military operated its own independent health delivery and education system. Military hospitals and medical schools were regulated by a separate Department of Military Health, which reported directly to the General Logistics Department of the PLA, thus exempting these institutions from the Byzantine structure of the civilian health system (with its multiple bureaus, departments, and ministries of health corresponding to local, provincial, and national levels of government). With a smaller and more streamlined administrative system, the military hospitals were able to capitalize more aggressively on economic opportunities enabled by Deng's economic policies. Although the military's Department of Health controlled the prices of basic medical services for military personnel, it allowed hospitals to charge higher fees for new medical technologies and medical treatment for civilians. Like their civilian counterparts, military hospitals thus pursued high-tech medical interventions as lucrative income sources.

One of the key strategies hospitals employed for acquiring new medical techniques involved sending personnel abroad for advanced training. The Naval General Hospital thus sent Huang to the United States in 1997 to pursue postdoctoral research at New York University. He started out conducting research on gliomas, a type of brain tumor. After meeting Wise Young, then the director of neurosurgery research at New York University, Huang switched his focus to mechanisms of repair in spinal cord injury. The regeneration of damaged spinal cord neurons had long been considered an impossibility by doctors, but basic research results in neuroscience were beginning to dislodge this conventional wisdom. Young, who was in the process of setting up the Keck Center for Collaborative Neuroscience at Rutgers University, encouraged Huang to follow him to New Jersey to study a special type of nerve support cell located in the olfactory bulb. As I noted in chapter 2, scientists in Canada, the U.K., and Spain had conducted basic laboratory experiments suggesting that olfactory ensheathing glial (OEG) cells potentially played a role in repairing damaged spinal cords. Huang pursued this research in New Jersey by studying whether injecting OEG cells into the damaged spinal cords of rats produced any functional changes. He published his results in the Naval General Hospital's academic journal, reporting in Chinese that the injured rats he had transplanted with OEG cells showed varying degrees of functional recovery, with some even regaining the ability to use their hind limbs (Huang et al. 2001).

At this point, Huang faced a juncture in his career. Although he was still on the payroll of the Naval General Hospital and expected to return to his post in Beijing upon completing his research training, Huang had begun to put down more permanent roots in New Jersey. His wife and teenaged son had accompanied him to the United States, eager to transform his professional boon into an opportunity for the entire family. They had even purchased a single-family house in the New Jersey suburbs, complete with a backyard grill to enable the neurosurgeon to re-create the Uyghur mutton kebabs he had acquired a taste for during his youth in Xinjiang province. But as a foreign-trained neurosurgeon, Huang was unable to operate on American patients. Laboratory research was his only pathway forward in the United States, and he would be relegated to working with rat models if he chose to remain.

Eager to translate his laboratory findings into clinical use and enticed by a promotion to vice-chair of the Naval General Hospital's neurosurgery department, Huang decided to return alone to Beijing in 2000. His most significant challenge involved finding a ready supply of cells suitable for human transplantation. Working together with the obstetrics and gynecology department at his hospital, which performed abortions as part of its routine birth planning services, Huang procured olfactory bulbs from fetuses aborted in the second trimester. He adapted the cell culturing techniques he had learned at Rutgers University for obtaining rodent OEG cells, developing a similar protocol for isolating and growing OEG cells from human fetal tissue.

While the politics of abortion would have rendered this arrangement impossible in the United States, Huang's interdepartmental partnership raised no moral qualms among hospital personnel at the Naval Hospital and was even considered an innovative use of discarded "medical waste." Under the one-child policy established in 1979, abortion has become normalized throughout China as a routine and even mandated part of birth control (Greenhalgh and Winckler 2005; White 2006).[20] While these birth planning policies were heavily contested and ultimately modified in rural areas during the 1980s (Wasserstrom 1984; Greenhalgh 1994; Anagnost 1995), they have become entrenched among urban parents anxious to cultivate "high-quality" little emperors who will be competitive on the world stage (Greenhalgh 2003; Anagnost 2004; Fong 2007). Even many rural couples eligible to have a second child have chosen not to, citing the rising costs of child-rearing and growing female empowerment (Zhang 2007; Shi 2011). Abortion is regularly utilized not just as a coercive means to eliminate unauthorized pregnancies but also as a desired tool to reduce "imperfect" or "defective" fetuses (Zhu 2013). Huang was thus able to secure a readily available supply of raw material for his experimental investigations.

In November 2001, he performed his first human OEG cell transplantation on a thirty-year-old Chinese woman who had suffered a C5 cervical spinal cord injury nineteen months earlier. Prior to surgery, the quadriplegic woman had lost tactile sensation and most muscle control in all four limbs; her arm movements were limited to bending her elbows. Huang reported that his patient regained tactile sensation in both her arms and legs following the experimental procedure, and she subsequently was able to move her wrists for the first time since her injury (Huang 2002). Buoyed by these promising results, Huang performed his second OEG transplantation on a twenty-eight-year-old man from Inner Mongolia with a similar-level injury. This patient achieved even more spectacular results after surgery: he regained the ability to move his formerly paralyzed fingers and could now grasp objects with his hands and even brush his teeth (Zhao 2002).

A reporter for *Health News* (健康报 *Jiànkāng Bào*), a publication of the Chinese Ministry of Health, published the first media announcement of Huang's results in December 2001. The officially sanctioned news report proclaimed that Huang's clinical application of the fruits of basic science research was "the most important progress [最重要进展 *zuì zhòngyào jìnzhǎn*] in the treatment of complete spinal cord injury to date" (Chu 2001). Responding to intense interest among both medical experts and the general public in the potential of this new method for nerve regeneration and functional recovery, the nationally circulated newspaper invited Huang to write a report detailing the successful results of his first three transplantations (Huang 2002). An editorial accompanying

Huang's article characterized Huang's experimental treatment as "achieving a foundational breakthrough [零的突破 *líng de túpò*] in the clinical treatment of spinal cord injury" (*Health News* 2002).

A Chinese media storm quickly followed as reporters from the *Health Times* (健康时报 *Jiànkāng Shíbào*) (Zhao 2002) and the *Science and Technology Daily* (科技日报 *Kējì Rìbào*) (Tang, Wang, and Ji 2002) featured Huang's experimental procedure as front-page news. His fame spread across the country after China Central Television's (中国中央电视台 *Zhōngguó Zhōngyāng Diànshìtái*) popular *Road to Health* program highlighted his clinical successes in a national broadcast (CCTV 2002). The television program featured Dr. Huang and his Naval General Hospital colleague Dr. Xiu Bo answering queries from a *Road to Health* moderator and viewers who called in questions. By the time the program aired in February, Huang and Xiu had performed fourteen OEG transplantations and claimed that all fourteen SCI patients had experienced varying degrees of functional recovery. Another physician who had worked with him during this initial period proudly described how the show caused the phones at the station to ring off the hook for an entire month afterward as eager people flooded the lines with requests for more information.

Recognizing Huang's growing importance, the Naval General Hospital appointed him chairman of a newly created Second Department of Neurosurgery to accommodate the surge of patients with spinal cord injury seeking OEG transplantations. The hospital also granted him the coveted title of professor, allowing him to serve as an academic advisor for graduate-level medical students. Huang operated on a frenetic work schedule, performing more than two hundred OEG fetal cell transplantation procedures by the end of 2002. One of his subordinates chronicled the major developments in spinal neurosurgery at Naval General Hospital in 2002, producing what essentially amounted to a hagiography of Huang:

> Director Huang Hongyun began research on spinal cord disease early on . . . accumulating a wealth of experience. He then went to the United States to undertake related scientific research for more than two years, achieving many successes. In 2000, he turned down the high-paying salary of remaining an American expert, took upon himself the burden of leaving his wife and son, and came back to the motherland to return to Naval General Hospital. After returning to the country, he worked nonstop night and day to [translate] the fruits of the knowledge and research he learned more quickly into clinical applications, in order to release the suffering of patients. In basic and clinical research on spinal cord injury, he achieved breakthrough progress in using the method of olfactory ensheathing cell transplantation in the treatment of late-stage [chronic] spinal cord injury. . . .

> Director Huang Hongyun carries forward a "Never fear hardship, never fear exhaustion" fighting spirit and good medical ethics. Regarding his work he is

meticulous and diligent; his technique is excellent and perfect; he cares for patients in everything he does, considering everything for the sake of patients. Sometimes he conducts over 100 consultations during his expert outpatient hours, [seeing patients from 8:30 in the morning until 7 or 8 at night]. He performs one surgery after another, from 8:30 in the morning until 6 or 7 at night, [working with] two groups of doctors to do four or even six consecutive surgeries. . . . All of these have set hospital precedents. Although Director Huang Hongyun's own body is not too good, but he has never thought of himself, he always insists that clinical treatment is the first priority. On one occasion, he developed a high fever, but he continued to hold his outpatient consultations while attached to an IV. Sometimes when his heart feels uncomfortable, he will take a brief rest in the hospital ward, and then continue working.

The return for arduous work is countless achievements in scientific research and satisfied smiles from patients. A patient admitted to the hospital was unable to stand up, but after the surgery he was not only able to stand, but with the support of his family he could even walk in the room. When he was discharged from the hospital, he clutched our doctor's hand and said in a choked voice, "Thank you, thank you, I can't thank you enough!" (translated from Chinese by the author)[21]

This celebratory story of Huang's vocational calling as a tireless hero transforming the lives of the disabled echoes narratives about how Deng Pufang, the paralyzed son of China's paramount leader Deng Xiaoping during the 1980s, became the paradigmatic advocate for disability advocacy—what Matthew Kohrman has described as a "biomythography of statesmanship" comprised of a "complex brew of fact, elision, obfuscation, genre, discourse, and ideology" (2005, 36). In Huang's case, the chronicle of his career functioned as a creation myth or legitimizing charter that authorized the experimental fetal cell procedure in terms of the Chinese neurosurgeon's American research credentials, his work ethic, and the "satisfied smiles" of patients.

Huang's postgraduate research on OEG transplantation in the United States and triumphal return to Naval General Hospital exemplified the potential of "biotech pilgrimages" pursued by thousands of Chinese "sea turtles." While I coined this neologism to describe foreign patients' quests for fetal cell therapy in a bid to challenge popular media representations of medical tourism (Song 2010), the term "biotech pilgrimage" may even more aptly characterize the journeys of Chinese scientists and scholars who obtain graduate or postdoctoral training abroad and return—transformed by their experiences and eager to implement change back home. Propelled by their desire to capitalize on the latest advances in medical science, "sea turtles" such as Huang journeyed abroad to pursue specialized training. The successful ones returned home with newly acquired cutting-edge technologies that held the potential of transforming their personal careers, their home institutions' fame, and even their nation's global standing.

BUILDING A NEUROSURGICAL ENTERPRISE

Although the military medical system had provided him with the initial impetus and means to pursue experimental biomedical interventions, Huang faced increasing constraints in his ability to negotiate hospital beds and resources to expand his clinical practice. A growing backlog of domestic patients awaited OEG transplantation, while American spinal cord injury patients on the CareCure online discussion forum eagerly discussed the possibility of undergoing surgery in China. Unable to treat foreign patients at the Naval General Hospital, Huang began looking elsewhere for possibilities.

At the beginning of 2003 he negotiated a move to Chaoyang Hospital (朝阳 医院 Cháoyáng Yīyuàn), one of the largest public hospitals in Beijing. Located in the heart of Beijing's wealthy business district with the highest concentration of foreign embassies and expatriates, Chaoyang Hospital provided a more accessible operating venue for potential Chinese and foreign patients. The new position also offered Huang more flexibility in negotiating the terms of his employment. Chaoyang clearly considered Huang's move a key coup, announcing his appointment in popular medical newspapers to publicize the new institutional location of the breakthrough surgical treatment for spinal cord injury (Ma 2003a, 2003b). As the main affiliated hospital for the Capital University of Medical Sciences (首都医科大学 Shǒudū Yīkē Dàxué), the eager hospital appointed Huang a full professor with advising privileges for master and doctoral level graduate students. The hospital also created a Second Department of Neurosurgery so that Huang could become chairman of his own independent hospital department.

At Chaoyang, Huang began treating a steady stream of foreign patients in addition to his demanding domestic surgical schedule. The first foreign SCI patients—the American CareCure pioneers featured in the previous chapter—underwent surgery in September 2003, and the first ALS patients followed soon after. The foreign patients were given the best rooms and first priority at the hospital, while Chinese patients stayed in shared rooms with five to eleven other patients and made do with communal toilets. Despite their special accommodations, most foreigners still found the conditions of a Chinese public hospital barely tolerable. Although the foreign patients had private bathrooms in their rooms, many found the sewage smell seeping up from the open drains unbearable. Some were not even able to utilize these private bathrooms, with motorized wheelchairs too wide to fit through the narrow interior door frames.

As Huang encountered more American and European patients critical of Chaoyang's facilities, he aspired to provide a level of service equaling and even exceeding the quality of medical care in his foreign patients' home countries. His opportunity came when a top administrator at Chaoyang Hospital left to direct the expansion of a smaller medical facility on the outskirts of Beijing. As I introduced in chapter 1, New Century Hospital (新世纪医院 Xīn Shìjì Yīyuàn)[22] was the revamped identity of a former sanatorium for injured workers aspiring to become a state-of-the-art rehabilitation hospital. Located on the western outskirts of China's capital city in Shijingshan district, this state-owned medical facility was a sleepy, run-down institution built in the 1950s that consisted of decrepit buildings ringed by overgrown gardens. The rehabilitation institute was on the opposite side of the city from Chaoyang Hospital in both physical distance and metaphorical feel. Beijing's first subway line traversed the gap between the two hospitals, and riding from one end to the other provided a visceral example of the vast discrepancies in development even within China's capital city. Starting in Beijing's central business district, Subway Line 1 traveled beneath the landmark China World Trade Center, past the ritzy department store–lined Wangfujing shopping street, and between Tiananmen Square and the Forbidden City—the city's current and past centers of political power. Going west beyond the city center, the subway meandered past the Military Museum, the original headquarters of China Central Television, and still farther past the Babaoshan Revolutionary Cemetery. The subway line deposited remaining riders in the midst of the sprawling living quarters of the state-owned Capital Steelworks, comprised of row after row of grimy apartment buildings and a raucous jumble of restaurants, shops, and hawkers catering to steel workers and their families. Getting to New Century Hospital required an additional twenty-minute bus ride on rutted roads that circled past squalid clusters of one-story homes scattered on the edges of a training ground operated by the People's Liberation Army.

Typical of other state-owned health facilities, New Century Hospital faced growing budget deficits at the beginning of the new millennium that encouraged hospital administrators to remake the neglected health facility into a profitable institution that could provide advanced medical services and new technologies to more lucrative patrons. Huang's search for a suitable place to treat foreign patients thus provided New Century Hospital with an ideal opportunity for capitalizing on their ambitious plans. I will examine the significance of these institutional maneuverings as a tactical form of bureaucratic practice in more detail in the following chapter; here in the remaining pages of this chapter I demonstrate how Huang's move to New Century aligns medical entrepreneurialism with technonationalist agendas.

FOREIGN PATIENTS AND GLOBAL AMBITIONS

Huang initially attempted to split his time between his new neurosurgery center at New Century Hospital and Chaoyang Hospital, which gave him flexibility while maintaining the respect of being a full professor at one of the city's largest public hospitals. A purported power struggle among Chaoyang's senior neurosurgeons ousted him from the more prestigious hospital's ranks by the spring of 2005, however. Staff members who had come to New Century with him from

Chaoyang whispered that "one mountain cannot tolerate two tigers" (一山难容二虎 *yī shān nán róng èr hǔ*), even though Huang had generated significant revenues for the hospital.[23]

Relegated to the outskirts of Beijing in an obscure, second-tier hospital, Huang quickly decided to focus almost exclusively on treating foreigners—for whom the prestige of a Chinese institution mattered little. Unaware of the classifications and distinctions of an unfamiliar medical system, potential foreign clients placed more value on firsthand testimonials from other patients who had tried the procedure as they trawled the Internet for information. While Chinese patients were very interested in the OEG transplantation procedure during Huang's tenure at Naval General Hospital and then Chaoyang Hospital, many were perturbed by his multiple moves to decreasingly prestigious medical institutions (Huang later experimented with building partnerships with health facilities in other provinces, which I will discuss in chapter 6). As a skeptical self-described "old paraplegic" (老截瘫 *lǎo jiétān*) asked on a Chinese Internet discussion forum devoted to disability issues:

> In four years Huang Hongyun has switched four hospitals, and the final one is even outside of Beijing. What is the purpose of this? If he is winning glory for our country [为国争光 *wèi guó zhēng guāng*], blessing the people with a great deed [为民谋福的大好事 *wèi mín móu fú de dà hǎoshì*], then why does he always give people a sneaky feeling [偷偷摸摸的感觉 *tōutōumōmō de gǎnjué*]? (Yan 2006)

For a prospective domestic patient, these multiple institutional moves seemed suspicious and cast doubt on Huang's medical credibility. For Huang's foreign patients, however, a different semiotics emerged that emphasized his attentiveness to their care and comfort. Huang framed his transition to New Century as an opportunity to provide better facilities, including individual patient rooms with private showering and toileting facilities, televisions, air conditioning, and more. As Trophic, the American expatriate lawyer, described in his blog:

> It's nine-twenty in the evening and we've been here at the Workers Sanatorium since some time early this afternoon, one-thirty or thereabouts. "Here" is nothing less than the lap of luxury. Let me describe: a large room, big enough for two beds, a reading chair, a closet, a small desk—at which I'm writing as we speak—an upright two-gallon water-filter-cooler-heater (cold water comes out of one faucet, near-boiling out of another), a small refrigerator with, on top of the refrigerator case, a 21" (or larger??) TV and on top of that a DVD player. Beyond the large room is a wash-stand with two sinks and attached to that a large, wheelchair-accessible toilet-cum shower. Today I had the first really good wash since I arrived in Beijing two weeks ago. (Trophic 2004d)

As the subtext of Trophic's post suggests, providing better Internet access to foreign patients and their family members was a key part of the experience at Huang's new neurosurgery clinic inside the revamped worker's sanatorium. In addition to providing a digital "umbilical cord to hope" for the experimental pioneers so that they could stay connected to their family and friends back home, the blog posts and discussion forum threads served as a key source of international credibility and publicity for Huang and his experimental procedure.

Treating foreign patients at New Century was both an expedient and lucrative business decision. Since the Ministry of Health price controls applied only to Chinese patients, Huang was able to charge much higher fees across the board for treating foreign patients. While his Chinese patients paid approximately 30,000 yuan (approximately $3,750 U.S. in the early 2000s when Huang began performing the experimental procedure at Naval General and Chaoyang), Huang charged his foreign patients $20,000 U.S. This flat fee covered the OEG transplantation as well as all associated treatment and living costs during a patient's one-month stay in the newly built VIP ward that Huang developed at New Century (including all medical examinations and laboratory tests, a private hospital room with attached bathroom, twenty-four-hour medical care from nurses and physicians, medicines, post-surgical rehabilitation therapies, acupuncture, massage, meals, transportation, and accommodation and meals for one caregiver).

How did foreign patients and their caregivers justify spending tens of thousands of dollars on a potentially risky therapy? For some, cost posed no barrier to treatment: Huang's wealthiest patients arrived in Beijing on chartered jets, including a member of the Kuwaiti royal family suffering from ALS and the paralyzed son of a canned goods magnate from Mexico. Many generated support from their communities, such as Jeff, the firefighter from Colorado, whose colleagues auctioned off a Harley-Davidson motorcycle to help pay for his treatment. I met many others in Beijing who received tremendous support from their neighbors, church congregations, schools, and even pseudonymous online donors. Still others cashed out their life savings, refinancing their homes or tapping their retirement funds to finance their biomedical odysseys. Gary, an electrician from Wisconsin who had become paralyzed from the waist down after an abdominal aortic aneurysm, compared the expense of the fetal cell transplant with the price tag of a new car during a conversation we had together in August 2005 after his experimental treatment at New Century: "It costs no more than a new set of wheels, and everyone needs a new set of wheels once in a while."

To put Huang's surgical and hospitalization fees in further perspective, a study of patients undergoing a lumbar laminectomy (a surgical procedure similar to the one performed by Huang for his SCI patients) at a U.S. academic medical center found the average surgeon's fee to be $6,889±$2,882 in addition to an average inpatient hospital bill of $14,766±$7,729 for an average hospital stay of 3.5 days (Molina et al. 2013).[24] Although the overall fees are comparable, the cost per day for Huang's procedure comes out to $667 (versus $6187 for an analogous U.S. procedure)—an order of magnitude less.

While Huang's fees were quite reasonable compared to those of his American counterparts (and an overall better deal once total resources and extent of hospital-based care were factored in), he remained sensitive to accusations of undue profiteering: "Many people are criticizing me. They say that the reason I'm treating foreigners is to make money, that I look down on Chinese patients."[25] Huang defended his focus on foreigners as an eminently practical decision on medical grounds. In an ideal world, he explained to me in Mandarin over tea in his office on a bleak January afternoon in 2006, he would be able to treat everyone: "Chinese, foreigners, they're all pleading for help, and they all ought to be helped."[26] But Huang was a Chinese neurosurgeon operating in less than ideal circumstances. He relied solely on the income from his clinical practice to hire new staff, purchase better equipment, and conduct research on the efficacy of his experimental therapy. As one of the American CareCure pioneers had described, Huang's early efforts at Chaoyang Hospital were still in the "Model-T" stage of development, with the "Rolls-Royce" still far off in the future (Tim C. 2003d). Faced with what he described as the "limitations of existing circumstances," Huang wanted to make the biggest impact possible—which meant focusing on wealthier patients with access to better resources.

From a treatment perspective, Huang noted that foreigners had better access to rehabilitation facilities than did Chinese patients. He complained that many Chinese patients simply went home after their surgeries and languished in bed, unwilling or unable to continue the hard work of rehabilitating their atrophied muscles. At best, Huang's therapeutic intervention purportedly worked by awakening dormant nerve connections and improving the conduction of nerve signals—but lost muscle tone and dexterity still needed to be rebuilt through repeated exercising. Thus Huang felt that patients who engaged in intensive physical therapy following OEG transplantation stood to gain more extensive functional recovery.

Huang's motivations extended beyond practical financial and medical considerations. Defending his choice to focus on foreign patients in geopolitical terms, he pointed out that a Chinese doctor treating Chinese patients would never be able to command an international stage: "If I don't treat foreigners, people won't pay attention, they won't know what's happening in China. If I were just treating Chinese patients, do you think the editor of the *New England Journal of Medicine* would visit New Century? Would *Nature* send a reporter here?" Intrigued by and apprehensive about the steady flow of American patients coming to Beijing for treatment, leading scientific experts and journalists from around the world had indeed toured Huang's clinic and interviewed his patients. *Nature Medicine*, a subsidiary of the scientific journal, even featured Dr. Huang as one of China's top three "people to watch" in March 2006 (Cyranoski and Mandavilli 2006).

In an ironic twist, Huang explained his decision to treat foreigners rather than Chinese patients as a matter of glorifying China. Taking obvious pride in treating patients whom American neurosurgeons had declared incurable, Huang declared that his OEG transplantations demonstrated that China had surpassed the United States in advancing cutting-edge medical treatment: "The West hasn't been able to do it. I'm using Western medical methods to treat foreign patients. This proves that China is superior."[27]

Huang relished lecturing me on the intricacies of medical science and national pride in a transnational era, treating me as a fellow compatriot ensnared by the global politics of knowledge production:

> Science—even though the entire world can contribute and enjoy its accomplishments, it brings some politics with it. After I went abroad, I realized that America was even more patriotic [than China]. Americans, Europeans are attacking me. They don't want to admit that their patients have improved. They think that China is a backward [落后 luòhòu] place, that it can't possibly be ahead [优先 yōuxiān]. Why can't they bravely face the reality, and stand from the perspective of the patients?[28]

As Huang framed his motivations, "I'm doing this for the sake of China, for Western medicine. But the most important question is: What can this do to help patients?"[29]

Recognizing that his OEG transplantation technique was far from perfect, he saw his greatest contribution to the medical world as a conceptual one. He declared that he was challenging the conventional wisdom that gave up hope on curing spinal cord injuries and fatal neurodegenerative disorders:

> To go from zero to 0.1 is a huge breakthrough. Some people will dismiss your effect as very minimal. Yes, but this kind of small change has been unprecedented. I think that this is its value, to let people realize that the traditional concepts of the past are wrong. At every occasion I've repeatedly stressed that its value is not that it can suddenly restore the ability to walk, or that it can suddenly conquer this disease. Its significance instead lies in changing the traditional pessimism, the extremely pessimistic traditional concept. Only if we believe that this traditional concept is wrong will more people jump in, become interested, and conduct more research.[30]

Huang explained that his main goal was to "attract the attention of more scientific experts, so that more people can join in this research. Increasing our influence will be advantageous both for patients and for the development of science." He sincerely hoped that more doctors would start performing the OEG transplantations. So many patients wanted the surgery, and he lamented that he "would never be able to treat all of them."[31]

His tactical move to focus on foreign patients thus reflected local practical and financial concerns as well as larger geopolitical processes. For Huang, treating foreign patients was tied up inextricably with a healer's concern for his patients' well-being, an ambitious clinician's desire for renown, a director's concern for ensuring the fiscal survival of his fledgling enterprise, and a Chinese citizen's unabashed national pride.

THE LITTLE RED BOOK OF INDEPENDENT INNOVATION

Huang explicitly connected the development of his new neurosurgery enterprise based at New Century Hospital with the cultural imperative for scientific and technological modernization. Under the stewardship of then Chinese president Hu Jintao, this drive during the 2000s took the form of "independent innovation" (自主创新 *zìzhǔ chuàngxīn*). Huang unveiled this grand vision in print while commemorating the center's first-year anniversary at New Century Hospital. Calling together staff members for a center-wide meeting, he handed out small photocopied booklets sandwiched between red cardboard covers to the doctors, nurses, researchers, lab technicians, administrative assistants, and the center's resident anthropologist, who all crowded into the shared doctors' office in the northwest corner of the third-floor ward. Titled the "Beijing New Century Hospital Neurological Disorders Research and Treatment Center First Five-Year Development Plan 2006–2010," the little red booklet summarized the previous year's accomplishments and laid out guidelines for the next few years over the course of nine pages.

The content and rhetoric of the guidelines were self-consciously modeled after the Communist Party of China's Five-Year Plans, drawing inspiration from these national directives. The New Century Plan began by quoting a recent Party communiqué: "No less than our Party's 16th Central Committee's Fifth Plenum has noted: 'the development of science and technology should hold firmly to independent innovation [自主创新 *zìzhǔ chuàngxīn*], focus on making major strides, support development, and lead the way to guiding principles for the future'" (Huang 2006).[32]

Championing independent innovation in science and technology as "the essential motivating force of a country and a people's development,"[33] Huang framed his clinical use of the OEG fetal cell transplantation procedure in terms of this guiding principle:

> This innovative treatment method is an important source of China's contribution to the worldwide field of medical treatment, a rarely encountered achievement in our country's medical profession. This pioneering research fills an international gap and brings our country to the forefront of this field. From the perspective of our national honor [国家荣誉 *guójiā róngyù*] and our country's international medical status, the ability to attract a large number of patients from Europe, the United States, and other developed countries to our country to receive medical treatment is of historical significance, and the Chinese medical profession should be proud and filled with glory. (Huang 2006)[34]

Like the ode to olfactory ensheathing cells penned by one of his admiring subordinates, Huang's own medical manifesto situates the experimental therapy on a grand historical timeline. The focus here is on his revolutionary contribution as a Chinese citizen to medical knowledge worldwide, with his foreign patients serving as embodied evidence of his achievement. He explicitly invokes a tech-nonationalist trope to describe his ability to attract hundreds of patients from developed countries to receive experimental fetal cell therapy in China. Huang's bold vision encompassed everyone on his staff, instructing them that "each one of us should feel honored to participate in this collective work, truly feeling the pride and honor of being Chinese."[35]

CONCLUSION

Although the details of Huang's extraordinary career may not be easily general-izable, his story illuminates how a new breed of medical entrepreneurs leverages a global clientele in the context of cutting-edge regenerative medicine at a par-ticular historical moment in the fraught politics of China's health care reforms. In order to situate the analytical and historical significance of Dr. Huang's story, it is important to recognize that globalization and translocal interactions are not new phenomena in the history of Chinese health care. Historians have traced the influence of missionary medicine and Western scientific discourses during China's late imperial and Republican eras (Rogaski 2004; Yang 2006; D. Zhang 2006; Lei 2014), and anthropologists have focused attention on translocal med-ical connections during the more recent socialist era. In her ethnography about the "worlding" of Chinese medicine, Mei Zhan (2009) documents the successive ways in which knowledge about "traditional Chinese medicine" has been con-tinuously remade through engagements with translocal encounters. As Zhan notes, staging acupuncture and other medical successes in front of foreign vis-itors has long been a key strategy of the Chinese government's efforts to garner legitimacy and worldwide recognition for Chinese medical practices and health care policies.[36] Zhan's analysis of translocal knowledge production spans Maoist government efforts in the 1960s and 1970s to export preventive medicine in order to serve the proletariat of the world to the corporatization of acupuncture during the 1990s to ease the stresses of cosmopolitan urbanites in Shanghai and California.

Operating in the high-tech tertiary care sector in twenty-first-century Beijing, Huang's transnational neurosurgical enterprise and experiences embody the emerging culture of medical entrepreneurialism in late socialist China. Huang's neurosurgical career highlights the accelerating convergence of individual and state interests in promoting advanced technologies as well as the importance of leveraging foreign pedigrees and training opportunities abroad. While the transformation of health care into a business has encouraged enterprising Chi-nese doctors to experiment with lucrative biomedical interventions for foreign patients, prioritizing foreign patients was not simply a profit-driven scheme that capitalized on emergent market logic. Huang's experimental health care prac-tices also drew on enduring socialist ideals refracted through Communist Party rhetoric. The pursuit of advanced medical technologies by medical entrepreneurs such as Huang ultimately is not just about making money but also about professional ambitions and national pride.

Scholars of post-Mao China have noted the enduring influence of socialist ideologies and practices in processes that might elsewhere be framed in terms of neoliberalism (Rofel 2007; Zhang and Ong 2008; Kipnis 2008).[37] Even anthropologists who have embraced neoliberal frameworks for understanding emerging subjectivities in post-Mao China have situated their analyses in the context of broader questions of social belonging. Returning to Nikolas Rose's notion of the "enterprising self," we need to temper his claims about these calculating, self-disciplined, self-interested subjects to see how they invoke affinities with broader collective projects to resist market logics and challenge moral critiques.[38] In her analysis of job choice for Chinese college students as a technique of governing, Lisa Hoffman (2010) develops the term "patriotic professionalism" to highlight the centrality of patriotism in the development of professional subjectivity in late socialist China. In Hoffman's analysis, young professionals' cultivation of a self-enterprising ethos entailed a sense of responsibility to collective projects of strengthening the nation. Rather than engaging in a generalized patriotism, however, Huang draws on his professional identity as a neurosurgeon to capitalize on technoscientific innovation—and herein lies the specificity of medical entrepreneurialism as a cultural phenomenon predicated on technonationalism. As we have seen in this chapter, Huang invokes the trope of technonationalism to elevate his experimental therapy to international prominence, deflect charges of undue profiteering, and ultimately reframe medical entrepreneurialism as a moral duty in the service of both his patients and the glory of the Chinese nation.

As a highly trained doctor thinking resourcefully about how to take his work to the next level, Huang demonstrates how developing innovative therapeutic interventions offers the hope of personal and national salvation. For Huang, his ambitious neurosurgery enterprise not only capitalized on foreign patients as a lucrative source of income but also challenged the boundaries of medical knowledge and catapulted China into the limelight as he promoted a pioneering but potentially dangerous therapeutic intervention. International medical researchers have begun to discuss new hope for treating intractable disorders such as spinal cord injury and amyotrophic lateral sclerosis, but Huang is one of the few who have translated these potential visions into concrete clinical treatments. While the effectiveness of this experimental therapy remains highly controversial (a concern I will address in chapter 7), Huang himself has argued that his greatest contribution lies in overturning conventional wisdom about the "untreatability" of neurodegenerative conditions.

In the next chapter, I take a more intimate look at the institutional logics and machinations that have enabled Huang's medical entrepreneurialism to thrive.

CHAPTER 6

BORDERLINE TACTICS

IN THIS CHAPTER, I TAKE a closer look at how experimental medicine works in the institutional contexts of "socialism with Chinese characteristics." As the previous chapter documented, changes in the political economy of health care have encouraged hospitals and administrators to experiment with novel ways to meet the bottom line by pursuing the development of advanced biomedical technologies. Although some health policy analysts have characterized this worrisome phenomenon as the radical privatization or even complete dismantling of public health in China (e.g., Hesketh and Zhu 1997b; Blumenthal and Hsiao 2005), a finer-grained ethnographic analysis reveals that the supposed headlong descent into privatization consists of a more nuanced mixture of practices.[1] The uneven processes generated by late and post-socialist transformations in China have engendered proliferating practices that draw not only on new market opportunities but also on enduring socialist institutions.[2] This framework highlights the interplay between state control and self-governing practices, emphasizing the ways in which state agendas have selectively authorized the pursuit of self-interest.

How are enterprising clinicians negotiating the complex and incomplete marketization of China's health care system while working under ever more restrictive bureaucratic regimes of accountability? I use the case study of Huang's neurosurgical enterprise in order to illustrate how entrepreneurial clinicians have responded to proliferating political uncertainties and economic anxieties by experimenting not only with new biomedical procedures but also with resourceful bureaucratic techniques. These medical entrepreneurs leverage state rhetoric, maximize institutional flexibility, and exploit administrative loopholes in the spirit of "independent innovation." These experimental forms of institutional practice challenge and redraw the boundaries between public and private, legal and illegal, as well as ethical and unethical in contemporary China.

My analysis of these borderline institutional practices draws upon calls in recent anthropological scholarship for ethnographies of the state grounded in the everyday workings of bureaucracy. While earlier studies of bureaucracy tended to focus on the symbolic aspects of *talk* about bureaucracy (as in Michael Herzfeld's [1992] incisive analysis of how the ubiquitous "bureaucratic horror story" operates in the social production of bureaucratic indifference), more recent ethnographic studies have delved into the formal properties and material dimensions of bureaucracy itself. Akhil Gupta (2012) articulates the workings of a "disaggregated" state to analyze how bureaucratic inscription practices such as inspection reports and complaint forms systematically produce arbitrary outcomes that enact structural violence on India's poor. Matthew Hull (2012) deconstructs Pakistani state power through a semiotic analysis of "graphic artifacts" such as urbanization plans, petitions, files, signatures, and maps. These ethnographic studies underscore the importance of investigating "the state" not as a monolithic and unified entity but rather as a fragmented collection of agendas, institutions, and bureaucratic paperwork.[3] I take up these insights in this chapter to explore how bureaucratic practices intersect with the workings of medical entrepreneurialism in the highly complex and often confusing landscape of China's health care system.

Returning to our earlier discussion of medical entrepreneurialism in China, recall Judith Farquhar's discussion of the self-employed, fee-for-service *gètǐhù* doctors operating storefront clinics in a model rural township during the 1990s. Farquhar explicitly contrasted these enterprising private practitioners with salaried doctors working in state-run county hospitals, whom she characterized as holdovers from an outdated socialist era who "work[ed] for artificially low salaries, [were] discouraged from participating in the thriving gift economy . . . [and were] often treated as interchangeable functionaries by patients and administrators alike" (1996, 243). In Farquhar's analysis, an entrepreneurial spirit thrived only outside the walls of state-owned work units. But as political scientist Lü Xiaobo demonstrates in his analysis of organizational corruption, the predatory behavior of "bureau-preneurs" has played a key role in driving Chinese state-led economic development (2000, 274–75). Building on Lü's insights on "booty socialism," John Osburg (2013) fleshes out the lurid world of urban Chinese entrepreneurs in his ethnography of the private lives of China's new rich in the southwestern city of Chengdu during the 2000s. Unveiling the seamy strategies by which entrepreneurs "create embeddedness . . . with their clients, partners, and patrons in the government," Osburg details the socializing, banqueting, drinking, gambling, and sexual bribery practices that establish the "moral economies of elite *guānxì* [关系 relationship] networks . . . at the very heart of 'capitalist' development in urban China" (2013, 31–32). This vivid portrait of the increasing "collusion" and "enmeshment" between entrepreneurs and state officials highlights the consolidation of power through the cultivation of *guānxì* and gift-giving—a central theme in anthropological analyses of Chinese social relations (e.g., Yang 1994; Yan 1996). But I argue here that focusing on *guānxì*-building among business elites and state officials maintains a conceptual boundary between entrepreneurial and bureaucratic categories that obscures important processes in entrepreneurial subjectivity and state-making. Following Gupta's (1995, 2012) critique of the state–civil society divide, I eschew the conventional analysis of *guānxì*-building to focus on a particular category of subjects who blur the boundaries between state and society: ambitious health care professionals such as Dr. Huang working in state-owned hospitals in the new millennium.

These enterprising urban clinicians are contending with a different set of institutional logics generated by successive rounds of hospital reform, state defunding of health care, and the complex interactions of various "biobureaucracies" (Kohrman 2005, 3) governing health and well-being. In contrast to the rural *gètǐhù* doctors and moribund county hospitalists of the 1990s or even the wealthy businessmen of the 2000s, a different kind of entrepreneurial subject is emerging at the margins and interstices of urban health bureaucracy in twenty-first-century China. These medical entrepreneurs not only optimize socialist legacies, invoke patriotic values, and leverage advanced technologies (as I demonstrated in the previous chapter) but also manipulate bureaucratic tactics[4] in the process of hedging against regulatory uncertainty and building transnational enterprises that attract patients from around the world.

WEARING A RED HAT

Like other public hospitals in China at the beginning of the new millennium, New Century Hospital faced growing budget deficits that encouraged hospital administrators to seek out novel sources of income. While prestigious hospitals institutionalized stratified service tracks that index patients' degrees of political and economic privilege, smaller medical facilities such as New Century took an even more radical approach toward profit generation. By reinventing themselves as real estate brokers, these hospitals "leased departments" (出租科室 *chūzū kēshì*) or "outsourced departments" (外包科室 *wàibāo kēshì*) to entrepreneurial doctors and others looking to expand their businesses. Unlike Beijing's top hospitals, where famous experts could attract a flood of patients from far-flung provinces willing to pay a premium for privileged access, second-tier hospitals such as New Century lacked the reputation and human resources to build their own lucrative VIP wards or "special needs" outpatient centers (特需门诊 *tèxū ménzhěn*). Many thus looked to external sources to attract patients and generate revenue by renting out extra space to medical entrepreneurs.

The tactic of operating "a hospital within a hospital" (院中院 *yuàn zhōng yuàn*) drew upon a common practice among Chinese entrepreneurs known as "red-hatting" (戴红帽子 *dài hóngmàozi*), in which private companies partnered with public enterprises as a cover for their business activities (Wank 2001, 79; Song 2011, 147). By leasing underutilized real estate to private health care providers, struggling public hospitals capitalized on the socialist valorization of public property and status. This symbiotic public-private partnership benefited both sides. Private entrepreneurs profited from using the name and institutional legitimacy of the hospital in order to conduct their business, while the relevant hospital administrators received monthly "management" and "rental" payments, a share of the profits, and presumably a shower of *hóngbāo* (红包) (red packets of money) and other "gifts" to smooth out the transactions. The medical entrepreneurs conducted their own health-related activities within the public hospital—from recruiting patients and hiring personnel to setting fees and collecting payments—with little to no oversight from the contracting hospital. This institutional practice effectively produced an independent "private hospital" operating under the umbrella of the larger public hospital. While the PRC State Council (1994) formally declared such conduct illegal, savvy medical entrepreneurs circumvented these regulations by partnering with a network of medical institutions and local governments. Hospital administrators and entrepreneurs thus gained institutional credibility and legal recognition as "academic partners" of lucrative joint ventures stimulating local economies.

Without the capital funds to buy their own equipment and cultivate their own experts, New Century administrators sought to rent out their facilities to already established physicians such as Huang Hongyun. With a proven track record that had attracted the attention of domestic and foreign media outlets ranging from CCTV to the *Chicago Tribune* and even prestigious scientific journals such as *Nature* and *The Lancet*, Huang had the potential to bring patients from around the world to the wards of New Century Hospital. As a second-tier public hospital, New Century Hospital looked to raise its profile by appointing the neurosurgeon to serve as the chairman of a newly established Department of Neurosurgery. To entice the headline-generating neurosurgeon to set up shop in 2004 at the virtually unknown institution at the fringes of the city, New Century administrators simultaneously allowed Huang to create his own independent medical research institute and refurbish a wing of the hospital to serve as a new VIP ward for foreign patients.

Huang's partnership with New Century Hospital thrived by manipulating the boundaries between public and private in a characteristic example of redhatting. In practice, the neurosurgery department and the "Beijing New Century Hospital Neurological Disorders Research and Treatment Center" (北京新世纪医院神经疾病研治中心 Běijīng Xīn Shìjì Yīyuàn Shénjīng Jíbìng Yánzhì Zhōngxīn) were identical: they shared the same employees, the same equipment, and the same director operating in the same physical space on the third floor of the hospital. But on paper, the two organizational entities provided Huang and hospital administrators with the institutional means to maneuver around bureaucratic obstacles and legal impediments, to the benefit of both parties. Huang's appointment as the chairman of the hospital's neurosurgery department provided him with a legal mandate to conduct clinical activities under the hospital's name. As the director of his own independent medical research institute, however, Huang bypassed many of the bureaucratic restrictions that had constrained his opportunities for expansion at his previous medical institutions. He now had the power to hire new staff members, purchase equipment, and set treatment fees without having to obtain approval from the hospital administration. In return, he paid the hospital "maintenance" and "scientific cooperation" fees.

While these tactics were deployed most spectacularly by elite medical entrepreneurs such as Huang, the practice of leveraging public status and private profit extended to health care workers at all institutional levels. Dr. Liang, a neurosurgeon who had worked with Huang at Naval General Hospital, was now the *èr bǎshǒu* (二把手, literally "second handle" or second-in-command) of the New Century neurosurgical enterprise. Despite working long hours at New Century Hospital, Liang continued to make the tedious commute back to Naval General each night in order to retain the military institution as his official *dānwèi* (work unit). Liang thus hedged his bets by maintaining one foot in the "iron rice bowl" (with its guaranteed employment and steady if meager salary) and the other foot in a more profitable but risky venture. Even those without official employment status still tried to secure the stability of working at a public institution while benefiting from the lucrative potential of Huang's experimental enterprise. Sunny, a middle-aged woman from rural Sichuan province, had worked for several years as a janitor in the neurosurgery department at Chaoyang Hospital. Impressed by her work ethic and cheerful disposition, Huang invited her to come with him to New Century as an all-purpose hospital aide. Instead of informing the head nurse at Chaoyang that she was quitting to take a higher-paying position, Sunny told her employer that she was going back home to her natal village for a family visit. Because Chinese rural-to-urban migrant workers often return home for extended periods, particularly around the annual Spring Festival holiday, Sunny calculated that this would enable her to return fairly easily to the more stable public institution in case the situation at New Century did not work out.

TRIUMPHAL EXPANSIONS

The autumn of 2005 was a triumphal moment in New Century history. Approaching a full year of operations in their new location, the staff orchestrated multiple celebrations in honor of the New Century Neurological Disorders Research and Treatment Center's first anniversary. The momentous occasion inspired Dr. Wang to write his extravagant eleven-stanza poem praising the "miracle of olfactory ensheathing cells" (嗅鞘细胞的神奇 *xiùqiào xìbāo de shénqí*).

Both the hospital and Huang's enterprise flourished under their tactical partnership. Financial matters were always a sensitive issue, and despite Huang's willingness to let me observe the workings of his neurosurgery enterprise on nearly every level, he never disclosed the exact amounts he paid hospital administrators for the privilege of running his own research center. But his neurosurgery center was clearly a profitable venture for the hospital, providing enough revenue to finance a major renovation of the buildings and grounds. Material signs of the lucrative partnership proliferated throughout the hospital complex: sparkling glass doors replaced the grimy vinyl flaps obscuring the main entrance, while wood paneling and glowing light-boxes supplanted the peeling paint and rusting metal signs. The hospital also began constructing a state-of-the-art rehabilitation facility to replace the cavernous canteen.

Recognizing Huang's successes in attracting patients, hospital administrators evicted the second-floor tenants (an unprofitable department of endocrinology) and bestowed the additional wing on the neurosurgeon so that he could expand his clinical practice and develop more extensive laboratory facilities. The addition of the new ward infused a sense of unlimited potential in the expanding horizons of the neurosurgery clinic—what Gary, the electrician from Wisconsin, described as "the road to hopes and dreams." The potential of the OEG transplantations to revolutionize medical treatment captivated the imaginations of staff members, patients, and caregivers alike: Sunny, who eagerly offered to lug the heavy suitcases of incoming patients; Dr. Liang, who went for months without seeing his own baby daughter and instead stayed late into the night to check on patients; Leo, the SCI-advocate-turned-cure-crusader who set up his own business to help would-be fetal cell pioneers make the journey to China; Gerald, the British carer who taught enthusiastic English lessons to Chinese nurses; Lillien, an American nurse practitioner and mother of a T12 paraplegic who painstakingly answered the flood of emails from other families desperate for more information; even the anthropologist, who compiled a patient support handbook to help those coming from abroad to navigate the chaos of Beijing. Caught up in the promise of fetal olfactory glial cells, we lavished our energies and care into improving the center.

On a warm autumn day in 2005, we thus found ourselves orchestrating an extravagant party to celebrate the opening of the new second-floor neurosurgery ward. Young Chinese security guards maneuvered an enormous roll of red carpeting past an elderly Japanese woman taking hesitant steps down the long corridor. Teacher Yan directed several nurses pushing stainless steel medical carts laden with oranges, watermelons, and floral arrangements around two bemused Italians in wheelchairs who had rolled out of their rooms to witness the spectacle. Although officially retired, Yan was quite a formidable presence as the former head nurse of the busy neurosurgery service at Beijing's Chaoyang Hospital. She could quell an obstinate surgeon with a single disapproving look. Yan had been persuaded to come out of retirement to help set up this new neurosurgery venture in western Beijing, and she now presided over the clinic's daily operations.

At the end of the freshly painted hallway, one of the taller neurosurgeon trainees carefully lined the windows of the communal activity room with translucent blue film embellished with dolphins and tropical fish. As a nurse exclaimed in Chinese about how lovely the new decorations looked, I overheard two American patients wondering why the staff had blocked out the view of the surrounding mountains with a "tacky" plastic sheet. In the central office, an administrative assistant placed an order for twenty large pizzas from Bàng! Yuēhàn (棒约翰) (literally "Excellent! John," the Chinese transliteration for the American pizza delivery chain Papa John's). Although the cheese would congeal and the crusts would turn soggy during the hour-long journey from Beijing's Central Business District to this small hospital on the western edge of the city, the pizzas would still be a special treat for the clinic's foreign patients and their accompanying caregivers.

No expense was spared in preparing for the grand celebration of the neurosurgery clinic's first-year anniversary and expansion to a new ward of the host hospital. While the clinic staff would later celebrate on their own with a lavish Chinese-style banquet, multiple rounds of toasting while imbibing fiery 100-proof *báijiǔ* liquor, followed by late-night karaoke singing, their visions of what constituted a suitable party for foreigners followed a different script.

Angel was the master of ceremonies for the evening's momentous event, and she nervously practiced her introductions in anticipation of her first big role as the center's patient support coordinator. The twenty-two-year-old from nearby Hebei province had graduated from Chengde Medical University's first cohort of "English nursing" majors two months earlier—a new program that sought to prepare Chinese nurses for the growing influx of foreign patients in China as well as capitalize on the rising trend of Chinese medical professionals seeking employment abroad. Angel's enthusiasm was contagious and she easily recruited several European caregivers to help her prepare for the festivities. On her own initiative, she had organized a series of practical care sessions to help New Century patients and family members living with neurodegenerative conditions, and tonight marked the official inauguration of her fledgling patient support association. Flirtatious yet earnest, the pretty college graduate relished a grateful patient's description of her as "a beautiful angel from heaven." She had thus chosen Angel as her English name, and she worked long hours to live up to the demands of her new identity and first job.

As Angel and Teacher Yan finalized their preparations, other clinic staff invited patients to come out of their rooms into the hallway, helping those with more limited mobility into wheelchairs to join the festivities. On Angel's cue, we proceeded outside to the garden—a parade of neurosurgeons in blue scrubs, nurses in white smocks and starched hats, laboratory technicians in casual summer clothes, administrative staff in colorful blouses and floral-printed skirts, and a range of patients and family members hailing from around the world. English was the default lingua franca among our diverse group, although on this particular day I also heard Farsi, French, German, Greek, Italian, Japanese, Romanian, Tagalog, and Turkish.

Posing for photos, Chinese neurosurgeons and nurses flashed double-handed victory signs together with their smiling patients: fifty-four-year-old Abdul from

Bangladesh, forty-five-year-old Kiki from Greece, sixty-four-year-old Guido from Italy, twenty-five-year-old Neslihan from Turkey. Several patients had large gauze bandages taped to their shaved heads, lingering signs of their recent surgical encounters in the hospital's operating room. All of them had come to Beijing in order to undergo experimental fetal cell transplantation in the hopes of regaining lost neurological function.

Over sixty people gathered around the red-carpeted clearing fringed with bamboo and cypress trees to await a speech by the man who had brought all of us together at New Century: Dr. Huang Hongyun. Not one for much pomp and circumstance, the plainspoken fifty-year-old neurosurgeon urged everyone to enjoy the feast the staff had prepared. But before we could eat, Gerald, the co-author of the Sweet N Sour blog, stepped forward with a surprise. Explaining the significance of the fetal cell transplantation surgery in freeing patients from the diseases that had trapped them, Gerald thrust an open cage containing two speckled pigeons into the neurosurgeon's hands. The first bird burst out of its metal prison and soared into the sky to the delighted cries of both hospital staff and guests. But the other bird stubbornly clung to the inside of the cage, refusing to leave. "He like here," blurted one of the nurses in English, inducing a chorus of laughs from the crowd. Doctors and patients called out suggestions as Dr. Huang tried to coax the recalcitrant bird out. "I want you be free!" he shouted with an emphatic shake of the cage. In the end, the neurosurgeon reached into the cage and pulled the bird out. Released from its prison with a bit of extra help, it too soared into the air to the cheers of the audience who had gathered to celebrate the first anniversary of the New Century Neurological Disorders Research and Treatment Center.

ESCAPING RECTIFICATION MEASURES

Even as foreign patients flocked to New Century and staff members celebrated the opening of the new second-floor ward, Huang and hospital administrators faced increasing pressure from shifting state priorities. Although government policies throughout the 1990s had pushed the expansion of high-tech health services, the profit-oriented practices of Chinese hospitals angered both rural and urban Chinese citizens who found health care increasingly unaffordable. From rampant overprescription of expensive medicines and unnecessary testing to outright corruption in the form of direct kickbacks from pharmaceutical companies and monetary gifts from patients, the Chinese health care system's lopsided expansion under the mandate of market socialism was increasingly criticized as the "failed health care reforms" (失败的医疗卫生改革 *shībài de yīliáo wèishēng gǎigé*). A report issued by China's State Council has acknowledged these issues with surprising public candor: "Since the Reform and Opening Up, China's health care system has undergone significant changes. In certain aspects we have made progress, but the problems that have been exposed are even more serious. Overall, the reform has not succeeded" (People's Republic of China State Council Development Research Center 2005).

Much of the critical attention focused on the worsening health inequalities that plagued rural primary care. However, the technology-intensive tertiary care sector concentrated in affluent urban centers also came under fire. In particular, Chinese journalists excoriated private "hospitals within hospitals" (院中院 *yuàn zhōng yuàn*) as "black-hearted institutions" (黑心院 *hēixīn yuàn*) that "advertised mutton but sold dog meat" (挂羊头卖狗肉 *guà yáng tóu mài gǒuròu*) as they used the name and fame of legitimate public hospitals in order to conduct often unsavory business (Li 2004). These proliferating abuses prompted the Ministry of Health to launch the "Special Rectification Program to Crack Down on the Illegal Practice of Medicine" (严厉打击非法行医专项整治工作方案 *yánlì dǎjí fēifǎ xíngyī zhuānxiàng zhěngzhì gōngzuò fāng'àn*) in 2004. This nationwide campaign specifically targeted the practice of "hospitals within hospitals" operated by unqualified individuals, prohibiting medical institutions from contracting out medical wards and services to non-medical personnel. The rectification measures also addressed the issue of "red-hatting" by explicitly forbidding nonprofit medical institutions from leasing or outsourcing hospital departments (People's Republic of China Ministry of Health 2004).

Despite these regulatory efforts, the lucrative "hospitals within hospitals" phenomenon remained entrenched throughout the 2000s. The Chinese media uncovered repeated instances of these questionable practices. In 2005, Xinhua News Agency reported on rented clinics that fabricated diagnoses and prescribed expensive remedies for male sexual problems (Xinhua News Agency 2005b). That same year, reports surfaced about private pharmaceutical dispensaries that masqueraded as public dermatology clinics (Wang 2005). In a particularly flagrant example, as reported by China Central Television, the private Wansui Pharmaceutical Group continued to lease more than fifty-eight hospital wards in twenty provinces and municipalities across the country even after the crackdown, using these public health facilities as a front for marketing their products to unsuspecting patients. An undercover investigation by a CCTV reporter revealed that purported doctors working in a Wansui-operated orthopedic department in Jiangsu province did not possess medical licenses, diagnosed false medical problems, and urged patients to purchase expensive pharmaceutical products manufactured by Wansui (CCTV 2005).

Although Huang's partnership with New Century could be interpreted as an example of a "hospital within a hospital," the complex institutional ties they had created resisted easy pigeonholing. Huang was a legitimate neurosurgeon with a license to practice medicine in Beijing, and he held an official clinical appointment at New Century. Furthermore, even though his neurosurgery department functioned as an independent research unit, Huang's "scientific collaboration" (科学协作 *kēxué xiézuò*) with New Century had not been formally registered as a distinct institution. On paper, their relationship thus did not fall under the scope of the Ministry of Health's "rectification measures" since the hospital was not "leasing" or "outsourcing" wards to unqualified outsiders. Of course, Huang had considerably more latitude than most department chairs, and he compensated the hospital handsomely for these privileges. These bureaucratic tactics thus enabled Huang and New Century administrators to dodge the specific charges of the Ministry of Health's campaign through 2005.

Bureaucratic maneuverings such as these are colloquially called *cābiānqiú* (擦边球), a Ping-Pong metaphor for a ball that brushes the edge of the table. Suggesting a borderline move with contested legitimacy, the metaphor of an "edge ball" conjures up the challenges of playing a tactical game that navigates a precarious line between a skillfully placed ball and one that is ruled out-of-bounds. In the case of the national crackdown campaign, these borderline *cābiānqiú* tactics enabled the ambitious neurosurgeon and hospital administrators to dodge charges of engaging in the illegal practice of medicine. But the regulatory landscape was constantly shifting and their bureaucratic machinations proved less successful in hedging against municipal-level "rectification measures."

DUMPLING DOLDRUMS

My footsteps reverberated in the darkened corridor as I made my way through New Century Hospital's central artery. Usually bustling with nurses pushing metal carts and anxious family members running between the registration desk and the pharmacy window, the hallway was empty today. Even the pajama-clad rehabilitation patients—long-term hospital residents who staked out the elevator entrance in their wheelchairs as they took long drags on their cigarettes—had signed out of the hospital in anticipation of the national holiday. It was the eve of the Spring Festival in 2006, and I hurried past the silent examination rooms to help wrap dumplings for the few foreign patients, their caregivers, and Chinese staff members who had remained in Beijing. The empty corridors hadn't surprised me. As the most important holiday in Chinese culture, Spring Festival marked the beginning of the lunar new year. Government offices and businesses shut down for an entire week. Nobody liked to spend the biggest celebration of the year trapped in a hospital, and Chinese medical facilities generally stopped admitting patients in the period leading up to the seven-day national holiday. Hospitals operated on a skeleton crew as doctors, nurses, and administrative staff traveled home; even seriously ill patients tried to obtain temporary discharge papers so they too could spend the holiday with their families. Although the fetal cell clinic had a backlog of patients numbering into the thousands, I assumed that Dr. Huang had reduced his experimental transplantation schedule so that his staff members could take time off. But I soon discovered another reason behind the holiday slowdown.

On my way upstairs to the office I shared with two Chinese doctors, I encountered a sweaty Driver Zhang slurping down some noodles in an empty patient room. Usually busy shuttling foreign patients and their overloaded suitcases back and forth between the airport, Zhang and a few other staff members who lived in Beijing had taken advantage of the lighter holiday schedule to rejuvenate the second-floor ward. After nearly four months of heavy use by a steady stream of patients undergoing fetal cell transplantation surgery, the formerly new ward no longer sparkled like the red-carpeted VIP area that had opened with much fanfare in September. So under Teacher Yan's orders, Zhang and his colleagues had spent the previous several days scraping down the walls of the empty ward. They were now repainting the rooms a bright baby blue—to match the plastic dolphin screens that decorated the windows of the activity room.

Sidestepping the used paint brushes and overturned buckets scattered in the hallway, I retreated into my office to escape the paint fumes. Both of my officemates had already headed home for the holidays. Dr. Alan, the neurosurgery department's chief neurologist, had left the previous day on an overnight bus to Shandong province to join his family. By now he was probably wrapping dumplings together with his wife and eight-year-old daughter, who often sent him text messages reporting her latest exam scores. Dr. Brian, the young neurosurgeon who had taken care of cantankerous Frau K., had a much longer road to travel. His wife and three-year-old son lived in remote Gansu province in the shadow of the country's satellite launch center, which had catapulted China onto the world stage in 2003 with the successful launching of a Chinese astronaut into orbit. Dr. Brian's journey took two full days on a train followed by another night on a bus, and at best he was only able to go home once a year during the Spring Festival. His own son had not recognized him during his previous visit home, and he nervously wondered whether the new clothes he had bought his son would fit. The other neurosurgeons had agreed to cut short their own vacations to give their colleague a few extra days with his family.

Angel, the patient coordinator, called me over to invite the foreign patients and their families to participate in the Spring Festival tradition of making the crescent-shaped dumplings. As we speculated about whether the Americans or Europeans would make more shapely dumplings, she admitted that this was the first Spring Festival celebration she had spent away from home. Her parents had protested their only child's absence from the family table this holiday season, but she told them that the patients needed her. We walked up and down the neurosurgery ward knocking on the doors of occupied patient rooms, enticing out a middle-aged woman from California whose teenage son had been injured in a biking accident a year earlier. Another mother from Denmark joined us together with her thirty-three-year-old son, who had been paralyzed over a decade earlier when he jumped into shallow water at a beach and had suffered excruciating pain ever since the accident. We also rounded up a retired state trooper from Montana who had been injured while serving in Afghanistan with the U.S. National Guard, the veteran's adult son, the daughter of an elderly British man with ALS, and four generations of a Spanish family who had traveled to China to support

Alfonso, a fifty-year-old man with rapidly advancing ALS. Despite the vigilance of his father, mother, sister, brother-in-law, wife, daughter, granddaughter, and a round-the-clock watch of nurses and neurosurgeons, Alfonso had stopped breathing a few days earlier. The hospital staff managed to resuscitate him, but not before he had slipped into a coma. Although his condition had stabilized, the Spaniard had not regained consciousness and was now hooked up to a ventilator. Sophie, the head nursing administrator, had assigned herself overnight duty for New Year's Eve and set up a small desk in Alfonso's room so that she could keep continual watch over the comatose patient through the night.

By the time our procession arrived in the activity room at the end of the ward, Teacher Yan had already finished preparing the ground pork and chive filling with the help of Sunny. Although the middle-aged Sunny had only a few years of elementary school education, her cheerful disposition and surprising strength made her a favorite among foreign patients, even though they could only communicate by smiles and gestures as she delivered fresh fruit to the wards, replenished the supply closets, and helped nurses transfer patients. Both Sunny and Teacher Yan had followed Dr. Huang from Chaoyang Hospital in Beijing's central business district to the little-known New Century Hospital on the outskirts of the city. Huang relied on these loyal staff members to carry out the everyday details of ensuring the foreign patients' comfort during their monthlong hospital stays.

The dumpling-wrapping event seemed more like a dirge than a party, despite the constant crackle and boom of firecrackers filtering in through the windows. Although Angel once again served as Dr. Huang's master of ceremonies, her speech lacked the spirited enthusiasm that had animated her introduction of the Second Neurosurgery Ward for Foreigners just a few months earlier. I joined the small group of resident neurosurgeons and off-duty nurses in showing the foreign visitors how to make Chinese-style dumplings (figure 6.1), and they half-heartedly joked that my misshapen dumplings were a glaring sign of my American upbringing. Even Dr. Huang seemed preoccupied as he demonstrated his wrapping technique to the group, fusing the flattened circle of dough around a glob of meat filling with a single deft squeeze of his fist. Teacher Yan and Sunny had set out an expansive array of fruit, snacks, cold cuts, sodas, and wines to accompany the dumplings, but the festive meal could not cover up the undertone of anxiety running through the room. I thought that the staff was worried about Alfonso's precarious situation, but later on that evening Angel updated me on what had happened during the previous week while I had taken an out-of-town trip. The Beijing health bureau had shut down a third of New Century Hospital's clinical departments, including Huang's neurosurgery clinic, and the fetal cell transplantation procedures now had to be done in another city in a different province. The muted atmosphere of the neurosurgery clinic did not just stem from an ailing patient or an ordinary holiday slowdown; it turned out that the entire hospital had run into bureaucratic trouble.

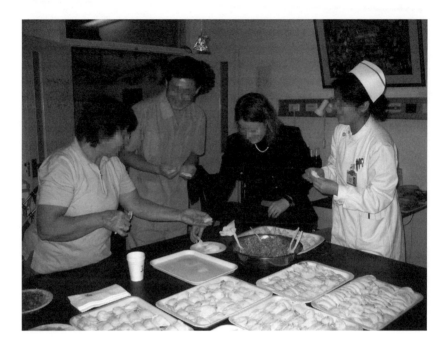

Figure 6.1. Spring Festival party at New Century Hospital, January 2006 (photograph by author).

CROSSING THE LINE

The Beijing Municipal Department of Health had paid a surprise visit to New Century just before the Spring Festival. Since the weeklong national holiday shut down most of the administrative functions across the country, very few crackdowns took place during the start of the new lunar year and Beijing residents could get away with activities not tolerated otherwise, such as setting off firecrackers in the city center. The weeks leading up to the holiday were another matter, however, as government bureaucrats, police officers, and other state employees hustled to meet quotas and take care of lingering business. More skeptical observers suggested that extra fines were imposed because corrupt officials wanted to line their pockets with additional cash in time for the holidays.

The municipal health inspectors who visited just before the 2006 Spring Festival charged the hospital with overstepping its clinical mandate. Citing hospital administrators for failing to register the new specialty services they had added over the previous few years, the municipal inspectors ordered the hospital to suspend Huang's neurosurgery operations as well as six other departments they deemed unauthorized. The municipal officials based their determination on New Century's classification as a Level 2 institution under the national Ministry of Health's three-tier hospital ranking system.[5] As a second-tier medical facility not designated to offer the comprehensive services of a top-tier tertiary care hospital, the former worker's sanatorium was only permitted to perform medical services related to its rehabilitation mandate. Approved clinical activities included general internal medicine, general surgery, physiotherapy, and traditional Chinese medical treatments such as acupuncture and massage. Seeking to raise the struggling hospital's profile, however, New Century's new administrators had added specialized services such as Huang's neurosurgery center through bureaucratic finesse. Rather than creating new departments (which would directly violate their clinical mandate), New Century administrators had sought to "enlarge the scope" (扩大范围 *kuòdà fànwéi*) of existing departments. Although the hospital had named Huang the chairman of neurosurgery, they never officially registered this new service as a separate department. On paper, Huang thus performed his experimental cranial and spinal surgeries under the authorization of New Century's *general* surgery license. In addition to Huang's neurosurgery activities, hospital administrators had also stretched the boundaries of their existing internal medicine department by adding cardiology, nephrology, and several other specialty services.

Akhil Gupta's (2012) analytic of the "disaggregated state" is particularly instructive for the Chinese context, with ethnographic attention to bureaucratic practices challenging stereotypes about centralized control and unified coherence. The Beijing Department of Health's investigation deemed that New Century had overstepped its bounds by establishing these new services as separate clinical departments—even though the hospital had sought to avoid this problem through a clever paperwork maneuver. While these bureaucratic tactics succeeded in circumventing national-level rectification campaigns, they failed at the local regulatory level with municipal inspectors who were physically confronted with the materiality of new hospital wards. The municipal officials noted that New Century's additional services operated as de facto clinical departments, citing the fancy brass plates and other signage throughout the renovated building that named these new services as separate departments and established them in distinct spaces within the hospital.

To place New Century's administrative woes in broader perspective, such bureaucratic troubles were hardly the isolated actions of an aberrant institution. The central government's emphasis on expanding health services and developing advanced medical technologies during the 1980s and 1990s had stoked the ambitions of hospital administrators and doctors throughout the country. This entrepreneurial medical culture was particularly pronounced among Level 2 hospitals such as New Century. Their "between and betwixt" status (不上不下的身份 *bùshàng bùxià de shēnfèn*) (Z. Wang 2006) gave these institutions the opportunity to encroach tactically onto the territory of the more prestigious Level 3 hospitals. Municipal and provincial regulators previously overlooked these borderline bureaucratic tactics during Deng Xiaoping's era of "Reform and Opening Up" and his successor Jiang Zemin's continued support for entre-preneurs and business activities. But under Hu Jintao's leadership in the 2000s, the central government took a more explicit stance against profiteering in health care and other sectors by targeting the predatory behavior characterizing local and regional levels of government. Unlike his predecessors' focus on decentral-ized economic development, Hu's ideological framework emphasized "building a socialist harmonious society" (构建社会主义和谐社会 gòujiàn shèhuì zhǔyì héxié shèhuì) in an effort to address the country's growing social and economic in-equalities. Faced with popular discontent over the escalating cost and inaccessi-bility of medical services, health officials in the Hu regime conveniently blamed the opportunistic expansion tactics of Level 2 hospitals for creating an "embar-rassing situation of recklessly scattering pepper over noodles" (撒胡椒面的尴尬局面 sā hújiāo miàn de gāngà júmiàn) (Z. Wang 2006)—a colorful metaphor that referred to the improper distribution of limited health resources. Provincial and municipal health departments around the country called for a more rigorous assessment of the classification system, cracking down on cābiānqiú tactics that had been permissible just a few years earlier. Beijing's Department of Health even proposed getting rid of the Level 2 hospital category altogether by demot-ing the majority to community health centers and transforming the rare few into full-fledged tertiary care centers (Z. Zhang 2006).

The staff members of the (formally unregistered) New Century Neurological Disorders Research and Treatment Center seemed relatively nonchalant about these new bureaucratic entanglements. Angel speculated that "greedy and cor-rupt officials" (贪官污吏 tānguān wū lì) probably carried out more investigations just before the Spring Festival so that they could generate more gifts from those hoping to smooth over the approval process. Invoking a double-negative in the hospital's defense, Teacher Yan explained that the situation at New Century was "not illegal" (不是不合法 bùshì bù héfǎ). She speculated that it was only a small bureaucratic snafu that would be resolved after "giving a few gifts" (送点礼 sòng diǎn lǐ) and "taking care of the formalities" (办手续 bàn shǒuxù). One of the young neurosurgeons on call noted that the holiday slowdown period was the perfect time to suspend operations, giving the hospital an opportunity to ren-ovate the operating room while they waited for the approval to come through.

MAKING TEN THOUSAND OUTSTANDING BACKUP PLANS

Three months later, the hospital's operating room was still "under renovation," and Huang still had not received approval to resume his surgical procedures. Perhaps a reasonable amount of time in other countries, this was atrociously slow in a city where hundreds of buildings were constructed in less than five years for the 2008 Olympics. In a further blow, New Century administrators had decided to repossess the second-floor ward. They gave the neurosurgery department less than eighteen hours to move out, announcing that another department would be occupying the second-floor space by the following morning. I first heard the news when I passed Sunny carrying a load of pillows, sheets, and blankets up the stairwell. I joked that she seemed to be doing inordinate amounts of laundry that day, and she urgently beckoned me into the supply room. In a distraught whisper, she explained that she had to move as much as she could from the second-floor rooms up to the third floor. Shaking her head in bewilderment, Sunny noted wistfully that she had to leave behind the blue dolphin window shade, which had been glued onto the glass.

I ran downstairs to the second floor, startling my officemate, Dr. Alan, with a vehement outburst. How could the hospital take away the ward after Teacher Yan, Driver Zhang, and the others had worked so hard to repaint all of the rooms? Dr. Alan reassured me that we would probably be able to keep our office, the communal activity room, and a few patient rooms. But he couldn't address the larger existential questions we both grappled with: What did these administrative changes mean for the future of the department? What would happen to the patients? Noting that over half of the ALS patients scheduled for surgery had died waiting before they could even board a plane to China, Dr. Alan worried that even a delay of one day, one week, or one month could be fatal for patients.

As the staff carried supplies and decorations between floors and wheeled confused patients to new rooms, Huang calmly made some phone calls in his office. Aware of his clinic's precarious administrative position, the resourceful neurosurgeon had already planned a backup system even before the Second Neurosurgery Ward for Foreigners expanded to the second-floor ward of New Century Hospital. Facing an increasing backlog of patients seeking his fetal cell transplantation procedure, Huang had been looking continually for ways to expand his neurosurgery center. An American businessman and his Israeli partner had approached Huang early in 2005, seeking to collaborate with the neurosurgeon on a for-profit health venture they had set up in Qingdao. The businessmen promoted Qingdao as an ideal place to host convalescing foreign patients. A short one-hour flight directly southeast of Beijing in Shandong province, the city was one of China's largest seaports and well-known domestically as a scenic vacation spot with clean beaches and fresh sea air. Deng Xiaoping designated the city as a Special Economic Zone (经济特区 *jīngjì tèqū*)[6] in 1984, and the domestic and foreign investment that followed this preferential status established Qingdao as one of the economic powerhouses in the region. The city also had a significant history of foreign influence,[7] and the businessmen suggested that the colonial architecture and Bavarian atmosphere would help Huang's European and American patients feel more at ease.

Huang had tried unsuccessfully for months to acquire additional space at New Century to accommodate more patients. Although he ultimately decided against collaborating with the American and Israeli business partners, the encounter inspired Huang to look elsewhere for options. He pursued the idea of establishing a secondary clinic in Shandong province, which he still considered his "native home" (家乡 *jiāxiāng*) despite having lived elsewhere his entire adult life. During the summer of 2005, he began treating a few patients at Wanjie Hospital, a private facility in Qingdao whose name literally meant "Ten Thousand Outstanding."

The Qingdao hospital was owned and operated by the Wanjie Group Limited, a collectively owned enterprise (集体所有制企业 *jítǐ suǒyǒuzhì qǐyè*) based in Shandong. The business had started out in the 1980s as a village-run enterprise (村办企业 *cūn bàn qǐyè*) that produced chemical fibers. Within a decade, the phenomenally successful Wanjie Group had established itself as one of China's "Fortune 500 companies" and was even called "the number one private enterprise in Shandong province" (Xiu 2007). With support from the Ministry of Health and the State Economic and Trade Commission, the Wanjie Group expanded into high-tech health services during the 1990s and sought to "use the top-rate quality medical equipment in Asia" and "attract China's top-rate experts" (Xiu 2007). The enterprise opened a succession of Sino-foreign joint-venture private hospitals (中外合资民办医院 *zhōngwài hézī mínbàn yīyuàn*), establishing the flagship facility in the founder's hometown in Shandong, another in Qingdao, and the third in Beijing. The Wanjie hospital system went on a massive shopping spree for the world's most advanced equipment, purchasing China's first Leskell Gamma Knife,[8] China's first positron emission tomography (PET scan) facility,[9] and a host of other advanced diagnostic and treatment technologies. Wanjie's emphasis on high-tech interventions was a perfect match for Dr. Huang's cutting-edge neurosurgical procedure, and they agreed to form a "joint venture" similar to the partnership he had set up with New Century. Huang became the director of the Qingdao Wanjie Hospital International Neurological Center (青岛万杰医院国际神经中心 *Qīngdǎo Wànjié Yīyuàn Guójì Shénjīng Zhōngxīn*) in the summer of 2005. The hospital provided Huang's new center with an entire floor of luxury patient rooms, and Huang received full operating privileges at the facility's state-of-the-art surgical center.

New Century administrators belatedly offered Huang the second-floor ward only after he had already initiated a partnership with Wanjie Hospital. As one of his resident doctors snorted, they were "afraid that the juicy piece of meat would be snatched away" (怕肥肉要调走了 *pà féi ròu yào diào zǒule*). Huang accepted New Century's tardy proposition, but he also continued to develop his new relationship in Qingdao. Starting in August 2005, Huang began carving time out of his busy schedule at New Century to conduct surgeries once a week at Wanjie. He would fly into Qingdao late in the evening, perform three to five fetal cell transplantation surgeries the following day, and then catch the last flight back to Beijing. Foreign patients who agreed to be treated in Qingdao received earlier appointment dates, and a steady trickle (consisting mostly of Europeans with ALS who were understandably anxious for treatment) thus made the hourlong flight to undergo fetal cell transplantation at the satellite clinic. Huang also decided to send his experienced Beijing staff members over to Qingdao in monthlong rotations to train the new nurses and doctors he had recruited in Shandong. He also invited a few Wanjie staff members to Beijing so they could experience how the New Century neurosurgical enterprise operated. By the time of the Spring Festival administrative crackdown on New Century, Huang was thus able to keep his neurosurgery center functional by shifting his operations over to Qingdao. When he convened an emergency meeting on February 17, 2006, to discuss the situation with his Beijing staff members, Huang simply informed them: "Let's put the emphasis on surgery at Qingdao."

PROLIFERATING INSTITUTIONS

Dr. Huang's use of Wanjie Hospital in Qingdao as a satellite clinic was a key tactic that enabled him to weather the sudden loss of operating privileges at New Century. Through processes of red-hatting and the implementation of backup plans to relocate his base operations, Huang's bureaucratic maneuvering was a dramatic example of how entrepreneurial doctors have operated in China's unstable politico-economic environment during the era of market socialism. Red-hatting was a particularly useful tactic for medical entrepreneurs testing out experimental therapies. I observed this practice in several other regenerative medicine clinics located in different cities along China's prosperous eastern seaboard (Song 2011).

Beike Biotechnology Company, for example, offered stem cell therapies through a distributed network linking laboratories and hospitals in different areas of the country. While Huang had rejected the overtures of the American-Israeli business team, Beike had embraced their help in recruiting more foreign patients. Beike was headquartered in Shenzhen, China's first designated Special Economic Zone (经济特区 *jīngjì tèqū*) located just across the border from Hong Kong, but the company collaborated with medical facilities in other cities. Like Huang's alliance with New Century, Beike Biotech's partnership with these second-tier public hospitals entailed paying "cooperation" fees to house its clients in VIP rooms, utilize nursing services, and collaborate with local physicians. Local crackdowns on hospital operations thus have little effect on the operations of a distributed network such as Beike. Because they are merely renting space within a partner hospital, these biotech entrepreneurs can easily move to a new location should any problems arise. As a Beike client from Florida described in a blog post documenting his hospital-hopping treatment in China:

> Today was a very hectic day. We were leaving for Qingdao because The Dr's here in Shenzhen don't really want to do the surgical injection on me, and I want it done. Qingdao is where I am having surgery where they will cut in to the back of my neck and inject the stem cells directly in to the injury site. (Jerry 2006)

As Jerry's entry suggests, when faced with problems or challenges at one site, Beike representatives could easily make arrangements with a more cooperative site to satisfy the demands of their customers. In Jerry's case, doctors in Shenzhen, who had been contracted by Beike to perform the stem cell injections in patients' private rooms either intravenously through the bloodstream or into the spinal fluid via a lumbar puncture, balked at performing the more risky laminectomy, which would involve exposing his spinal cord under general anesthesia in the operating room. Jerry thus traveled over 1,600 kilometers to a hospital in another province willing to perform the procedure. As his experience illustrates, while professional qualms of medical personnel or oversight by hospital administrators or even regional health bureaus may regulate unauthorized practices at one site, they have the unintended consequence of shifting questionable activities to another node in Beike's diffuse network.

REGISTERING NEW NAMES

Returning to the case of Huang's experimental fetal cell therapy, these institutional maneuverings had a differential effect on prospective domestic versus foreign patients. As I pointed out in chapter 5, Chinese patients interpreted Huang's multiple institutional moves as a sign of possible duplicity. Foreign patients, who lacked an understanding of the complex classificatory system of Chinese health facilities, framed these moves as evidence of Huang's solicitude in procuring better amenities for them.

These institutional maneuvers were not just bureaucratic matters but also moral choices that produced life-altering consequences for many patients and health care workers involved in these experimental fetal and stem cell therapies. In responding to the New Century administrative crackdown, Huang and his staff exploited another "edge ball" tactic of creative interpretation that differentiated between "small" and "big" surgeries—a distinction that had a crucial impact on the type and quality of care administered to patients visiting the two clinics. Huang interpreted the crackdown at New Century as an order to stop performing major neurosurgical operations in the official operating room. He thus transferred SCI patients to Qingdao, since the fetal cell transplantation procedure for these types of injuries was a "big surgery" (大手术 dà shǒushù) that required a fully equipped operating room. The procedure involved putting the patient under general anesthesia for two to three hours to allow the neurosurgeons to make an incision in the midline of the patient's back, dissecting through skin and muscle to reach the vertebral spinal column. The surgeons would subsequently remove a small portion of bone from the vertebra (a procedure known as a laminectomy) to create a space for injecting the olfactory ensheathing glial cells.

Although Huang had largely shifted his surgical emphasis to Qingdao during the crackdown, I discovered that some ALS patients were still receiving fetal cell transplantations in Beijing. As one of his attending neurosurgeons explained to me, these patients needed only "little surgeries" (小手术 xiǎo shǒushù) that could be performed safely in the comfort of the patients' own rooms. Rotating the tips of his index fingers against both sides of his forehead to underscore his point, the Beijing-based neurosurgeon emphasized that these types of cranial surgeries involved drilling small holes into the skull under local anesthesia and then transplanting the fetal cells with a syringe into the motor cortex of the brain—a minor or "little" procedure from the perspective of this neurosurgeon accustomed to cutting through layers of muscle and connective tissue during major spinal surgery. This "borderline" tactic of treating ALS patients at New Century was not merely a matter of semantics or convenience for Huang and his clinical staff. Pointing out that many of his ALS patients suffered from compromised breathing and weakened immune systems, Huang argued that it would be immoral to subject them unnecessarily to additional plane flights and exposure to outside pathogens. He thus framed his choice of treatment site for ALS patients as an eminently moral decision that prioritized patients' well-being over petty bureaucratic wrangling.

Huang continued to exercise other administrative tactics as insurance against erratic and unpredictable operational disruptions. In addition to heading the contested "Beijing New Century Hospital Department of Neurosurgery" (北京 新世纪医院神经外科 Běijīng Xīn Shìjì Yīyuàn Shénjīng Wàikē), establishing the "Beijing New Century Hospital Neurological Disorders Research and Treatment Center" (北京新世纪医院神经疾病研治中心 Běijīng Xīn Shìjì Yīyuàn Shénjīng Jíbìng Yánzhì Zhōngxīn), and operating the "Qingdao Wanjie Hospital International Neurological Center" (青岛万杰医院国际神经中心 Qīngdǎo Wànjié Yīyuàn Guójì Shénjīng Zhōngxīn), Huang also created a proliferating number of administrative entities, each of which had its own legal and political status. In March 2006 he registered a "private non-enterprise work unit" (民办非企业单位 mínbàn fēi qǐyè dānwèi) named the "Beijing City New Century Neurological Regeneration and Functional Recovery Research Institute" (北京市新世纪神经再生和功能重建研 究所 Běijīng Shì Xīn Shìjì Shénjīng Zàishēng hé Gōngnéng Chóngjiàn Yánjiū Suǒ). This was his first attempt to create a legally recognized entity independent of a larger medical institution, and he hoped that this new administrative tactic would help protect his staff and equipment from the vagaries of internal hospital politics. He soon discovered that the rules governing these nongovernmental, "people-run" (the literal meaning of 民办 mínbàn) organizations were even murkier than the bureaucratic shuffling he had endured at state-run New Century Hospital. In particular, the start-up money he had invested—supposedly held by the local government in the name of his private organization—disappeared into the coffers of the district office with scant information on how it would be utilized.

Huang thus decided to establish another type of business organization known as a "collectively owned enterprise" (集体所有制企业 jítǐ suǒyǒuzhì qǐyè). In December 2006, he registered the new "Beijing Hongtianji Neuroscience Academy" (北京虹天济神经科学研究院 Běijīng Hóngtiānjì Shénjīng Kēxué Yánjiù

Yuàn) with an initial capital investment (注册资本 *zhùcè zīběn*) of ten million RMB (approximately \$1.5 million U.S.) and designated his wife as the company's legal representative (法定代表人 *fǎdìng dàibiǎo rén*). Huang described this new enterprise in the registration papers as a "collectively owned, high-tech neuroscience research work unit" (集体所有制高科技神经科学研究单位 *jítǐ suǒyǒuzhì gāo kējì shénjīng kēxué yánjiū dānwèi*) guided by the national policy of "independent innovation" and devoted to "making greater contributions to national development, scientific progress, and human health" (为国家发展、科学进步、人类健康做出更大贡献 *wèi guójiā fāzhǎn, kēxué jìnbù, rénlèi jiànkāng zuò chū gèng dà gòngxiàn*). Comprised once again of the same researchers, clinicians, and administrative personnel working from the same location inside New Century Hospital, Hongtianji Academy nevertheless enabled Huang to maintain a legally independent, for-profit enterprise wholly under his personal control.

While Huang was responding to the Beijing Department of Health's crackdown by shifting his surgical focus to Qingdao and experimenting with administrative classifications, New Century administrators were also trying to implement their own bureaucratic techniques to regain their lost departments. The Spring Festival closure of seven "unauthorized" departments prompted New Century hospital officials to adopt a new name for their institution: the "Beijing *City* New Century Hospital" (北京市新世纪医院 Běijīng Shì Xīn Shìjì Yīyuàn). Although seemingly trivial, the addition of the word "City" to its name allowed the hospital to re-register at the Beijing Ministry of Health as a new administrative entity. By restarting the registration process from a clean slate, hospital administrators easily obtained authorization for its seven additional departments—including Huang's neurosurgery center. New Century Hospital's renaming practices were fortuitous for Huang. As an additional example of the uncertainty in the lives of Huang and his staff, the Qingdao operation closed down without notice in December 2006 when the privately owned hospital was sold off by its bankrupt parent holding group, Wanjie Jituan. Dr. Huang's staff received only one day's notice prior to the closure. The Qingdao doctors scrambled to rescue their supplies and begged another clinic to host their patients until they were medically stable enough to be transferred back to Beijing.

CONCLUSION

As we have seen in chapters 5 and 6, these experimental forms of health care are turning China's urban medical system into a laboratory for entrepreneurial tactics. From red-hatting to creative naming practices, these "borderline" tactics are emblematic of how medical entrepreneurs are maneuvering at the edges of legality in China's unstable politico-economic environment. The uneven transformation of health care into a business, combined with a complex regulatory landscape, has encouraged doctors such as Huang to respond to proliferating political uncertainties and economic anxieties by experimenting not only with new biomedical procedures but also with novel bureaucratic interventions. Seeking to secure their careers and their futures, these health care professionals deploy myriad entrepreneurial tactics ranging from exploiting administrative loopholes to capitalizing on technological advances in order to deflect government scrutiny and attract new patients. This emergent form of medical entrepreneurialism optimizes socialist legacies, invokes patriotic values, and manipulates bureaucratic practices in order to hedge against regulatory uncertainty and build transnational enterprises that serve patients from around the world.

For Huang Hongyun, his "cutting-edge" neurosurgical innovation represented his life's work—his means of making a living, his hope for helping patients, and his ambitions for changing the very foundations of medical practice in China and abroad. As one of his resident doctors explained to me, "It wasn't easy for him to build this department and he's not going to give it up." To protect his innovative medical technique, Huang deployed a multitude of ingenious administrative tactics ranging from red-hatting at New Century, setting up a satellite clinic in Qingdao, and manipulating different municipal bureaucracies to create a host of shadow organizations. These pluripotent administrative entities allowed Huang to expand the scope of his clinical and research activities, claim legality for new activities, and cut his losses when challenged or threatened.

As Huang's case illustrates, a different kind of entrepreneurial subject is emerging at the limits of urban medical practice in twenty-first-century Beijing. Operating on different registers and at different scales, this budding form of medical entrepreneurialism leverages (post)socialist bureaucracy itself in order to circumvent regulatory uncertainty while building transnational enterprises that attract a global clientele. Rather than privileging processes of privatization, marketization, and democratization—what Katherine Verdery has characterized as "that troika of Western self-identity" (Hann, Humphrey, and Verdery 2002)—my analysis of borderline health care practices illuminates the complex intersections of entrepreneurialism and bureaucracy in a non-Western context characterized by uneven state control. Through a careful ethnographic examination, I have demonstrated the ways in which enterprising Chinese clinicians maintain, remake, and challenge the conceptual and material divides between state and market, public and private, and legal and illegal in order to navigate a changing moral and regulatory landscape. The Ping-Pong metaphor of the precarious "edge ball" captures how entrepreneurial medical professionals have stretched bureaucratic rules to find gray zones between these dichotomies. Their survival tactics enable them to protect what matters most to them—while simultaneously changing the rules of engagement in medical practice.

PART III

HETEROGENEOUS EVIDENCE

CLINICAL OUTCOMES

Condition	Number of Patients Treated
Spinal Cord Injury 脊髓损伤	566
Amyotrophic Lateral Sclerosis 肌萎缩侧索硬化	436
Cerebral Palsy 脑性瘫痪	62
Multiple Sclerosis 多发性硬化	16
Ataxia 共济失调	10
Other Central Nervous System Diseases 其他中枢神经系统疾病	38

1128
Total number of patients treated from 2001–2008

= 10 Patients

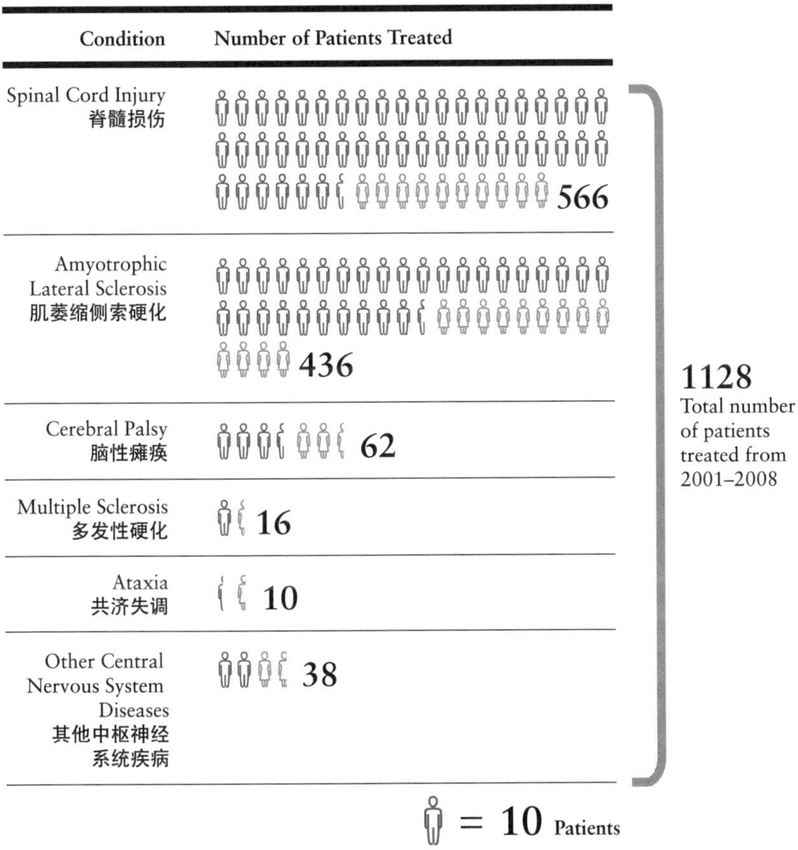

Figure 7.1. Clinical data for 1,128 patients treated with olfactory ensheathing glial cell therapy (chart designed by Oikeat Lam). Neurological conditions and gender distributions compiled from data published in the *Chinese Journal of Reparative and Reconstructive Surgery* (Huang et al. 2009, 16).

SEEKING TRUTH FROM FACTS

AS THE PROLIFERATION OF FETAL cell therapies suggests, the transition from laboratory bench to hospital bed is happening at an accelerated pace in contemporary China, with increasing numbers of new treatments being tested on patients. Researchers and regulators in the United States and Europe have lambasted Chinese practitioners for moving too quickly into human therapies without subjecting their treatments to the rigors of evidence-based medicine. Without proof in the form of placebo-controlled clinical trials, the critics charge, Chinese clinicians are deemed charlatans preying upon the desperation of patients. Medical entrepreneurs such as Huang are particularly susceptible to accusations of quackery as they negotiate the overlapping and at times competing motives of helping patients, advancing science, and making a profit.

The charge of medical fraud carries particular resonance in China. While the focus on evidence-based medicine is new, charges of quackery are not. Writer and social critic Lao She (老舍) satirized Chinese medical services in the 1930s in his short story "A Brilliant Beginning" (开市大吉 *kāi shì dàjí*), describing a group of charlatans posing as physicians who tried to make a profit by performing fraudulent injections (Lao 2011).[1] Since the reintroduction of private enterprise during Deng's Reform and Opening Up era, the country has been plagued by tales of counterfeit goods, from bootleg DVDs and pirated software to imitation handbags and fake cigarettes. The epidemic of fake and shoddy products produced in China has been particularly problematic in the medical realm, affecting domestic and foreign patients around the globe. Transnational scandals have included Chinese cough medicine laced with diethylene glycol[2] and exported abroad, which fatally poisoned more than one hundred Panamanians in 2006 (Rentz et al. 2008). Counterfeit heparin,[3] a blood thinner produced in China for the pharmaceutical giant Baxter, was linked to nearly a thousand cases of serious injuries reported to the U.S. FDA (Harris and Bogdanich 2008). Even infant formula has not been exempt from the tampering of unscrupulous manufacturers seeking to increase their profit margins.[4] The label "Made in China" has thus become synonymous with suspect imitations that are not just poor quality but have even injured or killed thousands worldwide. Regulators, trade officials, and journalists have blamed the problem on corruption, cutthroat competition, and a lack of regulatory oversight that have encouraged manufacturers to cut corners in the race to the bottom line. Given this context of global suspicion for Chinese products, it is not surprising that experimental biomedical treatments in China have been interpreted as ploys by profiteering medical entrepreneurs. Yet thousands of patients from more than eighty countries have been convinced to undergo fetal cell transplantation in Beijing. Although critics have been quick to dismiss these biomedical odysseys as a matter of desperate patients duped by false hopes, the nuanced deliberations and complex experiences of the people I met in Beijing and online deserve more careful consideration.

While the preceding chapters have examined the embodied motivations, social dynamics, and politico-economic calculations shaping their participation in these fetal cell experiments, the next two chapters take a closer look at the semiotics by which practitioners and patients recognize medical authenticity and charlatanism. The question "Does it work?" permeated my conversations with clinicians, patients, and family members involved with Huang's neurosurgery clinic. I provide ethnographic insight on how the clinic's Chinese clinicians (this chapter) and foreign patients (chapter 8) have interpreted signs of evidence, negotiated standards of proof, and resolved questions of efficacy in the transnational realm of experimental medicine.[5] I focus in this chapter on how Huang and his staff have contested international biomedical research protocols and devised new methods to assess the effectiveness of their experimental OEG cell transplantation surgery. These strategies included developing improved measurement scales to capture post-surgical differences in bodily function and feeling, inviting foreign doctors to witness clinical procedures for themselves, conducting follow-up studies with former patients, and attempting to publish scientific reports in internationally credible journals. By examining the ways in which New Century clinicians have evaluated the effectiveness of the fetal cell transplantation procedure, this chapter raises key questions about the ethics and epistemology of clinical experimentation at the "cutting edge" of biomedical practice in contemporary China. I demonstrate how new modes of validation are emerging as viable alternatives to the hegemonic discourse of randomized controlled trials that has dominated the quest for "evidence" in experimental medicine.

EVALUATING EFFICACY

Critics such as U.S. neurologist Bruce Dobkin have contested Huang's credibility on the grounds that he failed to perform a randomized controlled trial with defined entry criteria and blinded, predefined outcomes using reliable and relevant measurement tools. After an initial attempt to collaborate with Huang, Dobkin ended up lambasting the Chinese neurosurgeon in print for his "problematic methodology and scientific issues" (Dobkin, Curt, and Guest 2006, 9), characterizing Huang's "invasive cell implants for neurologic diseases" (6) as an "unsubstantiated clinical practice" (13). The Los Angeles–based neurology professor issued an unequivocal recommendation that "until international standards for scientific trial methodologies have been incorporated, clinicians are obligated to advise their patients to forgo Dr. Huang's procedure" (13).

Dobkin's critique must be contextualized within a broader historical framework that addresses how guidelines governing medical research in the United States have developed.[6] Researchers, clinicians, and pharmaceutical companies seeking to market a new medical intervention in the United States must first perform laboratory and animal tests to determine how the treatment works and whether it is likely to be safe for and effective in humans. In order to obtain approval to test the treatment in people, researchers must then submit an Investigational New Drug application[7] to the Food and Drug Administration. Both the conduct and evaluation of these clinical trials are monitored to ensure the protection of human subjects and the collection of reliable data on the safety and efficacy of the treatment under question. The focus on efficacy in the context of clinical trials is significant. As deployed by clinical researchers, "efficacy" refers to the measurable effects of a specific intervention under controlled conditions (Cochrane 1972; Higgins and Green 2011; IOM 2009). This is different from the effect that the intervention might have under ordinary circumstances in the real world, which in the field of biomedical research is described as "effectiveness."

This is not a trivial distinction, as discussions of biomedical "efficacy" set aside many of the real-world contexts under which a new intervention might be administered and taken.[8] The sociopolitical is one crucial context often neglected in considering biomedical efficacy. This is particularly evident when we look at how other disciplines have framed "efficacy." Anthropologists, for example, have explored broader questions of meaning and effectiveness in the context of social action. These approaches challenge the reductionist parameters of biomedical frameworks. Concerns about whether a medicine or healing practice "works" extend far beyond the narrow constraints of laboratory or clinical paradigms. As Sienna Craig (2012) highlights in the case of Tibetan medicine, efficacy is an intersubjective phenomenon negotiated between practitioners and patients in the context of specific "social ecologies." This expanded understanding of efficacy—as the capacity for producing a desired result or effect—takes into account the social and political contexts in which knowledge claims are made, by whom, and for what purposes.[9] The fact that clinical trial proponents have convinced regulators and the public to accept such a narrow definition of efficacy points to the ascendancy of laboratory-based methods in biomedicine today.[10]

Described by historian Ilana Lowy as a key technology in moving medicine from being an idiosyncratic "art of healing" to an exact science (Lowy 2000, 49), randomized controlled trials (RCTs) developed over the past half century as an objective way for doctors and drug manufacturers to evaluate proliferating drug therapies and provide proof of safety and efficacy. As the name suggests, RCTs involve the random assignment of research subjects to comparison groups. The intervention in question is compared against a standard (generally an inactive substance known as a placebo) given to a control group, which enables researchers to evaluate differential effects. RCTs have thus provided clinicians with a convincing method for establishing their own credibility, deflecting suspicion, and distinguishing themselves from fraudulent patent medicine peddlers.[11] Historian Harry Marks (1997) has documented how RCTs emerged through the process of "therapeutic reform" to become the key principle in experimental medicine. Broader shifts in the organization of medical practice and research in the United States contributed to entrenchment of RCTs—in particular the intensified involvement of the American government in biomedical research and the organization of health care after World War II, as well as the growth of academic medicine (Marks 1997).

The rise of the evidence-based medicine (EBM) movement in the 1990s to make health care a more rational and cost-effective practice (Guyatt et al. 1992) has further solidified the status of RCTs in clinical research and practice. Proponents have described EBM as a "paradigm shift" that "de-emphasizes intuition, unsystematic clinical experience, and pathophysiologic rationale as sufficient grounds for clinical decision making and stresses the examination of evidence from clinical research" (Evidence-Based Medicine Working Group 1992, 2420).[12] Medical historians have challenged this characterization of EBM as a groundbreaking phenomenon, noting a much earlier history of experimentation in medicine that emphasized the importance of compiling clinical data based on comparative observations since at least the eighteenth century in Europe (Tröhler 2005; Bynum 2006). Regardless of historical accuracy, proclamations about EBM as a scientific revolution in medicine have played a key role in elevating RCTs as the "gold standard" for determining the efficacy of new treatments.

CONTESTING SHAM SURGERY

The use of randomized, controlled clinical trials to test the efficacy of new treatments originated from a particular context: American pharmaceutical industry regulations during the twentieth century. But drugs are qualitatively different from surgical procedures. Surgeons historically have utilized very different methods for testing the safety and effectiveness of surgical innovations. Experimenting with new techniques on animals and then trying them out on patients has served as the dominant model through which surgeons have developed new surgical procedures. Clinical experience, intuition, and pathophysiologic rationale—the very methods that EBM proponents have sought to replace by standardized evidence based on scientific research—have long reigned as the key factors in clinical decision making for surgeons.

Not surprisingly, the vast majority of surgical procedures have never been evaluated in randomized double-blind clinical trials. Many surgeons have contested the philosophical basis of following clinical trial principles to evaluate surgical innovations. Unlike the "sugar pills" used in pharmaceutical clinical trials, a comparable "placebo control" for testing a surgical intervention often involves significant risk to the research subjects—especially when the "control" involves administering fake operations to patients. Mimicking the conditions of the actual treatment as closely as possible, sham surgeries are used in clinical trials to maintain double-blinding and minimize potential bias from patient and researcher expectations.

The few cases in which researchers have employed sham controls to test the efficacy of surgical interventions have been fraught with controversy. For example, during the 1990s American researchers studied the effectiveness of transplanting human embryonic dopamine neurons into the brains of patients with Parkinson's disease. Attempting to follow the stringent demands dictated by clinical trials, some of these studies randomly assigned patients to undergo either sham surgery or transplantation (Freeman et al. 1999; Freed et al. 2001). Participants in both groups received local anesthesia, had four holes drilled through the frontal bone of the skull, and had imaging studies performed on them (Freed et al. 2001). Although they underwent risky and invasive procedures that mimicked the actual transplantation procedure, patients in the control group did not get the actual injection of embryonic tissue.

The controversial deployment of sham surgery controls has incited much debate among North American doctors and bioethicists (Miller 2003). In an article titled "I Need a Placebo Like I Need a Hole in the Head," Charles Weijer, a Canadian bioethicist and physician, critiques the "scientistic bias" of clinical trials: "The clinician's office is not a laboratory any more than a research subject is a lab rat. Clinical care and human response to disease are simply too complex to be captured by such a simplistic model" (Weijer 2002, 71).

On the other side, supporters of surgical RCT have argued that these sham operations can be ethically acceptable as long as the benefits outweigh the risks of conducting the clinical trial—but who benefits and who is at risk in these determinations? In a 2005 survey of Parkinson's disease clinical researchers, 97 percent of respondents believed that sham surgery controls were better than unblinded controls from a scientific perspective for testing the efficacy of neurosurgical interventions. Furthermore, the survey designers noted that "half of the researchers believe an unblinded control efficacy trial would be unethical because it may lead to a falsely positive result" (Kim et al. 2005, 1357). In other words, a significant percentage of these researchers believed that sham surgery controls were not only scientifically superior but also ethically superior. But the problem with these abstract determinations of scientific and ethical superiority is that they fail to spell out for whom these interventions would be more scientific and more ethical—the participants in the control arm of the study getting a hole drilled in their heads? Future patients who would have evidence-based data on efficacy? Researchers attempting to advance their careers? The following section examines how these debates have played out in the context of Huang's experimental Chinese fetal cell therapy.

MISMATCHING TEMPORALITIES

Huang's critics have employed the same logic as supporters of surgical RCT to dismiss his experimental practice. In their case report of a seventy-year-old American woman with ALS who had undergone the Beijing OEG cell transplantation procedure, neurologists at Columbia University's Eleanor and Lou Gehrig MDA/ALS Research Center argued the following:

> Clinics that expose patients to experimental treatments for ALS with inadequate scientific justification or the construct of a well-designed clinical trial do a disservice to the ALS community. They put patients at risk without sound evidence that the procedures could be beneficial, they do not contribute to scientific understanding of the therapy, and they divert resources away from legitimate research, thereby delaying the development of truly effective therapies. Lacking in acceptable safety standards and sufficient evidence for the potential to provide benefit, these clinics perform procedures that fail to meet the standards for ethical research set forth in the Nuremburg Code and Declaration of Helsinki. (Chew et al. 2007, 316)

Claiming both the scientific and moral high ground, these American researchers charged Huang with gross scientific and ethical negligence. Their invocation of the Nuremburg code implied that Huang's OEG fetal cell transplantation procedure could be compared to the horrific experiments perpetrated by Nazi physicians on concentration camp prisoners in the name of advancing medical research.

But Huang and his advocates have inverted the objections of these detractors by arguing that the experimental fetal cell procedure provided a more ethical alternative to the clinical trial model of his American critics. With the support of patients and their families, Huang has challenged conventional clinicians for focusing on preliminary animal studies while neglecting patients who are suffering or dying now. This temporal challenge has resonated in particular with people diagnosed with ALS, whose life demands do not match up with research timelines.

As Stephen Byer,[13] a former Chicago-based marketing consultant and fine art investor who became a full-time patient advocate after the diagnosis of his son Ben in 2002, explained to me: "American and European neurologists have had [over 140] years to study ALS, and they still can't do anything for my son." The Byers first learned of Huang's procedure during a trip to Beijing in June

2004 to research a Chinese herbal compound[14] that showed promising results in the treatment of ALS. After meeting Huang in person and interviewing several patients recovering from the fetal cell transplantation, Ben seized the opportunity to undergo the experimental Chinese surgery—and also document the procedure for a film he was making about his condition (Byer 2008).

Like the Byers, many patients and family members who sought experimental fetal cell therapy in Beijing expressed anger and disillusionment with their neurologists back home. Jeff, the Colorado firefighter whose surgical experiences we followed in chapter 4, critiqued his American doctors' "inability to open and broaden their perspective on research and experiments." He noted that he and his fellow sufferers "share the common experience of diagnosis followed by a bottle of Rilutek,[15] a prescription for sleeping pills, and the instructions to complete a last will and testament."

Even when clinical researchers seek to develop treatments for ALS patients, their research timetables fail to match up with ALS patients' life demands. A former golf pro from Florida who underwent fetal cell transplantation in November 2004 described an ALS research symposium he had attended back home, which featured leading neurologists describing promising therapies in the pipelines. An audience member asked how soon these treatments would be available. The speaker replied with a lengthy explanation about setting up clinical trials, noting that it would probably take about five years to make the necessary preparations for ensuring a quality study. The ALS patient interrupted him to declare that he was talking to a room of dead people.

Not surprisingly, as a review of "medical progress" for ALS published in the *New England Journal of Medicine* observed, "The lack of effective treatment has caused many patients and their families to become activists, raising money for research and bypassing traditional granting agencies" (Rowland and Shneider 2001, 1696).[16] Describing these patient-led efforts as "guerrilla science," the authors urged nevertheless that "such approaches must first be attempted in animals to evaluate their safety and efficacy" (Rowland and Shneider 2001, 1696–97).

But faced with a catastrophic illness, many ALS patients are not willing to wait for the conventional course of biomedicine to wind its way through years of animal testing, double-blind clinical trials, and paper publishing before a vetted treatment becomes available. The ALS patients coming to New Century Hospital want help now, because they worry that they may no longer be around even a year from now. Next month they may no longer be able to use their legs. The month after that they may no longer be able to use their hands. Sooner or later, they will lose their ability to communicate. And by the end, they will no longer be able to breathe on their own.

Echoing critics of the research timelines for anti-HIV/AIDS drugs (Epstein 1996), ALS patients argue that since they are already facing a "death sentence," they should have the choice to engage in "guerrilla science" and pursue experimental therapy. Many of them are thus willing to subject their bodies to relatively risky experimental procedures in the hopes of staving off their unrelenting disease. In an email newsletter he circulated in June 2004 to those contemplating the experimental Chinese surgery, Stephen Byer captured the prevailing attitude among PALS who made the decision to undergo the fetal cell transplantation:

> Dr. Huang has not performed mouse or other lab animal tests, feeling, as many of us do, that such tests are not of direct benefit to humans, particularly those with a notably rapid advancing disease such as ALS. He regularly speaks of the questionable practice of extensive lab animal testing while people are dying and appears far more concerned with saving lives than proving theories on mice.

Huang's patients have championed him for placing them at the center of his work rather than concentrating on animal models of disease. But American critics have disparaged this focus on treatment over rigorous testing, noting that "such evasions are a classic mark of the charlatan" (Judson 2005). While American scientists see Huang's focus on alleviating suffering as evidence of quackery, patients see this as a badge of his dedication to their cause—and this divergence in emphasis demarcates the essential difference between clinical trials and experimental treatment.

Huang and many of his patients have explicitly rejected the principle of randomized placebo-controlled trials for surgical interventions. Whether taking place in China or the United States, clinical research has been plagued by the problem of therapeutic misconception (Sankar 2004; Henderson et al. 2007). Despite filling out laborious consent forms scrutinized word-for-word by institutional review boards, patients participating in a clinical trial often believe—erroneously—that the trial will benefit them directly. That clinical investigators are often doctors creates even more confusion. Although the ultimate aim of the trial may be to benefit the patient population, the patients participating in the trial have been selected to further the aims of science rather than to improve their actual condition. Thus some patients may receive nothing at all, while others may receive dosage levels known to be ineffectual. (This is particularly true of Phase I trials to evaluate the safety of a new drug or treatment.) The focus is on testing the drug, not treating the patient. This logic becomes even more fraught when shifting from pharmaceutical trials to testing a surgical intervention on a person facing an already demoralizing illness.

From an ALS patient's point of view, he or she cannot afford to get a placebo or a known ineffectual dose—even less so in the case of receiving a sham surgery for control purposes. Involvement in such a study literally asks the patient to sacrifice him- or herself for the greater good with no personal benefit whatsoever, and even take on significant risks in the case of testing a surgical intervention. This might be more comforting if there had historically been more progress on ALS treatment. Despite the thousands of research papers that have been published about ALS, however, neurologists have produced very little in terms of concrete results for patients. As an American ALS patient receiving treatment at

New Century Hospital noted, in a clinical trial "you don't even know if you get the stuff or not. You may be helping other people but you don't know if you're helping yourself." To subject vulnerable patients to the risks of surgery and only administer saline injections seemed particularly problematic to Huang and his supporters. While swallowing a sugar pill might pose little physical risk to patients, getting holes drilled into the skull was an entirely different matter.

As we drove to a banquet he was hosting for his staff at the restaurant of the Xinjiang Provincial Office in Beijing (新疆驻京办事处 Xīnjiāng zhù jīng bànshì chù) one evening in the spring of 2006, I asked Huang about the criticism he received for not submitting his procedure to the rigors of a clinical trial. He got so angry when I mentioned UCLA neurologist Bruce Dobkin that he pulled his car over to the side of the road and started pounding the steering wheel:

> Some people only know how to criticize.... Ok, Dobkin, so how would you do it? You say that I need to do a sham surgery comparison [假手术对照 jiǎ shǒushù duìzhào]. Are you capable of doing one? No you are not! This type of surgery is completely against Chinese medical ethics.

> Little Song, I already discussed this issue with you yesterday—let's say if some country permitted the use of sham surgical controls for the sake of so-called scientific ethics, I would completely despise that country! How could medical ethics have fallen to such an extent? To treat a person no longer as a human, to treat a patient not as a human, but instead to treat them as a machine or animal that we can conduct experiments on? This is very immoral! I think this type of vile medical practice should be eliminated!... To disregard a patient's wounds, to disregard the possible dangers and side effects, which perhaps may even be life-threatening—to disregard all of this! And all to achieve what? So-called scientific conclusions![17]

Huang was outraged by the suggestion that he should cut open a group of patients and only inject saline in their brains or spines in the name of science. Present-day discussions of clinicians injecting their patients with saline solution (in the name of scientific inquiry) oddly echo Lao She's satire of the 1930s entrepreneurs injecting hapless patients with hypodermic needles filled with jasmine and longjing tea. But in Huang's rendering, the American clinicians pushing for sham surgical controls are the medical quacks. Huang inverted the logic of his American critics, declaring sham surgical procedures to be morally reprehensible. He adamantly refused to conduct clinical trials in which a portion of his patients would be subjected to the dangers of a craniotomy without receiving the stem cell transplantation.

GENERATING A PAPER TRAIL

Although Huang rejected the practice of sham surgery as unethical, this did not mean that he abandoned medical science. Having witnessed his efforts over the past several years, I would argue that Huang has tried to carry out "evidence-based" research with the available resources at his disposal—albeit with abbreviated timetables and protocols that aspired to ideal scientific principles but often fell victim to expedient concerns. Since the very start of his fetal cell transplantation odyssey in 2001, Huang has sought to document, substantiate, and track the results of his pioneering experimental surgery. While I have previously discussed Huang's development of the OEG procedure both from the perspective of CareCure members (chapter 2) and in the context of his own career trajectory (chapter 5), I will now focus on the methodologies that Huang and his colleagues have deployed to substantiate their findings.

Since 2001, Huang has published more than thirty scientific papers in Chinese- and English-language journals on olfactory ensheathing glial cells. The form, content, and methodology of these papers have changed over time in response to his expanding audiences. Huang's first OEG paper—a three-page laboratory report written in Chinese—appeared in the academic journal of his home hospital upon his return to China (Huang et al. 2001).[18] Although this initial paper was based on laboratory experiments on animal models at Rutgers, Huang's return to clinical employment at the Naval General Hospital meant increased pressure to translate the previous years of basic science research he had been conducting in the United States into more immediate and practical applications for use in a Chinese clinical setting. Given the prevailing medical consensus on the inability of the adult mammalian brain and spinal cord to regenerate after damage, what explained these lab rats' unexpected functional improvements? Based on a postmortem examination of the spinal cord tissue of the rats that had demonstrated functional recovery, Huang reported evidence of axon regrowth across the injured area (Huang et al. 2001, 66). This was the holy grail of spinal cord injury research, which had slowly begun to challenge the longstanding dogma on the failure of central nervous system (CNS) regeneration (Horner and Gage 2000). Huang's brief paper did not include details on his immunostaining process or visual evidence of the rats' regenerated axons to substantiate his remarkable claim. But for Huang, who was at heart a clinician interested in the practical significance of his research efforts, the rats' improved functional ability was the crucial proof of the experiments' potential. With an eye toward his next steps, Huang proclaimed that OEG cells [嗅鞘细胞 *xiùqiào xìbāo*] are the better candidate for promoting nerve regeneration compared with other types of cells with regenerative capacities, holding very good applied prospects [应用前景 *yìngyòng qiánjǐng*] in clinical trials" (Huang et al. 2001, 67).

Huang followed this basic science paper with his first clinical case report the following year, describing a diverse group of twenty-three patients with spinal cord injuries he had treated with fetal OEG cell transplantation at Naval General Hospital (Huang et al. 2002).[19] He claimed that all of the patients in this first trial group showed improvements in both motor and sensory function. He published a much larger case series report a year later, documenting the results of OEG transplantation for 171 Chinese SCI patients (Huang et al. 2003a).[20] By this point, Huang had orchestrated his move to the civilian Chaoyang Hospital, the main teaching hospital affiliated with Beijing's Capital Medical University. He inaugurated his move by publishing this report in the academic journal of his new institution.

Huang's Chinese-language clinical reports attracted the attention of domestic journalists, who seized upon the potential for transforming the lives of patients with feature reports titled "There Is Hope for Spinal Cord Injury Treatment" (脊髓损伤治疗有望 Jǐsuǐ sǔnshāng zhìliáo yǒuwàng) (CCTV 2002) and headline news declaring "Paraplegic Patients Back on Their Feet Is No Longer a Dream" (截瘫病人重新站立不再是梦 Jiétān bìngrén chóngxīn zhànlì bù zài shì mèng) (Sha 2003). These television and newspaper reports, among others (cf. Zhao 2002; Tang, Wang, and Ji 2002; Liu 2002), generated a waiting list of patients numbering into the thousands from throughout China. But because Huang's initial clinical reports were published in Chinese by the local journals of the hospitals that employed him, their localized nature rendered them largely inaccessible to those outside China, including the international scientific community.[21]

In October 2003, Huang published his first English-language scientific paper on OEG transplantation (Huang et al. 2003b). The clinical data were identical to those in the Chinese-language report he had published in the Capital Medical University's academic journal earlier that year (Huang et al. 2003a). But because this version was written in English and published in a journal indexed in the Science Citation Index as well as MEDLINE, Huang suddenly began receiving an upsurge of interest from outside China. The publication of the paper also coincided with his treatment of the CareCure SCI pioneers Tim C., Handibob, and CJO—who were also the first foreign patients to undergo the OEG transplantation procedure.

Neuroscientists, clinicians, and journalists from the United States and Europe began boarding planes to Beijing, eager but skeptical to witness the groundbreaking experimental procedure that purportedly overturned conventional medical dogma that the central nervous system was incapable of regenerating. These visiting delegations included neurologists from the Miami Project to Cure Paralysis, representatives from the U.S. Embassy, the scientific journal *Nature*'s Asia-Pacific correspondent, and the *New England Journal of Medicine*'s editor-in-chief, among many others.

Various clinicians from the United States, Spain, and the Netherlands began to perform and publish independent assessments of patients who had undergone the Beijing fetal cell transplantation procedure, dismissing Huang's own assessments as biased and potentially flawed in execution (Guest, Herrera, and

Qian 2006; Dobkin, Curt, and Guest 2006; Chew et al. 2007; Giordana et al. 2010; Piepers and Van den Berg 2010). After examining the pre- and post-surgical status of a seventy-year-old American woman with ALS who had undergone the Beijing OEG transplantation procedure, Columbia University neurologists discounted Huang's efforts as unscientific on the following grounds:

> There is no evidence of defined enrollment criteria, a control group, blinded out-come measurements, or systematic collection of safety data, and no unbiased method has been used to discern positive or negative effects. These procedures cannot be considered credible research because they lack standardized impartial assessments of safety and efficacy. (Chew et al. 2007, 316)

Citing only two papers written by Huang, the Columbia University neurologists dismissed Huang's reports as anecdotal publicity rather than scientific research. This assessment conveniently overlooked the vast majority of the research pa-pers Huang had already published on the safety and feasibility of OEG trans-plantations. The Columbia University neurologists failed to examine papers by Huang that included a clinical case series report on the results of eighty-eight ALS patients who had received OEG transplantation (Huang et al. 2006a), a study on the interim safety of OEG transplantation for ALS based on magnetic resonance imaging (MRI) (Chen et al. 2006a), and two studies on the long-term safety of OEG transplantation for SCI based on three-year follow-up results as-sessed by MRI (Chen et al. 2006b; Huang et al. 2006b).

Since these papers were published in Chinese-language scientific journals, the Columbia clinicians' failure to account for them is understandable, if not excusable. Furthermore, the data from Huang's earlier papers could arguably be considered "unsystematic" since he did not establish a control group for comparison and selected participants based on a convenience sample of avail-able patients. But I would argue that it is wrong to charge Huang with failing to establish the safety and feasibility of his procedure. A demonstration of safety does not require a randomized controlled trial. Indeed, a simple registry track-ing patient outcomes would be sufficient for documenting adverse events. The Columbia clinicians' criticism of Huang makes a fundamental error: it con-flates the documentation of safety with methods for establishing efficacy. Call-ing Huang unscientific is also a rhetorical cheap shot at a Chinese physician who has made clear attempts to document and study his results. These flawed critiques ultimately reveal the unequal power dynamics characterizing global biomedical research.

FROM ANECDOTE TO DATA: DOCUMENTING
OUTCOMES THROUGH QUANTIFICATION

Although he realized that he was operating within an unequal playing field, Huang was determined to address critics who dismissed his results as mere "anecdotal reports" and "unsubstantiated clinical practice" (Dobkin, Curt, and Guest 2006, 5, 13). Even before the publication of these American neurologists' critiques, Huang and his clinical staff members had already begun conducting several studies with defined enrollment criteria, control group comparisons, and systematic collection of data on safety and efficacy (Huang et al. 2008; Chen et al. 2010). They also launched several ambitious projects to generate data on long-term outcomes for both their Chinese and foreign patients. Although he continued to refuse a sham surgery protocol, Huang devised several alternative methodologies to produce evidence substantiating the effectiveness of his fetal cell procedure.

In order to provide an objective basis for comparing functional change, New Century clinicians adopted internationally recognized assessment tools such as the International Standards for Neurological Classification of Spinal Cord Injury (ISNCSCI) of the American Spinal Injury Association (ASIA), which I discussed in chapter 3.[22] Initially developed in 1982 by American researchers attempting to achieve greater consistency and reliable data among centers participating in the National SCI Statistical Center Database, these standards were endorsed by the International Medical Society of Paraplegia in 1992 and have been updated multiple times by a committee of international experts (Kirshblum et al. 2011b). The ASIA classification standards[23] thus provided an internationally recognized, consistent method for categorizing the level of motor function and sensory impairment following spinal cord injury. Based on the conventional understanding that damaged neurons in the central nervous system cannot be repaired or renewed, a person's ASIA classification was not supposed to change once his or her condition stabilized. The New Century staff's careful documentation of their patients' ASIA classifications before and after the OEC transplantation procedure thus served as a key strategy for procuring potential proof of the experimental surgery's effectiveness.

In addition to using existing methods for assessing patients' neurological condition, New Century clinicians also developed their own assessment tools to document key changes they observed in patients receiving the fetal cell therapy. One of the crowning achievements of Dr. Alan, the chief Chinese neurologist, was to develop the New Century Hospital Spinal Cord Injury Daily Life Functional Rating Scale (NCHSCI-DLFRS). The NCHSCI-DLFRS measured functional outcomes that affected patients' everyday lives, including the ease of accomplishing activities such as eating, grooming, dressing, transferring to a bed, and using the toilet. The New Century scale also measured physiological sensations neglected by the ASIA scale, such as muscular tension, ability to sweat, and the degree of pain—issues that contributed to, or even defined, a patient's quality of life.

A patient's physiological status and quality of life could thus be quantified through these existing and new scales, enabling New Century clinicians to measure whether a given patient had experienced overall improvement following the OEC transplantation. The quantification of functional change also facilitated New Century clinicians' efforts to make comparisons between patients and construct extensive databases that could then be translated more easily into scientific publications and the production of proof that these surgical interventions worked. With strings of numbers rounded to the nearest hundredth of a decimal, complete with confidence intervals and p-values, the data generated by the New Century physicians provided a formidable shield against foreign critics' allegations of unscientific methodology. These numbers were generated from worksheets labeled with acronyms such as ASIA, ISNCSCI, NCHSCI-DLFRS, GMFM (Gross Motor Function Measure), ICARS (International Cooperative Ataxia Rating Scale), and CP-ADL (Cerebral Palsy Activities of Daily Living) as Huang and his staff expanded their treatment protocol to encompass additional neurological disorders. From a semiotic perspective, the proliferation of acronyms in the medical records of OEG cell recipients solidified the sense of objectivity accompanying the quantification process.

TRACKING CHINESE PATIENTS

Although the New Century clinicians devoted months to perfecting these various scales and measurement tools, their biggest challenge was finding patients willing to undergo these assessments. Tracking long-term postoperative outcomes for Chinese patients was a Sisyphean endeavor, not just for Huang but for many of the Chinese clinicians I talked with in hospitals across Beijing. As an internist at Peking Union Medical College Hospital explained to me, patients from throughout the country came to Beijing in search of treatment at the nation's top hospitals, often as a last resort after treatment at their local and regional-level hospitals had failed. Once they left the capital city (carrying their medical records back with them to their hometowns), these patients generally had no additional contact with their Beijing-based clinicians. There were few incentives on either side to remain in touch. The busy schedules of clinicians such as the Peking Union internist left little time in the workday to track down patients who had already received treatment. Patients who had already spent significant sums seeking treatment did not want to waste additional money on failed therapies or extraneous consultations. Carrying out clinical trials or even basic follow-up care was thus a difficult proposition in Beijing's clinical context.

Unlike the foreign patients, few of Huang's Chinese patients communicated directly with the head neurosurgeon. Most of them had signed up for the fetal cell transplantation through the typical bureaucratic channels at Naval General

Hospital or Chaoyang Hospital, going through the central hospital registration system before being transferred to Huang's neurosurgery department for treatment. Huang's institutional moves impeded his ability to access the medical charts of patients treated at these previous hospitals. He thus had to resort to other means of obtaining data, such as persuading colleagues at his former institutions to conduct chart reviews for him with the enticement of coauthoring research publications. Huang also tried to reconstruct his own set of patient charts. Starting in 2005, he began inviting former Chinese patients to return to Beijing for a free follow-up assessment. So even though Huang had decided to focus almost exclusively on treating foreign patients at New Century Hospital, the daily neurosurgical rounds generally included a few Chinese patients.

Brother Lu, whom we met in chapter 4, came to New Century Hospital for a follow-up assessment in March 2006. A slight but lively man in his early thirties with short cropped hair, Lu was a veteran of the experimental fetal cell therapy who had undergone the procedure at Naval General Hospital in 2002 in the hopes of bringing movement and sensation back to his paralyzed lower body. At Huang's invitation, he had returned to Beijing with his new wife, a vivacious woman who eagerly attended to his needs. Hu described the arduous process of getting from his home in Zhejiang to the capital city. The train ride alone took thirty hours, a difficult journey even for a man with a top-of-the-line wheelchair accompanied by a doting wife. Prior to the train ride, Lu and his wife had taken an overnight bus from his hometown to get to the nearest major train station. Embarrassed that the clinic was already paying for everything else, they presented only the receipts for the train to the hospital staff.

Lu explained that he had been "seriously ill" (很重的病 *hěn zhòng de bìng*) after being injured in a car accident in May 2000. At the time, he was unable to breathe on his own and had to rely on a ventilator. He slowly regained his ability to breathe during a three-month stay at the local hospital, but he remained unable to move his hands. He later saw a Chinese Central Television broadcast about Huang's surgery for spinal cord injury patients. Although the news report did not mention any specific details, he eagerly called the station and asked them for the name of the hospital where the surgeries were taking place. Describing the OEC transplantation he subsequently underwent at Naval General Hospital, he told me that the conditions were incredibly crowded and that he had to make many of the arrangements himself during his previous trip to the capital. Lu seemed quite pleased that he did not have to "dig out money from his own pocket" (掏钱 *tāo qián*) for the follow-up assessment. He was impressed by Huang's new facilities at New Century Hospital and even inquired about the possibility of undergoing a second OEC transplantation.[24]

Lu laughed about being too thin and showed me how his arm muscles had atrophied. He was missing the end of his middle finger and noted that his hands were weak. But before the OEC surgery, he explained, he was not able to move them at all. Now he could feed himself, but he still had trouble gripping things and could not write. As he scratched his head with his left hand, the head nurse Teacher Yan remarked that his hand seemed quite good and that he was doing very well compared with many of the other seriously injured patients they treated. Lu agreed: "In the past I could only lie on the bed watching the ceiling all day long. I could not sit up; whenever I sat up I would feel dizzy and light-headed, see golden stars in my eyes, feel nauseous, and vomit. After the surgery, I can now sit in a wheelchair for more than two hours and push myself around the entire yard."[25]

Cheerful and upbeat, Brother Lu was clearly thriving in spite of his paralysis from the waist down. He talked animatedly about owning a successful factory that employed twelve workers and produced tripods. He also gestured proudly at his pretty wife, declaring that they had gotten married two years after his successful fetal cell transplantation procedure. Lu's wife and his post-surgical sexual functioning later became the subject of much gossip among the New Century staff, as they discussed how a disabled man was able to convince such an attractive woman to marry him.

FOLLOWING UP: AN EPIC CROSS-COUNTRY JOURNEY

While Brother Lu was one of a few dozen Chinese patients who returned to Beijing for a free follow-up assessment at New Century Hospital, hundreds more did not make the onerous trip to Beijing. Despite Huang's offer to pay for all of their expenses, many other former patients failed to respond even after three rounds of invitations. Dr. Alan, the chief neurologist, speculated that some of the patients probably did not believe that the department would actually shoulder the costs, since this deviated from standard operating procedure among Chinese medical institutions. Furthermore, those unhappy with the results of the surgery could hardly be expected to waste their time by coming back. In order to fill in the gaps on their patient follow-up spreadsheet, Huang decided that New Century doctors would go out to visit the patients in their own homes. As he explained in a staff meeting at the end of 2005, "Because the majority of our former patients have difficulty traveling to the hospital for a follow-up assessment, we need to arrange for our doctors to go out to do this work."[26]

During the spring of 2006, the staff began preparations for a three-month "follow-up" (随访 suífǎng) expedition across eastern China, with the goal of "using the shortest route to interview the most patients" (用最短的路线去采访最多的患者 yòng zuìduǎn de lùxiàn qù cǎifǎng zuìduō de huànzhě). The goal of this suífǎng journey was to perform follow-up assessments on at least one hundred Chinese patients. This seemed like a modest figure given the nearly two hundred Chinese patients who had received OEC transplantations at Naval General between 2001 and 2002 and over three hundred patients at Chaoyang Hospital between 2002 and 2004. But the logistical challenges of locating these patients scattered across the country was proving to be a daunting task.

Teacher Yan brought a map of the country to the hospital to plot out potential routes. The neurosurgical trainees spent their off-duty hours marking the patients' homes on the map. In reviewing patient records, they discovered that most of the listed addresses were not detailed enough. Some entries only listed the name of a town, while others neglected to include an apartment number. The office staff thus devoted their energies to calling former patients to obtain more precise street addresses and to alert them that two doctors would be coming to give them a free checkup. In the process, they also discovered that a significant portion of the listed phone numbers were no longer in service. Angel explained that patients from other provinces avoided racking up long-distance charges by buying local cell phone cards to use during their sojourn in Beijing, which they would then discard upon returning home.

While the office staff struggled to plot out a viable route, the nurses put together a patient education pamphlet that featured translated testimonials from foreign patients describing their improvements after surgery. The small handbook also included advice about physical therapy and exercise routines to help patients strengthen atrophied muscles. Head Nurse Sophie explained that following the OEC procedure, patients needed to exercise in order for there to be any effect. Particularly for spinal cord injury patients, "the less you move, the worse it gets" (越不动越不好 *yuè bù dòng yuè bù hǎo*). Sophie noted how foreigners invented all sorts of contraptions to help themselves, praising their resourcefulness. She remarked that many of her foreign patients still had such positive attitudes despite their serious conditions, contrasting this with some of the rural Chinese "peasants" (农民 *nóngmín*) who tended to lie in bed doing nothing after getting sick or injured. The pamphlet was thus designed to "inspire Chinese patients to work harder."

Dr. Alan would be in charge of doing the follow-up neurological assessments (literally "assigning points" [评分 *píngfēn*]) while Dr. Gu would drive the vehicle and operate the video camera to create a visual record of postoperative changes. The deputized doctors spent several weeks poring over car advertisements and visiting dealerships—already a favorite pursuit among the clinic doctors, who were swept up in the nationwide car craze seizing China's increasingly wealthy urban residents. Envisioning difficult driving conditions outside the capital, Dr. Alan initially wanted to buy a jeep to help navigate the dirt roads along which many rural patients lived. Dr. Gu preferred something larger and more enclosed, anticipating that they might have to sleep in the vehicle overnight in more isolated areas without roadside inns. After heated debates over the merits of domestic versus foreign manufacturers, they ended up purchasing a Hyundai minivan manufactured by the Chinese state-owned Jianghuai Auto Group.

Eager to witness their data collection practices in action, I tried unsuccessfully to persuade the doctors to take me with them on their *suífǎng* journey. Invoking urban stereotypes about the "backward" (落后 *luòhòu*) and "uncivilized" (不文明 *bù wénmíng*) character of rural residents, Dr. Alan explained that it was "not safe" (不安全 *bù ānquán*) for a young woman to go on the trip. Dr. Gu agreed, noting that outside the city, the situation could be "very chaotic" (很 乱 *hěn luàn*). Although they framed the issue in terms of my personal safety, I caught the underlying subtext that my presence as a woman with a foreign passport would be too much of an inconvenience for two men traveling in a van all summer. I thus had to make do with tracking the doctors' progress retrospectively, through intermittent text messages and email updates during the times they had access to Internet cafés.

The challenges the office staff faced in piecing together incomplete street addresses and out-of-service phone numbers foreshadowed the troubles that Drs. Alan and Gu faced in the field. Despite extensive preparations for their *suífǎng* expedition, the doctors reported significant difficulties in locating former patients. From the dusty windows of their Hyundai minivan, they texted photos of empty houses that were marked for demolition, street names that had been changed, and even entire neighborhoods that had been razed to make way for new development projects. Local work unit leaders, public security bureau staff, and former neighbors were often not willing to cooperate, suspicious of these outsiders' intentions.

Of the patients they did manage to locate, Dr. Alan told me that many were disappointed by the outcome of the surgery: their high hopes for the experimental treatment did not match up with the actual results they had experienced. A few were lucky to live near county-level rehabilitation hospitals and continued to work on building finger dexterity, standing up, achieving independence, or broader life goals. But many more were bedridden, reliant on overburdened family members and friends to help them accomplish basic tasks and routines. Dr. Alan was not surprised by these disheartening results. Without access to the personal trainers and physical therapy equipment that many of Huang's foreign patients took for granted, Chinese patients lacking resources and support were perhaps doomed to experience deteriorating muscle mass and worsening neurological function.

VIDEOTAPING FOREIGN PATIENTS

Huang and the New Century staff ultimately found it easier to communicate with and follow up with their foreign patients. Despite living tens of thousands of miles away across oceans and entire continents, foreign patients tended to respond quickly to emails and were often eager to provide updates on their post-operative status.

Huang's ability to connect with his foreign patients hinged upon his dedicated patient coordinators. Bird (her own chosen English name) was one of his most talented employees and was acknowledged to have the best English ability by the entire staff. A graduate of the Beijing University of Traditional Chinese Medicine with a major in traditional Chinese medical nursing, Bird had rotated in the neurosurgery department at Chaoyang Hospital during her last year of school and was immediately hired after graduation by Dr. Huang to serve as the chief coordinator and liaison for his foreign patients. In the early phase of the OEG enterprise, the job involved being on call at all hours. She lived with the foreign patients and their families at their local hotel. She was also responsible for coordinating their test schedules and exams with each hospital department as well as making all of their eating and transportation arrangements.

Despite the frenetic pace of work, Bird looked back at the Chaoyang period with nostalgia, describing the close-knit community and warm relationships she had formed with the foreign patients and their families. Bird's empathy and ability to make an emotional connection with the foreign patients in Beijing stemmed perhaps in part from her own experiences of social and bodily dislocation. She was raised in Shanghai by her maternal grandfather, who had been labeled a landlord and repeatedly punished during the Maoist era. His wife had committed suicide before Bird's birth, unable to handle the humiliation any longer. For the first seven years of her life, Bird did not see her parents—they had been transferred to a rural area far away from the city, part of a generation of urban youth sent down to the countryside for reeducation through manual labor. Beyond the bad class label she had inherited, Bird faced the additional stigma of disease: she had contracted Hepatitis B at birth from her mother, an unfortunately all-too-common phenomenon across China.[27] She spent much of her childhood in hospitals and faced significant discrimination enrolling in school as a chronic Hepatitis B sufferer. Even her acceptance to nursing school had been a fluke. Although she had received a good score on the national college entrance exam, she should have been refused admission according to institutional guidelines. University officials had somehow overlooked her medical report and it wasn't until she had already started taking classes that they discovered her disease status. Her professors allowed her to continue taking classes, but they warned that she would not be able to find a job in the nursing profession following graduation. Bird was thus especially devoted to Dr. Huang, who had looked beyond her disease status to recognize her many other talents.

After moving to New Century Hospital, Bird began to spend more and more time in front of the computer rather than in the wards with patients. Facing a backlog of email inquiries from prospective clients and assessment forms for former patients, Huang put Bird in charge of electronic communications with patients. Her strong English skills made her the default front-line responder for any incoming email inquiries, although she still continued to be a key troubleshooter for day-to-day issues when patients and family members discovered a fluent and charming English speaker tucked away in the cramped department library.

Although Bird was supposed to focus on coordinating follow-up results for the foreign patients, she said her job involved much more than this. Whenever she wrote to patients, their replies would be filled with many other questions.

Bird confided that she found the emotional pressures of the job increasingly unbearable. On her first day back to work following the weeklong Chinese Spring Festival holiday in 2006, she opened her inbox to discover hundreds of messages awaiting her response. When I poked my head in her office around 7 P.M. to ask whether she would like to grab some dinner together, she burst into tears. Although she had not eaten all day, she said she had to finish replying to urgent emails before she could leave. Dr. Huang was in Italy for a medical conference and she needed to respond to the many patients who were hoping to meet him there. Other prospective patients, tired of the growing waiting list for the OEG procedure, announced that they had booked their own plane tickets and would be arriving in Beijing shortly. She was trying her best to persuade them to cancel their flights and wait for a scheduled appointment. Some former patients had also written to her to describe their worsening status. While she used to be able to dash off a cheerful email to an anxious patient, she now often found herself at a loss as to how to console patients. She described how she would spend an entire morning composing an email in an attempt to "comfort" (安慰 ānwèi) a patient but then delete the whole message in frustration because her response did not adequately address their suffering. Her colleagues counseled her just to use a "template" (模板 móbǎn), but she felt that she couldn't just use a generic form letter to write to patients whom she had met and befriended.

Bird's sensitivity and devotion to the foreign patients made her an excellent coordinator for Huang's ambitious follow-up goals (although the relentless workload and stress ultimately led her to quit the following year). She showed me an email she had written herself in English in response to Huang's plan to invite select foreign patients back to Beijing for a follow-up assessment. Her invitation was hard to resist, with its plea to help advance medical treatment and its concrete promise of a free and improved OEC transplantation surgery. The breezy recruitment letter contrasted sharply with the dry language of RCT informed consent forms and their litany of risks and benefits:

This is Bird flying from Beijing [New Century] Hospital (A big smile and a huge hug). How are you doing? I hope everything is going very well with you. We are still busy with more and more patients coming for the surgery, but we wouldn't feel happier than we see the hopes and the smiles in their eyes. Dr. Huang and all the other doctors are very busy also in doing more research for ALS and the treatment for ALS. . . .

Since that you were one of the 20 patients who had undertaken the Functional MRI, you became an important case for us that we need you to do us a favor and we do want to do something for you, too. . . . We are wondering that if we paid two round trip flight tickets of the economy class and a room with three meals a day for a week in Jade Palace Hotel, could you please to come back to Beijing to do this

Functional MRI, Pulmonary Function and EMG test again . . . (of course we will pay for the test, too).

We need you to come back to do this test again not only for continuing the research for a better way to treat ALS, but also we want to know about your progression of this disease. . . . I wish you would keep your condition stable as long as possible and I do pray for you everyday, however, if the functional MRI here showed that you do need the surgery again and you wanted to have it, too, we would do it sometime the month of April of 2006 or according to the progression of your condition, with the matched cells for you. . . . We will pay for the surgery. We will also pay the room and board for patient and one caregiver. This is the promise from Dr. Huang.

Please keep in mind we do care about you, and we do care about all the ALS patients. If you came back to do the Functional MRI test again, you would probably help a lot more ALS patients and you would probably help yourself, too. I'm awaiting for your quick response regardless of your decision.

Dan, a sixty-year-old ALS patient from Florida who underwent the OEC transplantation in March 2005, was one of the American patients who accepted Bird's offer to return to New Century for an all-expenses-paid follow-up assessment in October. When I initially interviewed him a week following surgery, Dan had been reading a Tom Clancy novel while reclining in the plush brown armchair in the New Century patient activity room. He joked about a recent night's sleep in which the bandage covering his surgical incisions had gotten stuck to his pillow. When he woke up in the morning, he discovered red blotchy stains on his pillow: "Holy mackerel! My brain's starting to fall out!" Dan had been diagnosed with ALS nine years earlier but thankfully the "progression has been so flat." He confided, "I look at some of the patients here who can't even walk or breathe . . . I almost feel guilty for taking a spot when other people are doing so much worse." Speaking in a clear, steady voice, Dan described how the OEC surgery had improved his ability to grasp objects firmly—which made it noticeably easier for him to write, cut food, and get dressed by himself. Reflecting on his experiences at New Century, Dan noted that it was all about "small victories." He told us how a fellow ALS patient from Belgium had walked down the hall the other day—before that Frank had only been able to take three steps. Dan said, "Friends back home ask what it was like, but it's really hard to describe in words. You have to just sit down face to face and see for yourself."

Dan's follow-up assessment six months later involved several components. First, one of the New Century neurosurgical trainees interviewed him to obtain a detailed history of the functional changes he had experienced following the surgery. The trainee took careful notes on any changes in sensory perception and functional abilities, including the ability to move various body parts, urination and bowel movements, sweating, and sexual function. Dr. Alan then attempted to quantify and corroborate this narrative account by using two internationally recognized ALS rating scales to assign specific point values to these various functional arenas. The New Century clinicians also performed a pulmonary function test and an electromyography (EMG), which recorded the electrical activity produced by his muscles. In addition, they sent him to a larger Chinese hospital to undergo a functional MRI scan.

The linchpin of the assessment involved recording Dan's ability to perform everyday tasks. While Dr. Gu operated the video camera, Dr. Alan asked Dan to write his name with a pen, unscrew the cap of a water bottle, and pour the water into a bowl. After screwing the cap back on, he pretended to take a sip from the bottle. The neurologist then asked Dan to put on a hospital shirt and button it up by himself. Following Dr. Alan's instruction, Dan then lifted a paperback book above his head, taking turns with both arms. Finally, the neurologist asked Dan to walk along the hospital corridor and up and down a staircase.

In reviewing Dan's videotapes with the New Century clinicians, I noticed that his postoperative movements were much more confident and self-assured than they had been prior to the surgery. In the videotape taken before his surgery, Dan's hands wobbled so much that he could not write out the letters of his last name. He also had difficulty buttoning up a shirt and needed Dr. Alan's hand to stabilize him while walking down the staircase. In the postoperative video, Dan strode confidently down the hallway in his red sweatpants and walked up and down the hospital's central staircase without any assistance. The New Century clinicians and Dan interpreted these video recordings as evidence for the effectiveness of the OEC surgery.

Dan subsequently decided to return to China to undergo a second transplantation procedure. His decision reflected his confidence in both the safety and effectiveness of Huang's experimental therapy. Huang also sweetened the deal by waiving the cost of the second operation, which was based on new research he was conducting on whether matched cellular tissue improved functional outcomes for patients.[28] Enticed by the offer of a free and more "advanced" surgery and buoyed by what he considered to be concrete evidence of his postsurgical improvements, Dan thus boarded the plane from Florida to Beijing once again in July 2006.

CONCLUSION

This chapter has examined how New Century clinicians have responded to allegations of quackery while devising new standards of evidence. Although Huang contested the ethics of sham surgery, this did not mean that he abandoned scientific principles. Since the very start of the Beijing OEG cell odyssey in 2001, Huang and his colleagues have sought to document, substantiate, track, and assess the results of this pioneering experimental surgery. Having witnessed their efforts over several years, I would conclude that the New Century Neurological

Disorders Research and Treatment Center has made credible efforts to develop alternative forms of "evidence-based" clinical practice with the available resources at their disposal—but these attempts have had mixed results.

In urging Chinese citizens to "seek truth from facts" (实事求是 *shí shì qiú shì*), both Mao and Deng quoted this proverb to highlight pragmatism as a guiding principle. As the different challenges posed by conducting follow-up studies with both domestic and foreign patients illustrate, New Century's research timetables and protocols aspired to ideal scientific principles but often fell victim to pragmatic concerns. Establishing efficacy under the controlled conditions of an optimized clinical trial fails to account for the practical constraints shaping the everyday lives of clinicians, patients, and their families. In the case of Chinese patients, the problems Drs. Alan and Gu faced in trying to track them down illustrate the broader difficulties in obtaining reliable evidence for determining the effectiveness of experimental treatments in contemporary China. Returning to the mismatch in temporalities I discussed earlier between patient lives and research timetables, these challenges in locating patients expose the fault lines created by socioeconomic change as they intersect with the spatial and temporal dynamics of illness and injury. Paralyzed patients have been "left behind" in China's interior hinterlands, with little access to assistive technologies and rehabilitation services. The precarity of their situation marginalizes them even further as ambitious Chinese clinicians such as Huang turn toward more promising candidates able to comply with research protocols. As Bird's follow-up work demonstrates, the New Century staff ironically found that they could produce better data and results with their foreign patients, even when they lived tens of thousands of miles away. The experiences of the New Century clinicians ultimately open up questions not just about efficacy of fetal cell therapies but about the very purpose of biomedical research and practice in a transnational world. I continue this line of inquiry in the next chapter by analyzing the efforts of patients and their families to assess the effectiveness of experimental treatment.

I-WITNESSING

WHILE HUANG AND THE NEW Century staff members were busy devising new methods to document the effects of their OEG cell transplantation surgery, patients and their families also developed their own ways of assessing whether the experimental procedure worked. In this chapter, I focus on how fetal cell recipients and their families have engaged questions of efficacy in the transnational realm of experimental medicine. Prospective transplantation candidates carefully parsed online reports of others' surgical experiences and analyzed the credibility of Chinese neurosurgeons' claims, while postoperative patients monitored their bodies for signs of difference and parsed these changes online. I argue that the digitally mediated forms of knowledge they have produced offer a poignant challenge to what counts as expertise and data in the quest for "evidence" in experimental medicine.

SCIENTIFIC LITERACY IN THE INTERNET ERA

The role of evidence played a crucial factor in foreign patients' decisions whether to undergo OEG surgery. How much and what kind of evidence was necessary for prospective patients to place their trust in Dr. Huang's experimental procedure? As I began to show in chapter 3, this "evidence threshold" depended upon the interplay of scientific literacy, embodied illness experience, and degree of urgency for each potential fetal cell recipient. In her influential study of the cultural meanings and social effects of prenatal diagnosis in the United States, anthropologist Rayna Rapp (1999) demonstrated that scientific literacy is forged in everyday life, not just in formal classes or medical encounters. Since she began conducting her original fieldwork in the 1980s, the Internet has become a mainstream pillar of the American cultural landscape, with online discussion forums and social media networks becoming key arenas for incorporating scientific knowledge into everyday life. On CareCure, for example, members dissected reports on the properties of olfactory ensheathing glial cells published in scientific journals (Curt Leatherbee 2003b), compared protocols for various clinical trials using OEGs (mk99 2002), and even questioned the dangerous influence of "OEG hype" (paulsask 2003). As a CareCure moderator remarked, "It amazes me, I think a lot of us here know more about this kind of stuff than most Doctors do!!! It is great we have these forums to discuss this stuff" (Curt Leatherbee 2003c).[1]

As a columnist for the popular technology news website *Wired News* who had even dabbled in research of his own, Cure forum moderator Steven Edwards was particularly attuned to the importance of scientific proof. In considering the data available to CareCure members back in 2003, he noted:

> As someone has mentioned to me, my strengths are science and math . . . I make my decisions based on evidence and fact. If I could read Huang's paper,[2] my decision may be very different. . . . If I knew more about the results, had a spreadsheet that showed pre-surgery function and post-surgery function [e.g., C3 pre, T2 post, etc.], my mind could possibly be changed. Until I know more, I would say no. If the majority of C3s regained 4 or more levels of function, I would go for it. Or if the majority of people with similar MRIs regained good function, I would go for it. Basically Jeff, it boils down to "not enough information." I don't like making decisions when I only have partial information. . . . If I had the opportunity [statistically probable] to get my hands and fingers back, I would go for it. (Steven Edwards 2003b)

The key for Steven was having concrete data on the effectiveness of the surgery: not just hope but statistical probability. Following the cue of the scientists whose work he tracked, he wanted to see the published results of a peer-reviewed study documenting significant functional recovery before he would risk any disruptions to his fragile local anatomy.

Given the heterogeneous nature of online resources, however, Internet-mediated scientific literacy is not a uniform affair. Even CareCure, a relatively stable discussion forum compared to the rapidly disappearing blogs of ALS patients, demonstrated significant variability in the scientific literacy of participants. Designated "senior members" of the CareCure community like Steven, who had been part of Wise's SCI "experiment" since the previous incarnation of the website, often developed a keen sense for evaluating purported scientific advances in the basic biology and clinical treatment of SCI. But newly enrolled "junior members" often stumbled into the midst of discussions with no prior context beyond a list of Google links. Thus, even as Steven, Handibob, Leo, and mk99 eagerly debated the finer-grained physio-anatomical effects of OEG transplantation on CareCure, others lacked even basic information about the experimental procedure: "Could someone please explain what this surgery is for. Is there a website I can go and check it out. Thx" (Duke 2003).

The distinction between those who demonstrated serious scientific engagement with Huang's experimental procedure and those lured by media hype was often visually demarcated by the terminology they used to refer to Huang's procedure. Senior members of CareCure carefully deployed the technical term for the fetal cells used in Huang's treatment: olfactory ensheathing glial cells (often abbreviated as OEG or OEC to save typing effort online). Extracted from the olfactory bulb of aborted late-term fetuses, these OEG cells were definitively not embryonic stem cells (or even more mature adult stem cells) that could potentially develop into new neurons. Their promise lay in their potential to change the local environment of injury to encourage damaged nerve cells to regenerate. But the hype surrounding the more (in)famous variety of progenitor cells often led patients, reporters, and even other scientists and clinicians to conflate the fetal cells that Huang utilized in his experimental therapy with stem cells. Huang thus frequently received inquiries from prospective patients and family members about signing up for his "stem cell" therapy.

Concerned about maintaining his scientific standards and credibility, Huang adamantly policed the boundaries between OEG and stem cells—even turning away potential patients who inquired about obtaining "stem cell" surgery. As an ALS patient from Missouri whom I met following his OEG transplantation surgery in Beijing told me, his first attempt to contact Huang was an absolute failure. He had sent an email to Huang requesting to be put on the waiting list for stem cell surgery. Huang had promptly written back to tell him: "We do not provide stem cell treatment. Good luck with finding a hospital that does." In another example from January 2005, Huang posted a public response on CareCure to yet another misinformed inquiry about his "stem cell" surgery:

> I am very sorry that I never do stem cell surgery. Even I repeated this sentence more than several hundreds to the doctors, scientists, media, patients and their family. But some of them still mixed our OEC or OEG transplant with stem cell. Because OEC or OEG is totally different with stem cell, I really don't want people to misunderstand what we are doing. (hongyun 2005)

The naming of the cells in question not only served as a marker of patients' scientific literacy, it also played a key role in convincing prospective patients of Huang's scientific credibility as a legitimate neurosurgeon offering a carefully theorized, well-tested experimental therapy.

The intervention of recognized experts played an important role in the cultivation of scientific literacy among online social networks. When confronted with preliminary and often contradictory research data, even longstanding members of the CareCure community often relied on the interpretation of established experts in the CareCure community such as Wise Young. Indeed, so many members asked the resident CareCure neuroscientist for his advice that he eventually started a discussion thread at the end of December 2004 titled "OEG transplants: to have or not to have?" Wise's advice summarized the results of the examinations he had performed on dozens of Dr. Huang's patients, detailed the potential side effects and complications, and compared the surgery with other experimental therapies. Beyond the clinical details, he also reminded anxious members about the practical challenges involved: "Beijing is far away from the United States. It is a significant investment of time and effort" (Wise Young 2004). This expert-mediated evidence had its limitations, however, when the expert in question urged members to make their own informed decisions. As Wise concluded, "people will simply have to weigh the risks and benefits" (ibid.). Although he advised members to wait for improved techniques and published results, he did provide the CareCure community with assurance that Dr. Huang's surgery was relatively safe and appeared to produce at least some degree of sensory improvement. This endorsement of safety provided members with at least a basic degree of confidence in the foreign procedure and doctor—an important guarantee in an era when "all sorts of odd and ancillary experiments, outright scams and pagan ritualistic medicines [were] popping up across the planet" (vgrafen 2004). With Wise's backing, mk99 could argue with conviction that the OEG surgery "probably won't kill me and won't 'screw me' from future better therapies" (2003c).

SCRUBBING IN

Other families also utilized CareCure to evaluate the experimental therapy and establish contact with Dr. Huang but needed more visceral proof of the Chinese neurosurgeon's credibility before subjecting their loved ones to a risky surgical procedure in an unfamiliar country. Chris, an eighteen-year-old from Southern California, pulverized his T-12 thoracic vertebrae in a snowboarding accident in May 2003. The accident rendered Chris a paraplegic, unable to move or feel sensation below his hips or control his bladder and bowel movements. As a nurse practitioner married to a professor of anatomy and physiology, Chris's mother, Lillien, leveraged her family's considerable medical expertise to track down possible treatments for her son. Chris had already received the most advanced treatment regimen available in his area, including decompression surgery to remove damaged bone fragments pressing on his spinal cord, stabilization of his shattered vertebrae with a titanium cage, and an intensive physical therapy program. He was able to walk only with the aid of full-length leg braces to stabilize his knees, ankles, and feet. Although his American doctors were optimistic that he would be able to achieve functional independence, they told him that he would most likely need to use leg braces as well as a catheter for the rest of his life.

Not satisfied with this prognosis, Chris and his family continued to search for treatments that might enable him to regain greater mobility and resolve his bladder and bowel dysfunction. Lillien discovered Dr. Huang's procedure through an Internet search that landed her in the CareCure forum. Excited yet cautious about the information they were reading online about the fetal cell transplantation, Lillien and her husband traveled to Beijing in April 2004 to assess Dr. Huang's operation with their own eyes first. At the time, Dr. Huang was still working at Chaoyang Hospital, the public medical institution where the first foreign patients had undergone Dr. Huang's procedure in September 2003. As these initial CareCure pioneers described in ample detail, Chaoyang Hospital was ill-equipped to meet the expectations of American patients, despite (or perhaps because of) its status as one of Beijing's largest and busiest tertiary care hospitals.

Dr. Huang permitted Lillien to "scrub in" with him on a fetal cell transplantation procedure for an American spinal cord injury patient. While the Californian nurse practitioner observed Huang's surgical skills in the operating theater, her husband, an anatomy expert, carefully scrutinized the olfactory ensheathing glial cell cultures to assess whether patients were receiving cultured cells, not random tissue or debris. The firsthand opportunity to observe Huang in action—both in the operating room and in the laboratory—convinced Chris's parents of the legitimacy of his experimental treatment. Their discussions with foreign patients undergoing the surgery and observations of post-surgical recovery provided the Californian couple with proof that the procedure was both safe and effective. Their son underwent the OEG fetal cell transplantation in November 2004. Lillien has publicly endorsed the OEG fetal cell transplantation, writing letters in support of Huang and talking with researchers and journalists about their experience.[3]

During the course of my fieldwork at New Century Hospital, I occasionally encountered other family members who traveled to Beijing first before subjecting their loved ones to a risky operation. While most of them did not have the same professional training as Chris's parents, they too wanted to obtain firsthand evidence for the safety and effectiveness of the OEG fetal cell transplantation procedure. Given the significant costs and hassles of international travel, particularly for those serving as primary caregivers for loved ones afflicted with paralysis or neurodegeneration, these advance "scouting trips" were a luxury that only a small minority of OEG fetal cell recipients could afford on top of the tens of thousands they already needed for the actual surgical trip itself.

OEG SURGERY REPORT THREADS

What about patients and families who did not have the means to travel in advance to Beijing to conduct a pre-assessment of the safety and effectiveness of the experimental treatment? The majority of Huang's patients relied on the digital reports of other OEG fetal cell recipients who had gone before. This culture of information sharing was particularly evident on CareCure. Indeed, many of the CareCure members who underwent OEG cell transplantation felt duty-bound to report online the results of the momentous operation they had undergone. This was particularly the case for the first Americans to undergo Huang's procedure. Tim C., Handibob, and CJO took their responsibilities as leaders of the SCI cure movement seriously, recognizing their role in helping improve the promising OEG therapy:

IMO [in my opinion] dr huang is a near-saint, he appears just totally thrilled with the current results he's getting. he is only limited with his resourses. to those in the medical community that are awaiting a pretty package of data ontop of data, publish-able for their pompous journals, should come here to beijing and see what dr huang is doing with such limited resourses. the journals are important, yet huang is keeps plugging away with chinese patients on a daily basis, and improving on his own technique as he goes. plse consider; IMO, this therapy is in it's model-T stage and the RollsRoyce is down the road a piece. i have to believe that by allowing US citizens to participate in his work, dr huang hopes that we, Handibob and CJO included, help plant the seed (sorry for mixing metaphors) in the researchers of sci within other countries who have the resources to build upon the technology (not just criticize it). (Tim C. 2003d)

Even the Model-T version of the surgery was producing results for the Care-Cure pioneers. All three reported immediate gains after receiving the OEG transplants, much to their surprise. Handibob, for example, began experiencing improvements upon waking up from surgery. As he described on his OEG surgery report thread:

I woke up in the ICU and shortly after Dr. Huang came in to visit. He checked for any progress and this is the amazing part: immediately we noticed that I was able to sweat below my level of injury everywhere he checked was perspiring (of course it was about 100 degrees in that ICU). We also noticed that my breathing function was much improved I can feel the breathing all the way into my stomach, I also have noticed increased strength my left grip in my hand was very much stronger and my right hand was stronger but not as much as the left. I am able to wiggle all of my toes on the left foot and some in right foot. I have also noticed that my circulation is improved my legs are warm and the swelling is gone. I noticed that my right leg is tingling and that I can move it up and down and move my ankle side to side. I feel increased bladder pressure and have noticed that my trunk is stronger. I can drink from a bottle with my left hand without holding on to my wheelchair with my right arm . . . I am very excited about my progress and will keep you updated. (Handibob 2003c)

Although Tim was plagued by a slight fever and high blood pressure following surgery, he noted Huang's immediate efforts to measure his postoperative function. This urge to document the effects of the surgery was reflected in his own desire to document his bodily changes online for CareCure readers:

Despite my discomfort, Dr. Huang was quick to begin measuring my immediate sensory and motor function. My tricep muscles appear to be activated but still very weak. Also my ability to perspire has increased down to my lower back. My torso also feels stronger, yet it's still too early to tell. My sensory improved on my arms in areas where I didn't previously have sensory. I was told by Dr. Huang that I should expect more to follow, however, everybody's degree of recovery varies. I will continue to hope for the best, and keep everyone apprised. (I was not expecting any degree of immediate recovery, rather over a period of time as the cells regenerate. This remains the mystery.) (Tim C. 2003g)

Handibob's and Tim's speculations about the mechanisms of recovery and reports on their bodily status, interwoven with commentary from the CareCure community, became a paradigmatic example of the format of the OEG surgery report threads.

CJO, who underwent surgery five days after the others, also documented his experiences of severe headaches and fever. These negative signs sparked significant trepidation among his CareCure readership, both in terms of concern over CJO's personal welfare as well as unease about the safety of the procedure. Neuroscientist Wise Young mediated the apprehension building up online by explaining that the headaches probably stemmed from the removal of cerebrospinal fluid when the dura protecting the spinal cord cavity was opened during surgery to inject the cells (Wise Young 2003d).

Like the other two, CJO experienced immediate sensory and motor gains following the transplantation. Whereas he formerly had no hand sensation beyond some slight feeling on the outsides of his thumbs, CJO noted the following postoperative observations for his CareCure devotees:

> That first afternoon I began sweating and my legs and feet were noticeably warmer. The next day, my thumbs had sensation all over them—almost normal in some places. My index fingers now have a lot of sensation. . . . My left wrist extensor has a grade of 4 now. Pinch muscles are firing very faintly. Hard work ahead. Left tricep is firing to where I can almost straighten my arm; the right one fires too but is weaker. Dr. Huang claims he can feel grip muscles firing and that my middle finger flickers when he tells me to move it. Muscle function has improved more on the left; sensory more on the right. Two nights after surgery a nurse had to move an IV line from the top of my left foot to the top of my right foot. I could tell exactly where they put it on my right foot because I could feel some pain. Weird. Please remember anything that I have gained is due to an early recovery mechanism that cannot be explained. Good things are happening now, but the actual regeneration is a very slow process. Hard work, rehab, and 12–18 months of these little cells doing their work should be a hell of a journey. (CJO 2003e)

Wise Young had also noted this nearly instantaneous recovery during his visit to Naval General (Wise Young 2002b), and both he and Huang were puzzled by the phenomenon. They considered this surprise recovery an unexpected "bonus" side effect of the procedure, which was ultimately intended to encourage the remyelination or even regrowth of damaged neurons—a process that, as the first CareCure pioneers recognized, should take months.

EYEWITNESSING ONLINE

The Beijing OEG surgery report threads can be understood as public transcripts of these American patients' illness narratives, attempts to make sense of their experiences of suffering and treatment. While medical anthropologist Arthur Kleinman (1988) originally discussed the construction of illness narratives in the context of improving patient-physician interactions, the CareCure pioneers' online narratives unfolded in the context of an entire community of people grappling with spinal cord injuries. Transcending personal quests to heal their own damaged bodies, these publicly documented accounts enacted a collective testament for rejuvenating an entire community.[4]

While the initial discussions on CareCure about Huang's experiment focused on one main thread that followed from Wise's Beijing trip report, the CareCure pioneers' OEG surgeries launched a "stampede to China" that swamped the Cure forum with a frenzy of postings. These new threads included everything from detailed notes dissecting the properties of olfactory ensheathing cells to multiple pleas started by people desperate to get on the "Soon-to-Be-Infamous Huang List." Part of this proliferation of threads stemmed from the splintering of authority surrounding the China procedure. After coming back from China in December 2002, Wise initially reigned as the sole eyewitness and authoritative expert on Huang's procedure. But dozens of CareCure members (as well as Christopher Reeve) saw video clips documenting post-surgical patients' increased functional recovery with their own eyes when Huang delivered a presentation at the Keck Center at Rutgers University in September 2003. This increased the number of witnesses who could provide reliable information to fellow community members ravenous for more details.

The ultimate eyewitnessing (or I-witnessing, as anthropologist Clifford Geertz might say) came with the arrival of the first CareCure pioneers in Beijing. These fetal cell recipients were no longer just reading about but physically experiencing the quest for the cure—and documenting their experiences online. Like the anthropologist who derives textual authority from a convincing demonstration of having "truly been there" (Geertz 1988, 4–5), these CareCure pioneers derived their authority on the CareCure forums from portraying their bodily experiences as participant observers in the quest for the cure. For Geertz, who was analyzing ethnographic monographs published long after their authors left the field, this act of persuasion constituted an "offstage miracle" (5). For the CareCure pioneers in Beijing, their authority was co-constructed through active engagement with their online audience. The real-time updates from Beijing gave their online surgery report threads an unassailable credibility—what we might call i-witnessing in the digital age—that was strengthened by the collective interaction of the community. At their best, these were "blow by blow accounts" that documented the procedures as they unfolded on the ground.

As one of the most popular discussion genres on CareCure, these interactive testimonials connect the visceral with the virtual in the quest for a cure:

> These discussions of the actual experience and recovery of individuals who have gone for experimental and alternative therapies are unique. The community can share vicariously with the experience and judge for themselves the merits and risks of such therapies. There is a strong sense of altruism in the sharing of these experiences, so that others can benefit. (Wise Young 2002a)

In the course of my research, I documented at least fifteen separate Beijing OEG surgery report threads by CareCure members who underwent Huang's procedure since 2003. Several others posted results and updates in existing threads, bringing the number of CareCure members who documented their OEG surgical experiences online to at least thirty. While these subsequent threads did not attract as much sustained attention as the original three, they still contributed to the overall body of knowledge and expertise on CareCure about the experimental Beijing procedure.[5]

POST-SURGICAL TRAJECTORY #1: HANDIBOB'S GAINS

What happened to these surgical report threads after the fetal cell recipients returned home from China? Some threads petered out as their original posters lost interest in the SCI forum and logged on less and less frequently. This was often the case for junior CareCure members who had set up user accounts for the express purpose of contacting Huang. Other OEG fetal cell recipients found the flood of interest from prospective patients overwhelming. As we saw in chapter 3, iublondie, who initially welcomed personal inquiries about her father-in-law's experiences undergoing surgery in China, had to scale back on her participation as demands from other parts of her life became more urgent: her job, her pregnancy, her family. In CJO's case, he ultimately chose to delete his user account altogether after being inundated with requests for information. His posts remained accessible online through the CareCure forum, but like other "orphan" posts whose users actively abandoned them, they now were attributed to an anonymous "guest" and lacked a specific individual's identity.

For others who tried Huang's experimental therapy, particularly senior CareCure members, the i-witnessing did not end in Beijing. They continued to post updates about their bodily status, and their reports provide invaluable insight on how assessments of the experimental procedure changed over time for OEG fetal cell recipients living with chronic paralysis. Checking in with his fellow CareCure members every few months after his surgery in September 2003, Handibob detailed the small improvements he continued to experience following the experimental procedure in Beijing: increased strength in his triceps, better balancing on his torso, the ability to remove and put back his own leg rest supports, a newfound capacity to pass gas. Handibob also joked about regaining the ability to "drink and drive" (i.e., propelling his wheelchair through a crowd at a local football game while holding a Bud Light) and to take care of ordinary household chores again:

> The other day I was outside picking up small screws, bolts and other leftover construction material off the ground, just thought I'd try and next thing I know I've got a small pile picked up. Then I grabbed a broom and swept the driveway, man it was awesome. I've tried that many times over the years and never came close. I joked with my neighbors about not telling my wife, she found out anyways and immediately started talking about doing laundry. I said, I knew I should've kept my mouth shut, lol. (Handibob 2004b)

While these changes might seem insignificant to an outside observer, fellow CareCure members recognized that these incremental improvements had a profound impact on Handibob's daily life, from his ability to participate in his local community to his relationship with the woman to whom he had been married for over two decades. Handibob's focus on the everyday and his interpretation of the "efficacy" of the OEG fetal cell therapy thus align more with an anthropological understanding of the term that encompasses broader questions of meaning and effectiveness in the context of social action.

Handibob staunchly believed that his improvements stemmed from the combination of Huang's experimental surgery and an intensive physical therapy regimen he was undergoing at a newly opened rehabilitation center in Michigan. As he explained to the CareCure community six months following his surgery:

> Remember, Dr Huang originally wanted us to spend 6 months in China to have the surgery and then intensive physical therapy. My point is that you have to do both, anyone considering this procedure must commit to this if you expect to see any improvement. Also, I spent 14 months in therapy after my injury back in 1999 and we didn't see any of these gains back then. AND BELIEVE ME WE TRIED AND TRIED AND TRIED. (Handibob 2004a)

For Handibob, the ultimate proof lay in his personal experience of these bodily changes. While a scientist might seek out large-scale randomized trials with hundreds of study subjects for statistically significant verification of Huang's results, Handibob focused on the single most important subject for his purposes: himself. Sixteen months after his experimental surgery in Beijing, Handibob continued to detail the small changes he was experiencing. He also addressed skeptics: "And for all those wondering, I haven't lost any of my gains since the surgery, the so called placebo effect" (Handibob 2005).

Handibob's ongoing assessments corroborated with those of the majority of other CareCure OEG recipients. In a poll that Wise Young initiated at the end of August 2005 asking "How many people who have had the Huang Procedure in Beijing have improved?" twenty-four members responded (figure 8.1). The overall consensus (50 percent, or twelve members) was that the OEG procedure had produced some slight improvements in sensory and motor function, with four members claiming substantial improvements and eight claiming not much change at all. Nobody reported any loss in function.

Handibob returned to Beijing in May 2006 to undergo a follow-up examination at Huang's invitation. He posted the neurosurgery clinic's official assessment for CareCure readers to analyze (Handibob 2006), which tracked his progress before his experimental surgery, immediately following the OEG procedure in October 2003, and three years later at the follow-up examination. This report provided a detailed rundown of Handibob's changing scores on the ASIA scale, the New Century Hospital SCI functional rating scale, as well as his results on standardized pulmonary function and electromyography tests.

Trying to figure out "what does it all mean?" another CareCure member responded, "I get cross-eyed reading the numbers and comparing. are you better? in what ways and how much usable function?" (W. Justin Martin 2006). A Care-Cure moderator jumped in to explain the results, noting that Handibob "made huge gains" particularly in his sensory capacities (both in response to light touch as well as a deeper pin prick) and his motor function (Seneca 2006). For Handibob, his epic journey to Beijing to undergo fetal cell transplantation paid off in the concrete gains he experienced following the experimental procedure.

POST-SURGICAL TRAJECTORY #2: TIM C.'S PAIN

Tim C. endured a different postoperative path. While Handibob enthusiastically welcomed his increasing sensory capacity and motor function, Tim C. found his postoperative changes puzzling and problematic. Six months following his surgery in Beijing, Tim C. detailed a "dramatic improvement in sitting balance," increased sensation on various limbs in unpredictable locations, and several other "not noteworthy" changes. Attempting to account for the post-surgical changes he experienced, he noted that "my improvements are more measurable in random point scores, not levels as some may expect to see" (Tim C. 2004b).

With a background in engineering, Tim C. had envisioned tracking his post-surgical results in a methodical and systematic way. But he found that the changes he was experiencing were difficult to quantify:

> As far as the whole effort is going, being a refugee of engineering education and training, i truly expected to measure and track my progress, if any, in a very technical format. i anticipated being evaluated by my original physiatrist on a monthly, or something similar basis. For reasons i'll comment later, this is not happening. Instead, if and when we notice improvement, it's one dermatone at a time, if there can be such thing. (Tim C. 2004c)

Tim C. grew increasingly pessimistic about the experimental transplantation over time. As we saw in chapter 3, a "gain" in sensory feeling from the OEG surgery could ultimately result in more pain. Tim C. was initially reluctant to post anything negative, acknowledging that "the OEG interest is still strong and i don't want to reduce it in any way" (Tim C. 2004d). But in update after update following his initial reticence, he began to report excruciating pain that he ultimately linked to the experimental procedure:

> SEVEN MONTHS POST-SURGERY: i did have what i identify as level 4 neurogenic pain pre procedure, i also had digestive pain. Now, both have been amplified. especially the leg and hand burn. it's got me jumping out of my skin at times, and a decent pain med dependency to boot. Is it the result of the OEG or natural changes in a 19–23 month post sci? (Tim C. 2004d)

> EIGHT MONTHS POST-SURGERY: my nerve pain has significantly increased since my oeg transplant from dr huang. the pain includes extreme burning sensation of my limbs and buttox. i have no pain-free days, zero. (Tim C. 2004e)

> NINE MONTHS POST-SURGERY: on CC it is as if my name has become synonymous with pain. i'm still fighting the demons of burning sensations in my limbs and buttocks. i can confidently state that it has elevated since the transplant. (Tim C. 2004f)

> TEN MONTHS POST-SURGERY: My pain levels have irrefutably increased since my OEG transplant of last september. Sarcastically speaking, each increasing level as illustrated in the all too familiar pain chart cost me several thousand dollars each. (Tim C. 2004g)

Each of these accumulated assessments was made in the context of his original OEG surgical report thread, receiving sympathetic as well as grateful responses from other CareCure participants eager for material evidence regarding Huang's experimental therapy. While Handibob welcomed the increasing sensations he was feeling anew, Tim C. found his awakened nerve sensation unbearable. But as he pointed out, "KNOW news is better than NO news. . . . If it were me sitting on the sidelines while a steady flow of sci's soaked up Dr Huang's OEGs, I'd be devouring all progress info, positive or otherwise, like a shark in a feeding frenzy. Not sharing our true experiences does everyone here a disservice" (Tim C. 2004h).

Tim C. abandoned his OEG surgical report thread after these final posts in 2004, having definitively concluded that he had lost the "gamble" of OEG transplant. Several years later, he was no longer an active member of the Cure forum, noting, "I'm so sick of logging on here for 13 years to see a lot, a lot of nothing. Really depressing" (Tim C. 2015). But he continued to peruse and post elsewhere on CareCure, making contributions instead to the Pain, Care, Caregiving, and Life forums. While the OEG experiment failed him, the experiment in cybersociality remained a success for Tim C.

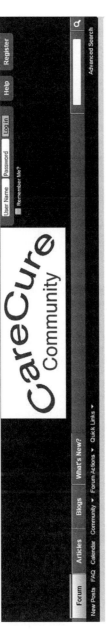
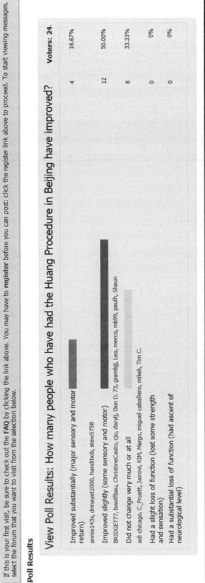

Figure 8.1. Screenshot of CareCure poll results: "How many people who have had the Huang Procedure in Beijing have improved?" (http://sci.rutgers.edu/forum/poll.php?pollid=736&do=showresults, accessed May 30, 2014).

POST-SURGICAL TRAJECTORY #3: UTRECHT MUSINGS

In discussing post-surgical results and assessments from the perspective of patients, I have thus far mainly focused on the surgical report threads of the Care-Cure fetal cell pioneers. This is no coincidence. As I discussed in chapter 3, the chronic nature of SCI enables CareCure members to engage in ongoing discussions of experimental therapy within the context of a robust and stable online community. ALS patients face a much more urgent timeline, with rapid neurodegeneration of their motor neurons often foreclosing their ability to maintain an online record of their post-surgical results.

But there have been a few exceptions. Although the disease claims most of its victims within three to five years after diagnosis, some live for a much longer time—most notably British physicist Stephen Hawking, who was diagnosed with ALS when he was twenty-one and has continued to have a celebrated career at the University of Cambridge over the past half century (Harmon 2012). Among the Dutch OEG fetal cell recipients, Loes Claerhoudt continued blogging for over a decade following her trip to China. As I discussed in chapter 3, Loes initiated her blog in January 2005 as a way to document her experimental surgical experiences in Beijing and keep in touch with friends and family members back home in Utrecht. She summed up her first intense month of blogging from abroad with an assessment of her postoperative condition:

> Re-measuring my lung function was also exciting (because it's so important!) To our delight, it confirmed my own feeling and perception. Soon after surgery (almost two weeks ago), I was able to breathe easier, had more air, no longer coughed and coughed and was not immediately out of breath after exertion. There was significant (some to quite some) progress on all parts (the test included six). And also the personal (and subjective) observation of the doctor was: "You breathe much easier, it costs you less trouble than before the operation." I am so pleased with this!!! The lung capacity must (and can) increase further in the coming months by building up my fitness. That also applies to the use and strength of my arms and legs. Walking, as I said earlier, has improved, but not spectacular yet. And progress in my arms has so far been marginal. But also that can be better targeted with therapy in the Netherlands, said the Chinese doctors. All in all, we left the hospital satisfied and grateful. Our efforts and those of everyone who has in any way supported us have turned out not to be in vain. Rather, we are delighted that we have been here! They were, let's be honest about it, heavy weeks. Everyone will understand that. You are in a different, very small world, almost 24 hours a day working on a mission: for God's sake let us come out better than before we came in. (Loes Claerhoudt 2005d)

Loes dedicated her initial posts following the experimental surgery to documenting her rehabilitation regimen and signs of bodily change. But as she moved further away from the monthlong liminal Beijing experience, her focus began to shift to other areas of her life. Apologizing for not updating her blog as frequently as she intended, she explained:

> Once again later than I intended, I am writing this blog post. There are several reasons for this. Life just continues after China. That's a good thing, of course. I immediately think of Patrick, who died a few weeks after returning, and also to the Englishwoman Barbara. She returned back home in a coma but has unfortunately died meanwhile. So that life goes on is a great thing, but also very annoying really. Trying to keep the household running, the boys' school work, the renovations, Harry who is back to working full-time again, and not to forget my [newspaper] columns. I also have to rehabilitate (that word still sounds good coming from my mouth!). That means practicing with my hands and arms, my feet and legs. I do this twice a week in the rehabilitation center. There, the practice goes well because the therapists accompany me. How they should exactly do that, is also new for them however. They and I don't know whether what we do is right. If my left arm deteriorates (which is the case), then we do not know whether this is due to lack of exercise, or the disease. I fear the latter, and that's also the second major reason that I'm not so eager to write: I just have a hard time dealing with it. (Loes Claerhoudt 2005e)

As the months and years stretched out from her experimental treatment in Beijing, the blog ultimately became a platform for her to describe her everyday experiences living with ALS—as well as everything else, including her thoughts on the Syrian refugee crisis affecting her hometown. Dreading a quick death, she instead suffered a slow decline over sixteen years. She mused about this unexpected timeline in one of her final blog posts before her death in October 2015:

> It's good that everyone can imagine the nightmare in which an ALS patient is ended up permanently. Just about all your muscles fail until death follows. Usually within a few years, but sometimes it takes longer. So I have lived for already sixteen years in that bad dream. "I'm glad that even so you still have so many years," I hear regularly. And that is true of course. The growing up of my children, for instance, I had never wanted to miss. As well as numerous other large and small events. But there is also a flipside. If I had foreseen that I would have lived this long, I would have perhaps done everything differently. (Loes Claerhoudt 2015b)

CONCLUSION

The fetal cell recipients' digitally mediated biomedical odysseys illuminate the ethnographic contours of hope in the face of devastating disability. The examples I have discussed in the preceding pages exemplify the potential of interactive online mediation for creating new forms of sociality and modes of knowledge production. For CareCure members connected to their virtual community by "the umbilical cord to hope and recovery," the online surgery report threads enabled them to become not only individual patients seeking to heal their own bodies but also contributors to the scientific quest for a cure. Although the exigencies of rapid neurodegeneration cut short the ability of many PALS to contribute to ongoing analyses of efficacy, the drive of OEG fetal cell recipients to document their experiences on public blogs stands as a testament to the importance of emerging modes of knowledge production.

The Beijing OEG surgery report threads and ALS blogs represent a different form of peer-reviewed, expert-mediated evidence—a digitally mediated "i-witnessing" based literally on the sweat of members who had gone to China. Unable to perspire below their neurological level of injury, many CareCure pioneers discovered that the OEG surgery enabled them to begin sweating for the first time since their injuries. A seemingly minor change, this small miracle enabled them to regulate their internal body temperatures—which meant they could now enjoy summertime barbecues with their families or watch their daughters' outdoor baseball games. As Handibob exclaimed several months after returning from Beijing as he sat at home in the sun without his shirt on: "I was perspiring everywhere I could touch, my belly my sides my back, even my armpits, WOW. This makes such a difference in keeping cool cause I live on a canal by a lake and I love to be in the sun, so this is awesome" (Handibob 2004c). The OEG pioneers' hard-earned sweat (together with other symbols of their guinea pig status) transformed these ordinary "lay" members of the CareCure community into experts who submitted their experience to their peers for support and examination.

These forms of "i-witnessing" reveal the crucial role of online discussion forums and blogs in mediating experiences of experimental surgery. As the post-and-reply format of the OEG surgical report threads highlight, the effectiveness of the experimental procedure was not just a singular physical event but instead a co-constructed, ongoing process that involved the visceral experiences of the fetal cell recipient and the meta-commentary of an online readership. In his detailed account of the transformation of AIDS research by social activism during the 1980s, Steven Epstein (1996) documented how the conversion of patients into activist-experts fundamentally changed the rules of engagement in biomedical research, from the interpretation of scientific results to the conduct of science itself. Empowered by digital communication technologies that transcend national boundaries, OEG fetal cell recipients in the new millennium are changing the scope of what counts as credible evidence as they pursue experimental medicine from cyberspace to China.

ON THE CUTTING EDGE

THE CLINICIANS AND PATIENTS WE have followed in the preceding eight chapters provide multiple perspectives on how hope intertwines with technology, travel, and the political economies of health care and medical research in a global era. The Chinese fetal cell therapies at the heart of these encounters open up important questions about the contours of experimentality and the possibilities for hope on the "cutting edge" of regenerative medicine. In order to address these questions, I return to the metaphor of "cutting edge" invoked at the beginning of this book to highlight the three ways this notion has framed my analysis.

The entrepreneurial spirit of technoscientific innovation is the dominant thread tying together the emerging practices coalescing around new information and biomedical technologies that I charted in Chinese hospital wards, laboratories, and blogs. As one CareCure member speculated, online patient forums could be read as an experiment in social organization and knowledge production, a novel attempt to jump-start scientific innovation by expanding engagement with information on a transnational scale. Through CareCure, people living with spinal cord injuries had a public platform to challenge prognoses, discuss the latest advances in clinical research, and investigate new nodes of experimental activity occurring around the world. Through authoring their own personal blogs or poaching threads on other forums, people living with ALS and other neurodegenerative conditions could reach out to an unprecedented network of others grappling with similar medical diagnoses, generate social and financial support, and cultivate new forms of documentation and symptom tracking online. OEG fetal cell recipients also placed themselves on the front lines of biomedical innovation by bodily engaging the experimental process of translating laboratory findings into novel forms of care. Some even joked about their status as "laboratory rats," acknowledging and even embracing the experimental as a new way of life. This understanding of "cutting edge" as scientific innovation also encompasses the self-promoting narrative invoked by Chinese clinician-scientists eager for renown and profit, the directives promulgated by government officials obsessed with bolstering economic development and patriotic pride, and the relentless logic driving the global expansion of medicine as a profit-making enterprise that I documented in the second part of the book.

While scientific advancement might be the ascendant framework for understanding cutting-edge fetal cell transplantation, the embodied experience of cross-cultural surgical intervention also forms an important part of this story of clinical experimentation. In this second sense, the notion of "cutting edge" ceases to be a metaphor when it comes down to visceral workings of surgical procedures. The slicing of a neurosurgeon's scalpel, the force of a drill bit boring into a human skull, the bodily incorporation of cells from aborted fetuses, and the punishing toll of international travel for people living with neurodegenerative disorders all provide important correctives to proclamations of a biomedical revolution of seamless information flow and transnational circulation. Online patient forums such as CareCure facilitate greater awareness of and access to potential therapies around the world, but these experimental forms of knowledge production and consumption cannot replace the embodied experience of undergoing risky operations in unfamiliar countries. The visceral "i-witnessing" of CareCure pioneers such as Handibob and Leo undergirds the legitimacy and credibility of their "blow-by-blow" online reports.

Following a third analytical trajectory, the "cutting edge" metaphor also alludes to the borderline nature of experimental activity occurring at the frontiers of ethics and legality. As I have documented throughout the book, Chinese clinicians and their foreign patients sought to leverage geopolitical differences in cultural, legal, and ethical norms to produce new horizons of hope for treating incurable neurological disorders. In pursuing regenerative therapies abroad, patients actively circumvented the regulatory restrictions and ethical qualms stymieing research efforts in their home countries. Their Chinese clinicians have taken advantage of these differences to capitalize on biological potentiality to sell reimagined futures, as the growing number of clinics offering experimental stem and fetal cell therapies in China attests. Yet as the changing fortunes of the New Century neurosurgical enterprise demonstrate, China is not what Western journalists have all too easily written off as the freewheeling and "morally bankrupt 'Wild East' of biology" (Dennis 2002, 335). Responding to a rapidly shifting regulatory landscape, Dr. Huang and his hospital staff members had to experiment with new institutional tactics in order to sidestep bureaucratic obstacles and keep their operation afloat. Strategically finessing bioethical universalism, these Chinese neurosurgeons also challenged blanket assumptions about clinical research design and developed new ethical guidelines to recalibrate the uneasy line between scientific innovation and medical quackery. Taken together, these three analytical approaches provide us with a more nuanced perspective for understanding the significance of hope and experiment on the "cutting edge" of regenerative medicine.

CHARTING THE FRONTIERS OF HOPE

Throughout the book, I have documented the ways in which the proliferating hopes generated by regenerative medicine are refracted by the grounded realities of experimental life. In these experimental contexts, hope operates as a temporal hedge against uncertainties of both biological and political natures, enabling patients and clinicians to suspend diagnostic death sentences, deflect bureaucratic arbitrariness, and perpetuate possibilities for the future. This approach provides a more nuanced understanding of the hope for cure and care on the part of the patients and their families, as well as the hope of Chinese medical entrepreneurs in achieving personal, financial, scientific, and national ambitions. Poised on the cutting edge—in the triple sense of the phrase—Chinese neurosurgeons and their foreign patients reveal the complex ways in which hope took flight in virtual forums, adhered on Chinese operating tables, and sedimented into post-surgical regimens of bodily care and maintenance.

Mobilized by virtual discussions about the potential of regenerative medicine in China, people from around the world arrived in Beijing to confront the practical logistics of navigating power wheelchairs between narrow door frames, the frustrations (and occasional mirth) generated by cross-cultural miscommunications, and other challenges of undergoing experimental medical treatment in a foreign country. Despite these ordeals, most of the patients and caregivers I encountered during their treatment in Beijing were infused with excitement about undergoing a potentially revolutionary procedure and meeting others on similar biomedical odysseys. I have described these journeys elsewhere as "biotech pilgrimages" (Song 2010). The liminal space and unique social configuration of the New Century Neurological Disorders Research and Treatment Center enabled like-minded people from around the world to gather together to compare notes about their experiences and challenge existing medical dogma. Patients emerged transformed from the operating theater, literally embodying their hope in fetal cells to change the course of their lives.

But the flush of optimism that had driven their transnational quests for therapy often began to fade after they returned home. While some such as Handibob and Loes Claerhoudt continued to document their bodily disposition for months and even years after the experimental procedure, others stopped updating their blogs or posting regular progress reports on CareCure. Giddy dreams about walking ultimately gave way to small incremental changes in functional abilities and the hard work of arduous exercise regimens.

The Chinese clinicians also dwelled in the gaps between expectation and reality generated by experimental activity. Driven by technonationalist dreams, Dr. Huang envisioned making a Nobel Prize–winning advance that would enshrine his legacy to his country and profession by transforming medical dogma about the irreversibility of neurological degeneration. Meanwhile, his clinical staff and trainees anticipated an institutional pathway to professional success, a lucrative source of income, and even a coveted Beijing residency permit. But their extravagant dreams for themselves and the experimental clinic adjusted in the process of encountering unpredictable regulatory regimes, the logistical challenges of tracking down clinical data to substantiate their claims, and the arduous demands of caring for patients suffering from rapid neurological degeneration.

Although the OEG transplantation offered tantalizing glimpses of better futures for both patients and their Chinese clinicians, this experimental therapy ultimately was no magic bullet. But this does not mean that these encounters at the cutting edge of regenerative medicine should be dismissed, even for those who deemed the Chinese therapy a failure. As Jeff, the Colorado firefighter with ALS who received OEG surgery in 2004, posted on his fire company's website a few months after returning home from Beijing:

> My fear is to take away hope from others but the fact is that I cannot honestly say that I experienced any measurable improvement. Additionally the trip was pretty difficult on me; the food, travel, time change. Despite what I have said in the two previous sentences, I am glad I went for two reasons. One, because it is about the fight for me. The doctors say to roll over and prepare to die and that is not an option for me. Secondly, we were blessed with a community and friends who raised the money for our trip, relieving us of the financial burden.

Despite his disappointment in the results of the fetal cell transplantation, Jeff's explanation points to the larger significance that his China trip held for him. As he declared elsewhere on his blog: "Remember, I have ALS, an incurable disease and it is as much about the fight as it is about winning. Someday there will be a cure and I am just trying to hang around until it's found." Although the Chinese fetal cell therapy ultimately did not help Jeff, it was part of the broader "fight for me" that transformed his family, colleagues, and community. Over a decade after Jeff's death, the members of Castle Rock United Fire Fighters Local 4116 continue to raise thousands of dollars each year through their "Fill the Boot" fund-raising campaigns for the Muscular Dystrophy Association.

This desire for agency and control in the aftermath of life-shattering diagnoses was one of the most important commonalities among the diverse group of patients, family members, and clinicians I met online and in Beijing. Faced with the limits of conventional medical dogma, they refused to acquiesce to resignation and hopelessness. Their affective orientation toward life and action offers us a powerful corrective to oversimplified narratives of exploitation and quackery that characterize media coverage of experimental fetal cell therapies. While some outside observers have dismissed these desires as "false hope," Jeff's explanation explodes the paternalistic assumptions of these oversimplified critiques. It is easy enough for uninvolved bystanders to write off these fetal cell experiments as a simple matter of desperate patients duped by medical charlatans peddling false hope with their sham therapies. But a deeper ethnographic engagement shows us what it means to live in the wake of neurological catastrophes and the ways we can continue to care for those whose afflictions have been deemed incurable.

WHEN EXPERIMENTS FAIL

We must consider whether the vibrant hopes in alternative technology-enabled futures run the danger of becoming tyrannical, as an expanding experimental logic urges patients and their family members, doctors, and scientists into a never-ending quest for the latest medical advance over the next horizon. At what point can medicine no longer treat and we must instead turn to care? At what point does the quest for the cure end and the work of everyday care begin?

During my fieldwork at New Century Hospital, I encountered a handful of patients whose conditions markedly deteriorated following the surgery. Those with breathing complications, particularly ALS patients grappling with rapid neurodegeneration, faced an uphill battle simply negotiating the ordinary challenges of going to a foreign country. Difficult travel conditions, coupled with Beijing's air pollution, unfamiliar food, and strange surroundings, made even their presurgical hospital stay a challenging prospect. I observed Dr. Huang on multiple occasions refusing to operate on patients whose conditions he determined were not stable enough to withstand the surgery. He also continually refined his procedure in the hopes of improving the safety and enhancing the effectiveness of the cell transplantation. In order to mitigate complications for those with compromised breathing, for example, Dr. Huang decided to inject fetal cells under local anesthesia for ALS patients—the so-called "little surgeries" characterized by another New Century neurosurgeon. Yet despite these precautions, complications inevitably occurred—as with any medical procedure. While no one I know of died on the operating table, several patients required extensive post-surgical care, including a handful who were ultimately transferred to intensive care units at other hospitals.

Alfonso, the ALS patient from Spain accompanied by four generations of his family, had one of the worst outcomes I observed at New Century. He unfortunately never recovered his ability to breathe independently after slipping into a coma a few days following the fetal cell procedure. He spent several weeks on a ventilator in Beijing, ultimately requiring an emergency medical evacuation. The Spanish embassy arranged for a physician from Spain to assess his condition and accompany him on the long flight home. Dr. Jay, a New Century neurosurgeon who had been named by the appreciative wife of an American patient, also accompanied the comatose Alfonso and his family. Still fuming about the supercilious attitude of his counterpart, Dr. Jay told me that the Spanish doctor repeatedly questioned his competency: "Whenever I gave anything to the patient, he would ask: Have you disinfected it? Is this clean? In his mind, probably everything in China has not been disinfected . . . I felt very humiliated."[1] Working with foreign patients and communicating with their physicians over the previous several years had given Dr. Jay a more nuanced perspective on the relative strengths and merits of different health care systems:

> I really do not believe that foreign doctors are necessarily all good doctors, just like doctors in China are not necessarily all poorly skilled doctors. Of course there are poorly skilled doctors in China, but there are also doctors with more sophisticated medical skills. It's the same in America and Europe. Their overall level is probably higher, but there are also poorly skilled doctors there. In developed countries in Europe and America, their doctors are more dependent on instruments and equipment. Because their equipment is very advanced, they are even more dependent on these things for doing any kind of checking. . . . So when [foreign doctors] encounter more primitive things, like pinching the leather ball [of the manual ventilator], I think they are not very smooth-handed.[2]

When it came down to the practicalities of caring for Alfonso on the twelve-hour flight home, Dr. Jay noted that the Spanish doctor failed in the most basic responsibilities:

> [The Spanish doctor] probably doesn't do much [manual ventilator] pumping in Spain; in developed countries they are used to using machines, but [in China] we often have to do it ourselves. When [the Spanish doctor] was pinching [the ventilator ball], he in fact wasn't very skilled . . . I watched him and he was pinching completely opposite to the patient. When the patient exhaled he pinched, and when the patient breathed he released [the ball]. So every time he pinched, the patient's son looked extremely nervous [and] had to keep wiping away his father's sweat. Because the patient was suffering, I was afraid to let [the Spanish doctor] pinch anymore. I told him, never mind, I'll do it myself. . . . When I left [Spain], the patient's family kept saying, "Chinese doctors are very good, Spanish doctors are not good."[3]

Instead of taking turns with his Spanish counterpart on the long transcontinental flight, Dr. Jay took over the hard work of pumping the hand-operated ventilator to keep Alfonso alive. Despite their dismay over the failure of the experimental surgery, Alfonso's family gratefully acknowledged the dedication of Dr. Jay and the other Chinese clinic staff who provided around-the-clock care for their loved one. The hard work of caring remained long after technoscientific advances had failed Alfonso.

BEYOND EXPERIMENT?

This book has documented the initial years of Huang Hongyun's neurosurgical enterprise, cataloguing the experiences of clinicians, patients, and family members during the heyday of domestic and international interest in his potential breakthrough therapy for neural repair.[4] Marked by an explicit orientation toward the experimental, this period captures the complex ways in which hope is produced and troubled online and through bodily engagements with emerging therapies transpiring on the cutting edge of medicine.

Dr. Huang's more recent efforts have focused on moving his therapeutic innovations out of the realm of the experimental and into the textbooks of established medical practice. He coined the term "neurorestoratology" in 2009, an awkward neologism in English that is more succinctly expressed in Chinese as "the study of neural repair/restoration" (神经修复学 *shénjīng xiūfù xué*). While Dr. Huang and his collaborators initially described neurorestoratology as one of the branch subjects of neuroscience on par with neurology and neurosurgery (figure 9.1) (Chen and Huang 2009), a few years later they were proclaiming this "newborn and emerging distinct discipline of the neuroscience family" as the "cross-point of all related disciplines" (figure 9.2) including neurosurgery, ophthalmology, pediatrics, physiotherapy, psychology, and even hyperbaric oxygenation and traditional Chinese medical science (Huang, Chen, and Sanberg 2012, S3, S5). From a side branch to the very center of the medical universe: the visual imagery is telling.

Dr. Huang and his colleagues provided legitimacy for this new field by establishing the International Association of Neurorestoratology (IANR), a medical society comprised of scientists and clinicians from around the world. With an ostensibly global platform that extended beyond any single clinical enterprise, the founding members of the association proceeded to organize annual conferences on neurorestoratology in different locations around the world (to date in Beijing, Amman, Bucharest, and Mumbai) featuring prominent researchers. They further bolstered their credibility and legitimacy by negotiating special issues and formal partnerships with scientific journals such as *Cell Transplantation: The Regenerative Medicine Journal* and ultimately establishing their own peer-reviewed, English-language *Journal of Neurorestoratology* as well as the *American Journal of Neuroprotection and Neuroregeneration*.

In tandem with his newly established "frontier discipline of the twenty-first century," Dr. Huang moved to yet another medical institution in 2011, partnering with a hospital in neighboring Hebei province beyond the scrutiny of Beijing's health officials. Although he faced increasingly stringent regulations in China's capital city, Dr. Huang explained his move according to a more palatable logic. On a practical level, Dr. Huang noted that New Century Hospital was undergoing extensive renovations to remodel itself into a premier rehabilitation facility, so it would not be a conducive location for foreign patients unaccustomed to the grime and noise of Chinese construction projects. More important, Dr. Huang emphasized that his new institutional home in Hebei province enabled him to establish a dedicated Neurological Center for carrying out what he called "Second Generation Comprehensive Neurorestoratology Therapy (version 2.0 or 2G-CNT), a multi-cell, multi-route, multi-process [in]

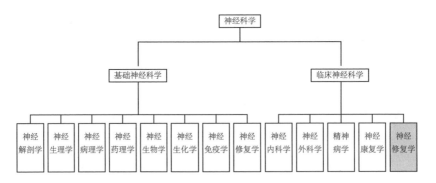

Figure 9.1. Neurorestoratology as a "branch subject of neuroscience" (Chen and Huang 2009, 367).

combination with multi-treatments" designed to achieve the best clinical out-come in conjunction with a 150-bed VIP ward (Huang 2014).

A cocktail of different cells delivered in multiple ways to multiple sites in the body accompanied by an assortment of postoperative supporting therapies, this revamped treatment protocol was touted by Huang (2016) as "reach[ing] the largest and the most effective neurological restoration by multi-route cell implantation and the individual optimizing cellular combination." Purportedly tailored to "the personal medical status of each patient," this next-generation therapy offered a sharp contrast to Dr. Huang's original insistence on the pu-rified nasal cells that marked his credibility as a researcher and launched the experimental revolution that I have documented in this book.

While this new approach capitalizes on continued patient interest in stem cell advances, the hodgepodge assortment of cells, transplantation sites, and tech-niques has raised red flags for those seeking more concrete evidence and rigorous standards of proof. But for Dr. Huang, neural repair had become an established fact rather than an experimental question. In 2015, he released a two-volume English-language textbook: *Theories and Techniques of Neurorestoratology* (vol-ume 1) and *Clinical Progress of Neurorestoratology* (volume 2). Although these volumes were not published by a reputable academic publisher with a rigorous peer-review process, Dr. Huang sought to gain credibility by listing two of the most prominent and well-respected neuroscientists in Britain and the United States as coeditors. His textbook move sought to formalize neurorestoratology as an established discipline, catapulting his evolving clinical practice out of the questionable realm of experimental activity.

*   *   *

While the original surge of patients from CareCure has subsided, Dr. Huang has continued to operate on foreign patients from around the world suffering from an expanding list of neurological conditions. Since his move beyond the borders

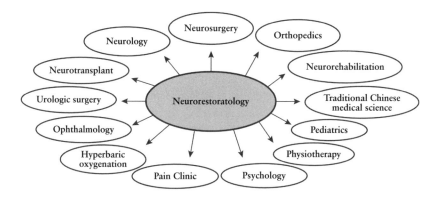

Figure 9.2. Neurorestoratology as the "cross-point of all related disciplines" (Huang, Chen, and Sanberg 2012, S5).

of Beijing, these patients have included a two-year-old girl from Romania with cerebral palsy, a nineteen-year-old woman from Indonesia with congenital spinal bifida, a forty-one-year-old man from Saudi Arabia suffering from neuropathic pain, and a fifty-year-old man from France with cerebellar ataxia, among dozens of other recipients of the next-generation neurorestoratology therapies.

Some of the New Century staff members chose to follow Dr. Huang out to Hebei, including Dr. Alan, Dr. Jay, and a few loyal neurosurgical trainees. Several others remained in Beijing to pursue alternative options: Dr. Huang's former second-in-command, Dr. Liang, completed his doctorate in neurosurgery and took a faculty position at a more stable university-affiliated hospital. My former acupuncturist roommate became a sales representative for a Japanese pharmaceutical company, parlaying her experience with foreign patients into a higher-paying career. Bird decided to give up a career in health care, flying back to Shanghai to explore new career directions.

Life ultimately ends, whether in planned-for or unexpected ways. But this does not preclude an enduring orientation to hope, care, and the future. Many of the fetal cell pioneers mentioned in the preceding pages died during the decade I have spent researching and writing this book: Jeff, the Colorado firefighter with ALS; Leo, the former mayor turned SCI cure crusader; Bob, the ship captain with ALS who joked about buying himself a coffin; Trophic, the American expatriate lawyer grappling with ALS in Russia; Loes Claerhoudt, the Dutch columnist with ALS who was able to see her children grow up. Their poignant yet grueling encounters with the experimental demand our acknowledgment of the complex ways in which hope endures online and through bodily engagements on the cutting edge of regenerative medicine.

The deaths that haunt this book—including the deaths of patients, the deaths of fetuses, the demise of medical institutions, and even the termination of particular forms of online communities and conversations—provide a more intricate texture to what might otherwise be a narrative of optimism. These darker overtones do not mean that these odysseys for regenerative medicine should be dismissed. Instead, these experiences show us how the metaphor of "cutting edge" central to the analytical framing of this book not only invokes the promise of scientific advancement and the embodied experience of surgical intervention but also illuminates the borderline nature of experimental activity occurring at the limits of ethics and legality.

GLOSSARY OF CHINESE TERMS

bàn shǒuxù　办手续	taking care of formalities; completing necessary procedures
Bǔnǎogāo　补脑膏	proprietary Chinese herbal medicine used by some ALS patients (literally, "mending brain ointment")
cābiānqiú　擦边球	edge ball (term used in Ping-Pong for a ball that lands at the edge of the table)
chī dàguōfàn　吃大锅饭	eating from the big pot (metaphor for egalitarianism)
chìjiǎo yīshēng　赤脚医生	barefoot doctors
chūzū kēshì　出租科室	lease a (hospital) department or ward
dài hóngmàozi　戴红帽子	red-hatting (tactic of private companies partnering with public enterprises to mask business activities)
dānwèi　单位	work unit
Dōngyà bìngfū　东亚病夫	sick man of East Asia
duōfā xìng yìnghuà　多发性硬化	multiple sclerosis
èrjí yīyuàn　二级医院	second-tier hospital
fùzhǔrèn yīshī　副主任医师	deputy director-level physician (the second-highest clinical rank for physicians)
gǎigé kāifàng　改革开放	Reform and Opening Up era (initiated by Deng Xiaoping in 1978)
gàn xìbāo　干细胞	stem cell
gāo gàn bìngfáng　高干病房	VIP wards for senior cadres or officials
gètǐhù　个体户	self-employed petty proprietor (literally, "one-body-household")
gòng jì shītiáo　共济失调	ataxia
gòujiàn shèhuì zhǔyì héxié shèhuì　构建社会主义和谐社会	build a socialist harmonious society (Hu Jintao's slogan)
guānxì　关系	social networks and relationships

guójiā shípǐn yàopǐn jiāndū guǎnlǐ jú 国家食品药品监督管理局	State Food and Drug Administration
hǎiguī 海归	Chinese returnees; homonym for "sea turtle" (literally, "return from the sea")
hóngbāo 红包	monetary gifts enclosed in red envelopes
huáqiáo 华侨	overseas Chinese
jīběn yīliáo fúwù 基本医疗服务	basic medical services
jī wěisuō cè suǒ yìnghuà 肌萎缩侧索硬化	amyotrophic lateral sclerosis (ALS)
jiǎ shǒushù 假手术	sham surgery
jiāxiāng 家乡	native place (hometown)
jīngjì tèqū 经济特区	Special Economic Zone (SEZ)
jìnxiū 进修	advanced studies
jìshù 技术	technology
jǐsuǐ sǔnshāng 脊髓损伤	spinal cord injury
jítǐ suǒyǒuzhì qǐyè 集体所有制企业	collectively owned enterprise
kējì 科技	science and technology
kēxué 科学	science
kēxué jìshù shì dì yī shēngchǎnlì 科学技术是第一生产力	science and technology are the primary forces of productivity (key concept from Marxism invoked by Deng Xiaoping)
kēxué jìshù xiàndàihuà 科学技术现代化	scientific and technological modernization
kòngbái duìzhào zu 空白对照组	blank comparison group (used in basic and clinical research studies to test safety and efficacy)
kuòdà fànwéi 扩大范围	enlarge the scope
liúchǎn 流产	abortion or miscarriage; the alternative term *duòtāi* 堕胎 refers specifically to abortion
luòhòu 落后	backward
mínbàn fēi qǐyè dānwèi 民办非企业单位	private non-enterprise work unit
mínbàn yīyuàn 民办医院	private hospital
nǎo xìng tānhuàn 脑性瘫痪	cerebral palsy
pēitāi 胚胎	fetus

píngfēn 评分		assigning points; evaluation or appraisal
ràng yībùfèn rén xiān fù qǐlái 让一部分人先富起来		let some get rich first (Deng Xiaoping's slogan)
sānjiǎ yīyuàn 三甲医院		top tertiary care hospital (the highest rank designated by the Ministry of Health)
shèhuì zhǔyì xiàndàihuà 社会主义现代化		socialist modernization
shénjīng xiūfù xué 神经修复学		neurorestoratology (term coined by Huang Hongyun to describe the study of neural repair and neurological restoration)
shìchǎng huà 市场化		marketization
shí shì qiú shì 实事求是		seek truth from facts (Chinese proverb quoted by Mao Zedong and Deng Xiaoping)
sì gè xiàndàihuà 四个现代化		Four Modernizations (agriculture, industry, science and technology, and defense)
sì jiù 四旧		Four Olds (old ideas, old culture, old customs, old habits)
suífǎng 随访		follow-up (on a patient)
tānguān wū lì 贪官污吏		corrupt officials
tèxū ménzhěn 特需门诊		"special needs" (VIP) outpatient centers
wàibāo kēshì 外包科室		outsource a (hospital) department
wèi guó zhēngguāng 为国争光		winning glory for the country
wèi rénmín fúwù 为人民服务		serve the people (slogan attributed to Mao Zedong)
wèishēng 卫生		health; hygiene; sanitation
wèishēng gǎigé 卫生改革		health reform
xiùqiào xìbāo yízhí zhìliáo 嗅鞘细胞移植治疗		olfactory ensheathing glial cell transplantation therapy
yīliáo 医疗		medical treatment
yǐnchǎn 引产		induction of labor by artificial means to stimulate uterine contractions
yī shān nán róng èr hǔ 一山难容二虎		one mountain cannot tolerate two tigers
yǒu zhòng guó tèsè de shèhuì zhǔyì 有中国特色的社会主义		socialism with Chinese characteristics
yuàn zhōng yuàn 院中院		hospital within a hospital
zhìfù guāngróng 致富光荣		getting rich is glorious (slogan attributed to Deng Xiaoping)

zhōngguó mèng　中国梦	Chinese dream (slogan attributed to Xi Jinping)
zhōngguó rénmín jiěfàngjūn　中国人民解放军	People's Liberation Army (PLA)
zhōngshū shénjīng xìtǒng jíbìng　中枢神经系统疾病	central nervous system disease
zhǔrèn　主任	director (an administrative appointment indicating a leadership role)
zhǔrèn yīshī　主任医师	director-level physician (the highest clinical rank for a physician)
zhùyuàn yīshī　住院医师	resident physician
zhǔzhì yīshī　主治医师	attending physician
zìzhǔ chuàngxīn　自主创新	independent innovation
zìzhǔ quán　自主权	autonomy
zǒu zī pài　走资派	capitalist roaders

NOTES

CHAPTER 1: INTRODUCTION

1. I have substituted pseudonyms for many of the patients, family members, medical personnel, and medical institutions mentioned in this book, depending upon the need to protect their privacy. In Jeff's case, his widow, Cyrilla, gave me permission to feature his story. For those patients and family members who have posted public accounts of their experience online or have been featured in the news, I cite their names as they appear in these publicly accessible sources and provide citations to link back to the original sources. At his request, I refer to the central Chinese neurosurgeon, Dr. Huang Hongyun, by his actual name.

2. There has been some dispute over the cause of Mao's death in 1976. In the final years of his life, he suffered from numerous health complications including congestive heart failure, a series of heart attacks, emphysema, and neurodegenerative disease (Li 1994, 26–27). Foreign media outlets such as the *New York Times* reported that he had died from complications related to Parkinson's disease, but the Chinese government never issued an official statement regarding the cause of death. Mao's personal physician, Li Zhisui, unequivocally describes Mao's neurological deterioration as the result of ALS, detailing his consultations with neurological experts in his controversial biography of China's paramount leader (1994, 581–83).

3. The price of the drug dropped from thousands to hundreds of dollars for a month-long supply when Sanofi's patent for Rilutek expired in 2013 and the U.S. Food and Drug Administration granted approval to several companies to market generic versions of the drug riluzole (Madsen 2013). But few of the ALS patients featured in this book have been able to benefit from this price drop; most have already passed away.

4. Scholars working at the intersections of medical anthropology and science studies have explored how these new biotechnologies are reconfiguring the boundaries between life and death (Lock 2002; Franklin and Lock 2003) and producing new sociopolitical formations enmeshed in market logics and speculative capitalism (Sunder Rajan 2006; Rose 2007; Helmreich 2008; Fortun 2008; Petryna 2009). While much of this work has focused on scientific developments in the United States and Europe, a growing number of anthropologists are examining the specific dynamics engendered by "Asian biotech" in the context of decidedly illiberal authoritarian states (Ong and Chen 2010) and divergent "frameworks of choice" (Sleeboom-Faulkner 2010). My book contributes to this scholarship by examining the social, moral, and politico-economic implications of experimental biotechnology in a new transnational context: the quest for fetal and stem cell therapies extending from online discussion forums to entrepreneurial medical clinics located in urban China.

5. Drawing on a Foucauldian framework to explore the role of the new sciences in re-shaping biopolitical subjectivity, Paul Rabinow (1996, 1999) articulates the concept of "biosociality" to emphasize how new social groupings are now orienting around genetic information. Other social scientists have emphasized the social welfare benefits and political entitlements accorded by membership in these newly con-stituted groups, examining the ways in which "biological citizens" draw upon their bodily status to make specific claims on the state (Petryna 2002; Rose 2007). An explosion of research has turned a critical eye on the biological reification of race in the post-genomic era, highlighting the unintended consequences of attempt-ing to achieve diversity in medical research (Lee, Mountain, and Koenig 2001; Epstein 2007; Fullwiley 2008), the dangers of "bioethnic conscription" in targeting specific ethnic groups for genetic research studies (Montoya 2008), the problem-atic assumptions and inferences made by genetic ancestry tests targeting African Americans (Rotimi 2003; Palmié 2007; Bolnick et al. 2007), and the pitfalls of using genetic data to mediate tribal membership claims (TallBear 2013; Bardill 2014).

6. Hannah Landecker, one of the first social scientists to recognize the importance of the cell despite the dominance of scientific narratives of the gene, has taken a dif-ferent approach to these issues that deemphasizes the human. Landecker's (2007) pathbreaking history of cellular biotechnologies examines the ramifications of var-ious techniques (such as cryobiology and cell synchrony) that transformed living cells into technoscientific objects, fundamentally altering what it is to be biological.

7. Although excitement surrounding stem cell advances has skyrocketed in recent years, research in regenerative medicine has a long-established history. Historian Jane Maienschein (2009, 2011) reminds us about developments since the beginning of the twentieth century in embryology, biology, and transplantation that long pre-date the current hype. The prestigious journal *Science* designated the cultivation of human embryonic stem cells as "Breakthrough of the Year" in 1999 (Vogel 1999), but the concept of a "stem cell" was deployed decades earlier as scientists tried to understand a grotesque kind of malignant tumor known as a teratocarcinoma (Pierce 1974; Sherman and Solter 1975; Andrews 2002). Arising spontaneously from germ line cells (male testes and female ovaries) in both mice and humans, this type of cancer generate tumors that contain a variety of cell types, including bone, cartilage, muscle, and brain, and even whole structures such as teeth. Unlike most tumors, in which the proliferating cells tend to remain undifferentiated, ter-atocarcinoma cells have the capacity to become many different types of tissues. By isolating cells from these tumors and growing them in petri dishes, scientists dis-covered that a single cell could give rise to all of the diverse cell types present in the tumor while continuing to regenerate themselves—crucial "stem-ness" properties that characterize early embryonic cells. Cultured cells isolated from teratocarci-nomas were thus called embryonal carcinoma cells. In her sociohistory of cancer oncogene research, sociologist Joan Fujimura describes the work on teratocarcino-mas as "outlier research" that ultimately "did not generate doable problems" (1996, 149–50)—that is, successful cancer research projects that were taken up by scien-tists and encouraged by funding agencies. Because these tumors did not involve changes in DNA, biologists could not explain them in genetic terms. Work on and interest in these tumors was thus relegated to the back burner as researchers, grant

administrators, government officials, clinicians, and patients jumped on the genetic "bandwagon" (Fujimura 1996, 2). Ironically, "epigenetic" research has become one of the hottest topics in biology today as scientists and others look beyond the gene for new solutions to pressing problems.

8. All stem cells can both replicate themselves and give rise to other cell types, but they differ in their capacity to differentiate. As their name indicates, embryonic stem cells are derived from early stage embryos just a few days after fertilization (when the zygote or fertilized egg has developed into a ball of cells known as a blastocyst). Embryonic stem cells theoretically offer the most hope for clinical application since they are capable of giving rise to any of the cells that make up the body. The cultivation of human embryonic stem cells from the start has been understood in terms of their potential not just for understanding human developmental biology but for transforming drug discovery and transplantation medicine (Thomson et al. 1998). But this biological potentiality has a dark underside: the spontaneous and uncontrolled differentiation of embryonic stem cells can lead to the formation of tumors. One of the biggest hurdles for embryonic stem cell researchers is controlling the differentiation process in order to produce the specific desired cell type.

   Given these challenges at the basic science level, most experimental stem cell therapies have focused on adult stem cells, which specialize in the generation of a smaller range of cells usually limited to the tissue type in which the adult stem cell is located. The term "adult" is somewhat of a misnomer, since these cells can also be derived from later-stage embryos or fetuses. The most common type of stem cell offered as therapy in China are hematopoietic (blood-forming) adult stem cells (Liao, Li, and Zhao 2007). These pluripotent cells are present in small quantities in umbilical cord blood as well as bone marrow, and they give rise to red and white blood cells, platelets, and other blood and immune cells. Because research with adult stem cells does not require the destruction of human embryos, political and religious conservatives have seized upon this form of research as morally desirable. Some Chinese clinics are capitalizing on the "ethically friendly" nature of hematopoietic stem cells as a key selling point for their experimental treatments while avoiding questions about the extent of these cells' biological "pluripotentiality" (Song 2011). Although these adult stem cells may be more "ethical" with respect to the human embryo, their biological properties and broader utility for regenerative medicine have been heavily contested within the scientific community. Some researchers have claimed that these adult progenitor cells can produce the differentiated cells of another tissue type (Bjornson et al. 1999; Lagasse et al. 2000; Krause et al. 2001), while others have raised serious concerns about whether and to what extent these adult stem cells can in fact "transdifferentiate" (Anderson, Gage, and Weissman 2001; Abkowitz 2002; Schwartz 2006).

9. Anthropologists have also examined the role of hope in a variety of other domains, most notably in Monique Nuijten's (2003) analysis of the Mexican state as a "hope-generating machine" for its peasant citizens, Vincent Crapanzano's (2004) discussion of "paralyzing hope" among white South Africans just before the end of apartheid (in contrast to more conventional understandings of hope as an active form of optimism oriented toward social action), and Hirokazu Miyazaki's (2004) focus on hope as a method of self-knowledge in evidential practices ranging from

compensation petitions by dispossessed Fijians to anthropological theory building. These approaches highlight the temporal dimensions of hope in generating desires about the future (Bloch 1986 [1959]).

10. Sunder Rajan (2006) demonstrates how these modes of "speculative capitalism" take on specific forms in different settings: while the promise of biocapital in the United States manifests itself as salvation and redemption for individuals and corporations, the Indian narrative highlights the nationalistic role of biotechnology in developing India as a global player in a postcolonial world.

11. Disappointment and failure also form an integral part of these "promissory horizons" in biomedicine and biotechnology. In exploring the "knowledge economy of expectations," sociologist Nik Brown (2003) traces the dynamic relationship between hyperexpectations and emerging disappointments characterizing the biotechnology revolution. Brown documents the costs of inflated promises for individual patients, whole populations, and even science itself. Anthropologist Cheryl Mattingly (2010) directs our attention to how hope is generated in the context of bleak prognoses and difficult life circumstances. Recognizing the everyday constraints posed by poverty, racism, and bodily suffering, Mattingly draws on Cornell West's (2008) evocative term "blues hope" to capture the paradoxical oppression and anticipation embodied in the African American experience. For Mattingly, the struggle for hope emerges as a "paradoxical temporal practice and a strenuous moral project" (2010, 3) produced discursively through specific narrative acts that shape the uneven processes of healing for a group of African American families seeking care for their chronically ill children. Anthropologists Karen-Sue Taussig, Klaus Hoeyer, and Stefan Helmreich (2013) have also highlighted the underside of hope embedded in biomedicine. Addressing not just the anticipation but also the anxiety generated by advances in the life sciences, these anthropologists have proposed using the term "potentiality" as both a key analytic and object of study for investigating utopian and dystopian visions about the promises and dangers of biomedical interventions.

12. See Salter and Salter 2007 and EuroStemCell 2014 for an overview of regulations governing stem cell research in various European countries.

13. In tracing the normalization of stem cell research in the United States over the past decade, sociologist Charis Thompson (2013) describes the "ethical choreography" that allowed stem cell research to proceed despite controversies surrounding the moral status of the embryo. Thompson notes that scientists have been able to "invent around ethical roadblocks" (2013, 5) to continue innovative work even in restrictive environments. One of the most stunning "invent-arounds" involved bypassing embryos altogether: the Nobel Prize–winning research on induced pluripotent stem (iPS) cells by Japanese scientist Shinya Yamanaka demonstrated that mature adult cells could be reprogrammed to behave like stem cells that can transdifferentiate into other cells (Takahashi and Yamanaka 2006; Takahashi et al. 2007). This development was framed as both an ethical and a biological breakthrough: researchers could avoid the ethical controversies surrounding the destruction of human embryos while simultaneously producing patient- and disease-specific cell lines. Despite the continuation of research efforts coupled with funding initiatives on the part of private philanthropic organizations and individual states such as

California, the prevailing popular rhetoric has continued to invoke fears of a "brain drain" and an American loss of competitiveness in the global science race.

14. While my research examines the clinical applications of stem and fetal cell research, Joy Zhang (2012) has focused on the basic science side of stem cell research in China. Zhang shows that stem cell research has so far failed to develop robustly in China because of "the conflict between a cosmopolitan prospect and China's conventional research environment" (2012, 107).

15. A growing body of recent scholarship has examined the rise of stem cell research and clinical applications throughout Asia, largely spearheaded by European social scientists. The most significant work has emerged from Margaret Sleeboom-Faulkner's multiyear initiative on "Bionetworking in Asia" at the University of Sussex, which has produced over a dozen articles featuring case studies from China (Rosemann 2013; Sui and Sleeboom-Faulkner 2015), India (Patra and Sleeboom-Faulkner 2013), Japan (Sleeboom-Faulkner 2011), and South Korea (Hwang and Sleeboom-Faulkner 2014), as well as cross-national comparisons (Sleeboom-Faulkner and Hwang 2012; Sleeboom-Faulkner et al. 2016). This work has been augmented by the BIONET (2010) project, a consortium of social scientists, bioethicists, scientists, and policymakers from China and Europe seeking to establish a set of best practices in the ethical governance of Sino-European life science research collaborations. Sociologist Joy Yueyue Zhang's (2012) monograph offers the only book-length treatment of stem cell research in China to date, drawing on interviews with scientists and regulators to illustrate the disjuncture between scientists' emerging cosmopolitan outlook and the structural constraints of China's conventional research environment. My book provides an important complement to this scholarship by addressing how these biotechnologies are translated from the lab to the clinical context. I leverage an ethnographic perspective based on long-term, situated fieldwork in order to show how stem and fetal cell therapies are humanized through poignant quests for a cure while becoming entangled in entrepreneurial frameworks of market medicine and global science.

16. While I focus on biomedical doctors in urban China, anthropologist Judith Farquhar (1996) has traced the ramifications of these politico-economic changes for traditional Chinese medical physicians operating private storefront clinics in a rural north China county town.

17. Leading scholars of contemporary China have examined both of these trends in ethnographic detail. In their edited volume *Privatizing China: Socialism from Afar*, Li Zhang and Aihwa Ong (2008) investigate how the proliferation of neoliberal values has engendered new self-governing practices among Chinese subjects. Arthur Kleinman and several of his former students and postdoctoral fellows trained in anthropology and psychiatry (2011) have examined the remaking of the person in contemporary China's changing emotional and moral context. See in particular Yan's (2011) analysis of the "ethical shift" from a morality of collective responsibilities to the justification of self-interest and an emphasis on individual rights.

18. When President Barack Obama issued an executive order in 2009 "removing barriers to responsible scientific research involving human stem cells," he explicitly framed his reversal of the earlier administration's restrictions in terms of shoring up American competitiveness in the global science race: "When government fails

to make these investments, opportunities are missed. Promising avenues go unexplored. Some of our best scientists leave for other countries that will sponsor their work. And those countries may surge ahead of ours in the advances that transform our lives. . . . This Order is an important step in advancing the cause of science in America. . . . By doing this, we will ensure America's continued global leadership in scientific discoveries and technological breakthroughs" (Obama 2009).

19. While these olfactory ensheathing glial (OEG) cells were not stem cells, the hype surrounding the more (in)famous variety of progenitor cells often led patients, reporters, and even other scientists and clinicians to conflate the fetal cells that Huang utilized in his experimental therapy with stem cells. Huang exclusively used OEG cells for his fetal cell transplantation procedure from 2001 until 2007 and made it his personal mission to educate patients, visiting clinicians, and journalists about the differences between fetal olfactory ensheathing cells (胚胎嗅鞘细胞 *pēitāi xiù qiào xìbāo*) and stem cells (干细胞 *gàn xìbāo*). Despite his continuing insistence on the correct classification of cell types, his patients' quests for a cure were often predicated on the hope and hype generated over stem cell research. After fielding repeated interest among his foreign patients in stem cell research, Huang later began experimenting with combination treatments involving other types of cells including Schwann cells, neural progenitor cells, and umbilical cord mesenchymal stromal cells (see Xi et al. 2013 for a preliminary report of this combination treatment for patients with multiple system atrophy).

20. Petryna makes her normative stance very clear: the use of vulnerable patients as experimental subjects is ultimately an exploitative abuse of power. The outsourced and globalized research enterprise is enriching predatory pharmaceutical corporations at the expense of local public health infrastructures and sustainable forms of care.

21. Between November 2001 and April 2016, at least 1,709 patients suffering from a range of neurological disorders from 83 countries received fetal cell transplantations from Chinese neurosurgeon Huang Hongyun. The following is a complete list of the countries/regions from which Huang's patients have come, with numbers of patients listed in parentheses except in cases where only one patient was treated: China (442), Romania (221), United States (219), Italy (147), Indonesia (51), Spain (40), Brazil (38), Netherlands (38), Belgium (29), Germany (29), Japan (28), Saudi Arabia (23), Canada (22), United Kingdom (20), Greece (18), Denmark (17), France (14), Algeria (13), Australia (13), Palestine (13), Syria (13), India (12), Turkey (12), Taiwan (11), Libya (10), Singapore (10), Sudan (10), Thailand (10), Iran (9), Croatia (8), Iraq (8), Oman (7), Sweden (7), Switzerland (7), United Arab Emirates (7), Kuwait (6), Norway (6), Serbia (6), South Korea (6), Vietnam (6), Jordan (5), Argentina (4), Austria (4), Cyprus (4), Egypt (4), Hong Kong (4), Hungary (4), Israel (4), Macedonia (4), Slovenia (4), Venezuela (4), Bangladesh (3), Ecuador (3), Ireland (3), Lebanon (3), Malaysia (3), Mexico (3), Morocco (3), New Zealand (3), Russia (3), Yemen (3), Kazakhstan (2), Moldova (2), Philippines (2), Portugal (2), Qatar (2), Tunisia (2), Afghanistan, Bahrain, Bolivia, Cambodia, Chile, Congo, Cuba, Finland, Jamaica, Kosovo, Mauritius, Mongolia, Myanmar, Nigeria, Slovakia, and South Africa. I have compiled these numbers from several different sources. Dr. Huang has not kept a master record of all the patients he has treated, partly for

administrative reasons since these patients were treated at several different hospitals. Instead, various staff members have kept overlapping records for assorted purposes. For example, Dr. Huang's secretaries have compiled various logbooks of foreign patients' appointments for surgery, while other administrative assistants have produced their own spreadsheets of foreign patients to track follow-up results. Each of the neurosurgeons kept their own records on the patients they managed, while the chief neurologist compiled several databases to compare detailed neurological scores for various types of patients. Note that the number of Chinese patients is underreported; a significant number were treated at hospitals where Huang has since left and he has been unable to access their medical records. Huang estimates that he has treated approximately 800 Chinese patients in total, but I only report here those whose records I could verify. Chapter 7 examines in more detail the challenges that Huang and his staff faced in compiling data and disseminating research results.

22. While Harris researchers coined "cyberchondriacs" in 1998 as a general term to identify anyone who goes online for health information, others have critiqued this description as pejorative and outmoded (Reid 2010; Fox 2010). Given that the majority of adults in the United States now utilize the Internet to research medical concerns and even perform self-diagnoses (Fox 2011; HarrisInteractive 2011), online health-seeking has become a mainstream feature of everyday life.

23. While some anthropologists have conducted fieldwork entirely within or among virtual worlds (e.g., Boellstorff 2008; Pearce and Artemesia 2009), most have followed their subjects across on- and offline experiences to highlight the interconnectedness of virtual and actual worlds (see Heath et al. 1999; Miller and Slater 2000; Wilson and Peterson 2002; Taylor 2006; Coleman 2010; Nardi 2010). Ethnographers have examined the role of computer-mediated communication in strengthening ethnic identity among members of diasporic communities (Bernal 2005, 2014; Burrell and Anderson 2008; Landzelius 2006; Lozada 1998), negotiating gender and sexuality in virtual worlds (Kendall 2002; Boellstorff 2008), shaping dating and courtship practices (Constable 2003; Gershon 2010), and jump-starting political activism (Kendzior 2011; Tufekci and Wilson 2012; Lindgren 2013), among other forms of cybersociality.

24. Although studying new forms of social media and online engagement seems to be a particularly timely and contemporary pursuit, it is important to note that these insights on medical cybersociality build upon longstanding research by scholars of science and technology studies who have investigated the role of patient associations in constructing collective illness identities as a basis for political mobilization (Brown and Zavestoski 2004; Landzelius and Dumit 2006; Epstein 2008). Various "disease constituencies" (Epstein 2008, 499) have transformed biomedical research and shaped public policy for a number of conditions, including HIV/AIDS in the United States (Epstein 1996), muscular dystrophy in France (Rabeharisoa and Callon 2004), breast cancer in Canada (Radin 2006), and rare genetic disorders in the United States (Taussig, Rapp, and Heath 2001; Novas 2006, 2007). Noting that much of this work on the politics and projects of patient groups has focused on such groups within North American or Western European contexts, Steven Epstein (2008, 525) has called for more studies of health movements that take place in other

countries, cross national borders, or are situated in a broader geopolitical context. This book takes up Epstein's call for more transnational research by examining how an American-based online discussion forum has mobilized the physically paralyzed to travel to China for experimental surgery.

25. Readers interested in seeing the original transcripts of these publicly accessible discussions can follow the citations to the relevant threads in the CareCure archives. In those cases where I have quoted from interviews that I conducted offline with CareCure members, I have asked whether they would prefer their private comments to be linked with their public CareCure identities or filed under separate pseudonyms. In the case of private electronic communications (such as password-protected members-only forums or personal email messages), I have obtained the writer's permission before quoting this material and safeguarded his or her confidentiality.

26. Although this book touches upon disability issues in China, I focus instead on the experiences of foreigners with neurological disorders in order to illuminate the transnational processes shaping their biomedical odysseys. For a fascinating analysis of disability as a key site for sociopolitical formation within post-Mao China, see Matthew Kohrman's *Bodies of Difference: Experiences of Disability and Institutional Advocacy in the Making of Modern China* (2005). Kohrman documents how the emergence of the biomedically informed Chinese concept of *cánjí* (残疾) is inextricably bound up in both the formation of state bureaucracy and the lived experience of bodily difference for Chinese people with physical disabilities. Unlike grassroots patient organizations such as CareCure, the China Disabled Persons' Federation that Kohrman examines is a formal appendage of the Chinese state. While the Chinese state plays a limited role in the first half of my book, I take up Kohrman's project of dissecting the inner workings of Chinese "biobureaucracies" in the second half of the book, which examines the experiences of Chinese clinicians offering these experimental treatments. While Kohrman's analysis focuses on the development of a state-controlled disability advocacy organization, I will examine the institutional entanglements generated by private entrepreneurs working in public hospitals in urban China.

CHAPTER 2: MOBILIZING THE PARALYZED ONLINE

1. As Arthur Kleinman emphasized in his study of health care practices in Taiwan, health care systems must be understood more broadly as local cultural systems comprised of three overlapping spheres: the popular, professional, and folk sectors (1978, 49–60). Formal treatment by medical professionals forms only a part of patients' experiences with health and illness. Informal connections among family members and friends often trump the advice of professional health providers. In his study of health-seeking practices among the Kongo of former Zaire, for example, John Janzen (1978) noted the crucial role of kin in directing the therapy management process for patients.

2. The development of technological infrastructure (which facilitated growing networks of interconnected computers) and the adoption of the World Wide Web (which standardized the way that information was accessed and displayed over the network) stoked the commercial growth of the Internet in the 1990s.

3. The ephemeral nature of personal websites is particularly problematic for the amyotrophic lateral sclerosis community, as patients succumb to the ravages of the terminal neurodegenerative disease and are no longer able to update their websites. I will discuss this issue in greater depth in the next chapter.

4. The CareCure Community claimed 323,463 members who had collectively posted 1,800,878 messages in 196,489 separate threads as of January 11, 2017. This membership statistic is based on the total number of account registrations, including those subsequently deleted by choice, removed by site administrators, or lost during platform upgrades. Thus only 31,366 members retain valid accounts according to a check of the forum's member list. To get a sense of the growth of the site, compare these numbers with usage statistics from nearly a decade earlier: 22,529 members and 830,216 messages as of May 4, 2008.

5. The CareCure website has been powered by different software platforms over the years. Each transition has required users to learn a new navigation interface, generating both consternation and new forms of engagement among its members. In its most recent manifestation, the site uses a commercial forum publishing software designed by the California-based company vBulletin.

6. This is a crucial difference from an electronic mailing list (listserv), another popular type of computer-mediated communication technology that operates by sending messages directly to a group of interested users' email accounts. Although most listservs (such as the popular H-Net mailing lists devoted to topics in humanities and social sciences) maintain websites that archive previous messages, users generally participate by subscribing to the mailing list. The primary mode of engagement thus involves receiving and sending messages distributed to the private email accounts of subscribers.

7. The CareCure website enables users to locate information based on an extensive set of search criteria. I used the search function to identify members attributed with a certain number of posts.

8. A "Members Only" section and audiovisual chat feature allow those logged into their accounts to hold more private conversations.

9. Some forum members found this explication of forum policy disturbing: "Yikes! Big Brother!" exclaimed senior CareCure member mimin from Israel (2007). Other forum members defended the administrators by pointing out that the presumption of privacy online was a fallacy: "For those who don't know, even if the admins did agree to remove content, that would not necessarily remove it from the Internet. Many don't realize that the very nature of the Internet is data storage, and often times that means being stored in more than one location. In addition to all of the search engines storing copies of the pages they find for varying lengths of time, many times you will find more persistent copies on sites such as The Internet Archives as well" (mvandemar 2007).

10. This statistic tracks the number of times unique site visitors have clicked on a thread. As we would expect, the "viewers" and "lurkers" far outnumber the active participants who actually type a response. For example, the "ChinaSCINet Update" thread was pinned second from the top of the Cure forum and had attracted 2,537 replies and 840,614 views as of January 12, 2017.

11. Users can also reorganize the display of threads according to other characteristics, including alphabetically by the title of the thread starter.
12. Tom Boellstorff's work on the online graphical platform Second Life highlights a very different process of virtual community formation, predicated on what he calls "synchronic sociality" (2008, 101). He examines how the simultaneous presence (and absences) of more than one person played a key role in fostering social interactions in Second Life. For the residents of Second Life, time "inworld" was experienced in discontinuous segments (e.g., logging on and off the program, experiencing delays known as lag caused by inadequate bandwidth or other communication technology failures, or taking short breaks from the keyboard to use the bathroom or spend time with actual-world family members). Boellstorff describes this discontinuous temporality as "the most consequential boundary-marker between the actual and the virtual" (2008, 102) that ultimately created a distinct experience of sociality online. For example, differentially experienced temporality created strange social interactions in Second Life as users had to accommodate others whose avatars (visual self-representation) were present on the screen but unresponsive because the people who animated these avatars were "AFK" (away from keyboard) and actually absent from the virtual exchange.
13. I maintain CareCure members' naming practices by referring to Wise Young by his first name throughout the book.
14. See http://www.youtube.com/watch?v=2SV6PrUiY3E for a video performance of ProfessirX's tribute song from his CD *A Soldier for the Cure* (video uploaded on May 16, 2007).
15. Like the United States, China has a separate medical system for its military force (known as the People's Liberation Army). With regulatory oversight carried out by a separate military health commission, Chinese military hospitals often have greater leeway than their civilian counterparts, which were governed by the Ministry of Health. The radical changes in financing brought about by Chinese leader Deng Xiaoping's opening and reform policies during the 1980s and 1990s have encouraged military hospitals such as Naval General to treat civilians in a lucrative bid to earn more money. I elaborate on these developments in the Chinese health care sector in chapter 5 on technonationalism.
16. The hippocampus (the brain's center for learning and memory) is the other region of the adult mammalian brain capable of generating new neurons.
17. Huang cultivated OEG cells from aborted human fetuses obtained through partnerships with obstetrics departments. I discuss the ethical questions and practical concerns surrounding the use of human fetal tissue in later chapters. Chapter 4 addresses how foreign patients grappled with these dilemmas, while chapter 5 examines the development of Huang's career and clinical therapies in greater detail.
18. Unlike Huang, Dr. Carlos Lima's team in Portugal uses olfactory mucosa (a mixture of OEG cells, neurons, and other support cells) harvested from patients' own nasal cavities. The two doctors also utilize different surgical procedures—Lima removes what he considers to be scar tissue in the spinal cord, while Huang prefers to keep the cord as intact as possible (Lima et al. 2006).
19. The myelin sheath is the insulating layer that encases nerve fibers and protects electric nerve impulses. Deterioration of the myelin sheath (demyelination) occurs

in many neurodegenerative diseases such as multiple sclerosis and Guillain-Barré syndrome. Spinal cord injuries usually damage both the myelin sheath and the underlying nerve fibers. Thus regenerating myelin (remyelination) may improve the transmittal of nerve impulses and may also provide a track to guide potentially regrowing neurons.

20. As a nurse who had worked with Huang at the naval hospital explained to me, "A mountain can only have one tiger." Fresh from three years of research experience obtained abroad and brimming with new ideas, Huang challenged the authority of his more senior colleagues. Hospital administrators responded by creating an organizational separation to appease the various factions. I discuss these developments in greater detail in chapter 5, which traces the trajectory of Huang's neurosurgical career.

21. The development of clinical treatments in the United States is generally divided into successive stages. Phase I involves assessing whether the experimental intervention is safe for human use. During this preliminary stage, researchers test the new treatment on a small number of people. Phase II involves testing the intervention on a larger number of people to assess its effectiveness and further monitor safety—this stage generally involves dividing research subjects into a group receiving the treatment in question and a comparison control group(s) receiving a placebo or an already established treatment method. Phase III involves still larger numbers of patients—these studies are generally done across multiple institutions to definitively establish the effectiveness of the treatment. In the United States, the federal Food and Drug Administration (FDA) grants regulatory approval to researchers to market new drugs or medical devices only after a successful Phase III study. The process of developing clinical treatments in China is currently in flux. The State Food and Drug Administration (国家食品药品监督管理局 Guójiā Shípǐn Yàopǐn Jiāndū Guǎnlǐ Jú) has adopted international guidelines that are even more stringent than the American FDA rules, but these regulations are not widely followed or enforced. I examine these issues in greater depth in chapter 7 when I address efficacy and the limits of experimental medicine.

22. I discuss these issues in greater depth in chapter 7, which examines Huang's efforts to collect systematic data on his experimental therapy.

CHAPTER 3: CYBERANATOMIES OF HOPE

1. She later changed her CareCure screen name to "Shannon."
2. A completely transected cord is rare. Most SCIs do not involve a complete severing of the cord but rather a bruising that results in tearing or destroying a portion of the nerve cells in the spinal cord. Even those injuries deemed "complete" generally leave some portion of the cord intact, although the damage is extensive enough to prevent any neural signals from getting past the area of injury.
3. As these medical and biological anthropologists have demonstrated, fluctuations in reproductive hormone levels are eminently suited for understanding how cultural and ecological contexts influence biology. I adapt the concept of local biologies to illuminate a different physiological realm: the neuroanatomical knowledge deployed by CareCure members.

4. The technical determination of a "complete" classification, technically called "ASIA Grade A," is based on a rectal examination. Only those without any evidence of anal sensation or sphincter contraction are considered complete. For those determined to be incomplete, enough of the spinal cord has remained intact to transmit at least some signals down to the base of the cord. The ASIA impairment scale distinguishes between three gradations of "incomplete," depending on the degree of sensation and function detected.

5. Despite his herculean efforts to promote cutting-edge research to cure spinal cord injury, Reeve ultimately succumbed to a more mundane problem related to basic everyday care for people living with paralysis. He died in October 2004 from complications related to an infected bedsore, which led to systemic infection, heart failure, and a coma.

6. Euphemism for rectal suppository.

7. I should point out that in an era of instant messaging expressed via emoticon shorthand, bloggers and other computer users blessed with the full use of both hands have also forgone the style conventions of more formal writing.

8. Americans like jshoham were not the only ones to utilize the CareCure forum in this manner. Lucas, a physician from Italy, made a public plea on the Huang contact thread on behalf of his mother: "Dear Dr. Huang. . . . I'm an italian doctor. I would like to see if my mother who has ALS can undergo your olfactory ensheathing cell transplantation. She would be a very good candidate. She was diagnosed on 2-02-04. She's the only mother that I've. I'm very afraid!" (Lucas 2004).

9. Several months after his experimental surgery in Beijing, he received a different diagnosis from his American doctors. They speculated that his symptoms were due to Parkinson's disease, although they did not rule out ALS (iublondie25 2005).

10. Although these personal blogs were once publicly accessible to anyone with an Internet connection, nearly all of the ALS blogs that I tracked from 2004 to 2007 have now disappeared from cyberspace. Since these blogs are no longer available to the public, I have substituted pseudonyms where necessary in order to protect the privacy of the PALS and their family members. For those PALS and their family members who chose to speak to journalists and are quoted by name in the public record, I have continued to cite their actual names.

11. Although I do not speak or read Dutch, I was still able to track these PALS and their family members online by running their websites through automated online translation tools such as Babelfish and Google Translate. I am also grateful for the translation help of multilingual historian Marjan Boogert, a graduate of Leiden and Harvard universities, and Susanne van den Buuse, a medical anthropologist at the University of Amsterdam.

12. The ephemerality of online information also poses a significant challenge for researchers. As I studied the visceral experiences and digital communications of people from around the world who sought experimental treatment in Beijing, I found myself compulsively taking screenshots of blog entries, copying and pasting chunks of information from websites, and printing out entire discussion threads, driven by the worry that I would not be able to find the information again. Although online search engines such as Google and Internet archivers such as the Wayback Machine create cached copies of websites as they trawl the World Wide Web, these archived

pages can only provide a partial and static snapshot of once-vibrant and interactive digital platforms.

CHAPTER 4: WHERE THE VIRTUAL BECOMES VISCERAL

1. Tim C.'s experiences appear in abbreviated form in Song 2010.
2. Hospitals with more than two thousand beds are quite common in major urban centers in China. The largest hospital in the country in 2015 was the First Affiliated Hospital of Zhengzhou University (郑州大学第一附属医院 Zhèngzhōu Dàxué Dìyī Fùshǔ Yīyuàn) in Henan province, with 8,000 patient beds and 19 million surgeries performed yearly (Zhengzhou University First Affiliated Hospital 2015). For comparison, *Becker's Hospital Review* reported that the largest hospital in the United States, New York-Presbyterian Hospital, had 2,236 beds and performed 77,900 surgeries yearly (Oh 2010).
3. These OEG surgery reports have attracted hundreds of replies and tens of thousands of views since the CareCure pioneers' trip to Beijing to undergo Huang's fetal cell transplantation procedure. Tim C.'s surgery report has received 253 replies and 38,688 unique views in the years following his experimental forays, Handibob's surgery report has received 310 replies and 62,210 views, and CJO's surgery report has received 200 replies and 24,467 views (statistics last updated October 18, 2015). Although these threads continue to attract readers into the present, their activity levels have fallen off dramatically. Between 2003 and 2005, these threads were located near the top of the Cure forum and attracted daily replies and inquiries. A decade later, these Beijing OEG surgery report threads do not appear until the 231st, 159th, and 250th pages, respectively, of the Cure forum (aside from the "stickies" pinned to the top by forum moderators, threads are arranged according to activity level with those receiving the most recent replies moving to the top of the list).
4. The label "pioneer" was used fourteen times across the three surgery report threads, compared with five mentions of the next most common term, "hero." I have analyzed the significance of the label "pilgrim" elsewhere (Song 2010), drawing on the concept of "biotech pilgrimage" to challenge the trope of "medical tourism" dominating popular media and even scholarly reports of the growing phenomenon of traveling abroad for medical care.
5. The list of CareCure members who contacted Dr. Huang publicly through this discussion forum grew to 524 posts between September 2003 and May 2012, and it has been viewed over 119,560 times. After Dr. Huang's secretarial staff posted their clinic's website address and contact information, many others have contacted Dr. Huang directly in private without announcing their intentions on the forum.
6. Most of Huang's Chinese clinical staff members adopted English names after they started working with foreign patients. Some like Bird and Dr. Brian chose their own names, while others like Dr. Alan and Dr. Pain were christened by their foreign patients.
7. While the emir himself was not at New Century Hospital, a delegation from the Kuwaiti embassy had accompanied a member of the ruling family seeking to undergo Huang's experimental procedure.

8. This option was not made available to Huang's domestic patients. While he was in town for his follow-up assessment, Brother Lu made inquiries about the possibility of obtaining a second OEG fetal cell transplantation. He pressed Huang's head nurse, Teacher Yan, about whether the New Century staff could take care of the arrangements for a second surgery, emphasizing that he would be willing to pay more for the convenience. He was particularly concerned about the fetal cell procurement process, given the difficulties he had encountered four years earlier. He also noted that making his own arrangements "wasted a lot of money" (浪费很多钱 *làngfèi hěnduō qián*). Hu was understandably crestfallen when Teacher Yan dismissed his concerns, telling him "this is something you need to take care of yourself" (这就你自己管 *zhè jiù nǐ zìjǐ guǎn*).

9. This document references different terms for and methods of abortion. *Liúchǎn* (流产) is a general term that encompasses a broad range of abortion methods and can also be used to refer to spontaneous abortions (miscarriages). 药物流产 (*yàowù liúchǎn*) refers to medically induced abortions while 人工流产手术 (*réngōng liúchǎn shǒushù*) refers to an early term abortion technique that utilizes surgical instruments to scrape the walls of the uterus (known as dilation and curettage in the United States). *Yǐnchǎn* (引产) refers to a later-term abortion technique that utilizes artificial means to induce uterine contractions and expel the fetus.

10. Sam Brownback actively worked during his tenure as Republican senator of Kansas (from 1996 to 2011) to advance his pro-life agenda, expanding restrictions on abortion and opposing the use of embryonic stem cells in research or treatment for human health conditions.

11. I would like to acknowledge Jean Langford's suggestion to think about Southern Baptists' invocation of sacrifice in terms of Lawrence Cohen's analysis of the biopolitics of (immuno)suppression. Her invaluable comments as a discussant for my 2005 American Anthropological Association panel titled "Marketing the Body" helped reframe my understanding of the ethics of fetal cell therapies.

12. Analyzing the concept of a "life unworthy of being lived," Agamben cites penal law specialist Karl Binding's radical support for euthanasia, in which Binding argues that "incurable idiots, either those born as such or those—for example, those who suffer from progressive paralysis—who have become such in the last phase of their life. . . . These men have neither the will to live nor the will to die. On the one hand, there is no ascertainable consent to die; on the other hand, their killing does not infringe upon any will to live that must be overcome. Their life is absolutely without purpose, but they do not find it to be intolerable" (Agamben 1998, 81).

13. Huang allowed observers to witness his surgical procedure, including other clinicians and medical journalists, as well as a few caregivers with medical experience who had traveled to Beijing to learn more about the procedure (such as a surgical nurse from California who was the mother of an eighteen-year-old former snowboarder). I also had the opportunity to scrub in and observe several surgeries for SCI patients.

14. This is a common type of spinal surgery used to decompress the spinal canal in order to relieve pressure on the spinal cord.

15. Huang and his clinical colleagues hypothesized that the bilateral corona radiata of the frontal lobes was an ideal cell transplantation site for diseases of the central

nervous system (CNS) such as ALS, multiple sclerosis, cerebral palsy, ataxia, dementia, and epilepsy: "Although they vary in etiology and pathologic findings, [these CNS diseases] ultimately affect similar elements in the brain such as neurons and nerve fibers of the cerebral cortex, spinal cord, cerebellum, pons, brain stem nuclei, red nucleus, substantia nigra, and basal ganglia. Thus, there might be a key point among these elements where cell graft should be delivered for cell-based therapy" (Chen et al. 2010, 189). They proposed the concept of a "key point for neural network restoration" based on their clinical experiences transplanting OEG cells in 1,255 patients with CNS diseases (Huang et al. 2009): "This site is where the frontal corona radiate pyramidal tract passes through, and represents a point at which numerous projection fibers, association fibers, and commissural fibers convergent [*sic*]. After transplanted [*sic*] into this important 'point' in the brain, the cells will initiate an extensive bidirectional remodeling in the entire neural network, including cerebrum, cerebellum, and spinal cord. Thus, the key point of cell transplantation should be of great importance in approaching the functional neurorestoration" (Chen et al. 2010, 189).

16. This is a company that manufactures drills and other power tools for home improvement.

17. While Jeff's blog was publicly accessible through the website of his fire department when I first read his account, it was taken down after he died in June 2006.

CHAPTER 5: MEDICAL ENTREPRENEURS

1. Scholars have likewise traced the development of nuclear power and weaponry in India in the context of Hindu nationalism and the rise of the right-wing Bharatiya Janata Party (Abraham 1998; Perkovich 2002).

2. 除四害 (*chú sì hài*), which included flies, mosquitoes, rats, and sparrows.

3. Unless otherwise noted, all translations of Chinese sources are my own. I have included the original Chinese for selected key phrases from published works. For unpublished research data including internally circulated documents and interview transcripts, I have included longer segments from the original Chinese texts in the notes since these cannot be cross-referenced independently.

4. They were announced at the historic Third Plenary Session of the 11th National Congress of the Chinese Communist Party.

5. Although the report officially prohibited "barefoot doctors who worked for rural production brigades" (农村生产大队的赤脚医生 *nóngcūn shēngchǎn dàduì de chìjiǎo yīshēng*) from engaging in private practice, it provided a loophole for those living in impoverished or sparsely populated areas to open up individual businesses according to local medical needs (People's Republic of China Ministry of Health 1980).

6. The report also specified that state-trained medical staff who disobeyed job assignment orders would not be allowed to engage individual medical practice (个体开业行医 *gètǐ kāiyè xíngyī*).

7. I invoke this phrase to underscore the contradictory nature of Chinese efforts to reform health care since the 1980s. In recent years, high-level Chinese officials such as Gao Qiang, former minister of health, have publicly acknowledged the failures of

these earlier market-based reforms and emphasized providing for the public good as the essence of "the road to health development under socialism with Chinese characteristics" (Zhou 2008).

8. The Four Modernizations were agriculture, industry, science and technology, and defense.

9. The stratification of health services did not originate with the Ministry of Health's market-inspired health reforms. During the Maoist era, high-ranking Communist Party cadres had access to exclusive medical wards. These VIP wards (高干病房 *gāo gàn bìngfáng*) were formerly the exclusive domain of political elites during Mao's era, but financially successful Chinese can increasingly buy their way into the ranks of the privileged and pampered. This trend has blossomed under the profit-driven priorities of "health care with Chinese characteristics," emphasizing high-tech medical services at corresponding higher prices.

10. Public health analysts have shown how the commercialization of high-tech medicine in China has led to the rampant overprescription of marked-up drugs, indiscriminate use of new medical technologies, a focus on acquiring new hospital equipment, neglect of public health and basic safety net programs, and widening rural-urban inequality (Hesketh and Zhu 1997b; Chen 2001; Blumenthal and Hsiao 2005). Anthropologists have also provided ethnographic insight into how commercialization and privatization have generated health crises for ordinary Chinese citizens, most notably the pernicious spread of HIV from predatory blood-selling practices in rural Henan during the 1990s (Anagnost 2006; Shao 2006). Anna Lora-Wainwright (2013) documents the destructive effects of rural-urban health inequalities in the ways in which rural families attempt to make sense of cancer and care for sufferers. The "rational separation of the flow of patients" may sound eminently reasonable on paper as a national policy directive, but it looks very different on the ground as the rural elderly forgo cancer treatment in urban hospitals and are driven to suicide to spare their families from the exorbitant expense of treatment.

11. Science (科学 *kēxué*) and technology (技术 *jìshù*) are usually conflated and discussed in Chinese using a single abbreviated phrase: *kējì* (科技).

12. The British invasion of the capital and destruction of the imperial summer palace Yuan Ming Yuan in 1860 forced the weakened Qing dynasty rulers to open key treaty ports along the eastern coast and even up the Yangzi River into China's interior, adopt English as the official language of communication, and allow the sale of opium (Spence 1990, 181). These humiliations convinced Qing scholars and military leaders such as Feng Guifen and Zeng Guofan of China's need to strengthen itself by learning Western military technology: "China was a hundred times larger than France and two hundred times larger than England, so 'why are they small and yet strong? Why are we large and yet weak? . . . What we then have to learn from the barbarians is only one thing, solid ships and effective guns'" (as quoted in Spence 1990, 197).

13. Visa regulations also played a significant role in ensuring return. In the United States, for example, PRC government-sponsored trainees received J-1 visas, which carried strict requirements about returning home. F-1 visas, however, provided privately funded students with an easier administrative opportunity to convert their status to permanent residency (Lampton 1986; Orleans 1988).

14. These categories reflect subjective orientations rather than objective types. Indeed, increasing numbers of *huáqiáo* are becoming *hǎiguī* as economic incentives beckon them back to China. Furthermore, many *hǎiguī* still employ the strategies of flexible accumulation, mobility, and citizenship that Ong (1999) highlighted in her analysis of *huáqiáo*. Examining the cultural logics of transnationalism, Ong noted that elite diasporan Chinese such as Hong Kong taipan often accumulated foreign passports and multiple residences as insurance to protect their families and investments.

15. For those unable to secure the necessary resources to study abroad, pursuing advanced studies (进修 *jìnxiū*) in higher-tier Chinese cities is another popular strategy. "Advanced study" is a formalized process established by major medical institutions to enable visiting physicians to pursue short-term training. The formal contract requires permission from both the sending and receiving hospitals. Applicants for advanced studies at Chaoyang Hospital, for example, are required to fill out an "Advanced Studies Application Form" stamped with the official seal of their sending hospital work unit in addition to providing a letter of introduction from the sending hospital. The sending hospital generally pays the host hospital a training fee and provides a living stipend for its employee, who is contractually obligated to return to his or her original institution at the conclusion of the training period.

    A significant number of *jìnxiū* students attempt to leverage their temporary studies into more permanent positions in the more desirable location, either by applying for advanced degree programs or by negotiating employment opportunities at other area hospitals. Not surprisingly, hospitals are often reluctant to allow their employees to pursue advanced studies at other institutions. Dr. Alan, New Century's chief neurologist, told me about his experiences in an interview on January 24, 2006. He explained the hurdles he had to go through in order to obtain permission from his home hospital in Shandong province to become an "advanced study student" (进修生 *jìnxiū shēng*) in Beijing. His Shandong hospital was originally not willing to provide him with a "certificate of work suspension" (停工证 *tíng gōng zhèng*), which the Beijing hospital required to process his application. Giving me a wink, Dr. Alan explained that they finally agreed to let him go after he "engaged in some activities and gave some gifts [活动活动送礼就同意了 *huódòng huódòng sònglǐ jiù tóngyìle*]." He also had to pay his home hospital a six-hundred-yuan "administrative fee" (管理费 *guǎnlǐ fèi*) in order to obtain the necessary paperwork. Like Dr. Alan, four of the five midlevel attending physicians who worked at the New Century neurosurgical enterprise had originally come to Beijing from other parts of China as "advanced study" students.

16. I provide a critical analysis of deceptive marketing practices utilized by Beike in Song 2011.

17. The medical academic degree system in China is complex and has gone through successive overhauls, with multiple tiers of health care providers and various pathways to accreditation (see Wu et al. 2014 for a succinct overview). The most prevalent model established since the beginning of the Reform and Opening era is a three-level system. At the basic level, medical students complete a five-year program and obtain the bachelor of medicine degree. Postgraduates may pursue increasing levels of clinical specialization, training, and/or research by completing a two- or three-year master's degree program. Further clinical training and/

or research can be pursued through a two- to four-year doctoral degree program. Some medical universities offer seven-year programs leading directly to a master's level qualification, while a few elite medical schools offer eight-year programs leading directly to the doctorate of medicine degree. Operating in tandem with the academic degree system, a residency training requirement was introduced in the 1990s to ensure adequate clinical training for medical graduates of all levels, but the quality of training has varied significantly across regions and even individual institutions in China.

18. As one conscripted medical expert reminisced on the school's fiftieth anniversary in 1996: "There was only the Gobi desert and peasants' fields when we arrived. . . . All of the school's teachers, students, and staff worked together handful by handful to move mountains of accumulated earth, rocks and debris, in order to impose order on the uneven terrain. . . . Under hard labor, some comrades even sacrificed their precious lives. Our generation of old comrades shed blood and sweat, enduring many trials in order to establish a solid foundation for the medical school. In the prime of our youth, we left our beautiful homes and superior work environments in order to go to sparsely populated Xinjiang" (S. Wang 2006).

19. Physicians are generally divided into four levels at both civilian and military hospitals in China: resident physician (住院医师 *zhùyuàn yīshī*), attending physician (主治医师 *zhǔzhì yīshī*), deputy director-level physician (副主任医师 *fùzhǔrèn yīshī*), and full director-level physician (主任医师 *zhǔrèn yīshī*). Additional distinctions include administrative appointments as deputy department chair (副主任 *fùzhǔrèn*) or department chair (科主任 *kēzhǔrèn*). Hospitals affiliated with medical universities also provide physicians with academic appointments corresponding to assistant professor (助教授 *zhùjiàoshòu*), associate professor (副教授 *fùjiàoshòu*), and full professor (正教授 *zhèngjiàoshòu*); professors are further credentialed as master's-level advisor (硕士生导师 *shuòshìshēng dǎoshī*) or doctoral-level advisor (博士生导师 *bóshìshēng dǎoshī*).

20. Although mandated birth planning has become routine across China, the national outrage over a Chinese woman's forced late-term abortion in 2012 suggests the contested role of state coercion in reproductive politics (Shi 2014). China formally ended the one-child policy in 2015.

21. Since this is an unpublished internal document provided to me by Huang and his staff, I provide the original Chinese text here for interested readers:

黄红云主任早年···进行脊髓疾病的研究，积累了丰富的经验，后又到美国从事相关科学研究两年多，取得了很多成果。2000 年，他婉言谢绝了美国专家的高薪留用，毅然舍妻离子，回到祖国，回到了海军总医院。回国后，为把学到的知识和研究的成果早日应用到临床，为病人解除痛苦，他夜以继日的做着临床治疗的各项前期准备工作。在脊髓损伤的基础和临床研究中，采用嗅鞘细胞移植的方法治疗晚期脊髓损伤，取得突破性进展···

黄红云主任发扬不怕苦、不怕累的拼搏精神和良好的医德医风，对工作一丝不苟，兢兢业业，在技术上精益求精，尽善尽美，事事处处关怀病人，为病人着想。有时专家门诊日接诊一百多，从早上八点半到晚上七八点钟，手术连台做，从早上八点半到晚上六七点钟，两组医生连续做四台甚至六台手术···这些都开创了医院的先例。黄红云主任自己的身体也不太好，但他从未想到自己，仍然坚持临床治疗第一线。有一次，他发高烧，一边输液，一边看门诊，有时心脏不舒服，他就在病房休息一会，继续工作。

辛勤的耕耘换回的是累累的科研硕果和病人满意的微笑。一位病人入院时不能站立,手术后不但可以站立,而且在家人的搀扶下,可以在室内行走了。出院时握着我们医生的手哽咽的说:"谢谢,谢谢,太谢谢你们了!"

22. For the medical institutions discussed in this book, I cite actual names (e.g., Naval General Hospital and Chaoyang Hospital) or use pseudonyms (e.g., New Century Hospital), depending on the need to protect confidentiality.

23. Pinpointing exact financial figures was always a sensitive subject, although one rumor circulating among his administrative staff members claimed that Huang's lucrative OEG transplantations contributed nearly one-fifth of Chaoyang's overall revenues in 2004.

24. An even more comprehensive nationwide analysis of over one million cervical spine surgical procedures for degenerative diseases performed in the United States between 2002 and 2009 identified average in-hospital costs between $10,034 (for a posterior cervical decompression procedure with an average hospital stay of 2.5 days) and $29,561 (for a posterior cervical fusion procedure with an average hospital stay of 7.4 days) (Oglesby et al. 2013). Note that these costs are exclusive of professional fees charged by the surgeons performing the procedures.

25. "很多人都在批评我…做外国人是为了赚钱…看不起中国病人" (interview with the author, January 25, 2006).

26. "中外都有求治的要求,都应该做" (interview with the author, January 25, 2006).

27. "西方做不到…用西方医学的方法来治外国患者,证明中国优先" (interview with the author, January 25, 2006).

28. "科学——虽然全世界可以共享,但是带一些政治…出国以后发现美国更爱国主义…美国、欧洲攻击我,不承认患者有改善,认为中国是落后的地方,不可能优先。为什么不勇敢面对事实,站在病人的角度?" (interview with the author, January 25, 2006).

29. "为国家,西方医学作…最重要就是能够为病人做什么?" (interview with the author, January 25, 2006).

30. "0 到 0.1 就是一个巨大的突破,有的人就否定你的作用很微小,是的,这种微小是前人没有的,它的价值我想就在这。让人们认识到这种东西,过去传统观念是错的,这是我在任何场合反复强调,它的价值是不是一下能恢复到走路,一下就克服这个疾病,不在于这个意义,而在于说改善传统的悲观,非常悲观的传统概念,改变是这个东西。认为这个观念是错的,人们才会更多投入进去,更多感兴趣,更多去探讨它" (interview with the author, March 17, 2006).

31. "吸引更多科学家,让更多人加入研究,扩大影响,对病人、科学发展有利…希望更多人回去做…治不完" (interview with the author, March 17, 2006).

32. "正如我们党第十六届中央委员会第五次全体会议公报所指出的:科学技术发展要坚持自主创新、重点跨越、支撑发展、引领未来的方针" (Huang 2006).

33. "科技自主创新是一个国家、一个民族保持发展后劲的根本" (Huang 2006).

34. "这是我国在世界医疗领域内开展的重要源头创新性治疗方法,在我国医学界实属少见。这一开创性的研究,填补了世界空白,使我国在这一领域处在国际领先地位。从国家荣誉和我国的国际医学地位来讲,能够吸引大批欧美发达国家的患者来我国就医,具有划时代的意义,是我国医学界为之自豪的荣耀" (Huang 2006).

35. "我们每个人都能在这个集体工作而感到荣幸,真正感到了作为一个中国人的自豪和骄傲" (Huang 2006).

36. In an arresting front-page story in the *New York Times* about his experiences receiving medical care in the People's Republic during the height of the Cultural

Revolution, American journalist James Reston (1971) reported on his experiences undergoing acupuncture to relieve post-surgical pain following an emergency appendectomy at the Anti-Imperialist Hospital in Beijing (Peking Union Medical College Hospital). Eager to showcase China's achievements in medicine and public health, the Chinese Medical Association subsequently invited a procession of foreign medical experts to visit following U.S. secretary of state Henry Kissinger's secret trip to China in July 1971 that reopened U.S.-China relations (which were subsequently formally reestablished with President Richard Nixon's official state visit in 1972). Many visitors were interested in the Chinese system as an alternative model for health care delivery, resulting in the publication of laudatory books such as Canadian neurosurgeon Kewal Jain's *The Amazing Story of Health Care in New China* (1973) and American medical experts Victor Sidel and Ruth Sidel's *Serve the People: Observations on Medicine in the People's Republic of China* (1973).

37. There has been significant debate over whether post-Mao China should be considered "neoliberal" or even "post-socialist." Despite the Chinese party-state's explicit rejection of neoliberal values, anthropologists Li Zhang and Aihwa Ong have argued that "the cross between privatization and socialist rule is not a 'deviant' form but a particular articulation of neoliberalism," which they describe as "socialism from afar" (2008, 2–3). Other anthropologists have challenged whether these practices should be characterized as "neoliberal." Andrew Kipnis, for example, points out that the features theorists have identified as quintessentially "neoliberal" (e.g., governing from a distance, calculability, and the promotion of an enterprising self) can in fact be found in a wide range of governing cultures (2008, 283–84). In particular, he notes that the qualities of self-discipline and self-cultivation have been foundational touchstones in both Confucianism and Maoism, two governing philosophies that can hardly be mistaken for Western neoliberalism. In identifying the emergence of "desiring subjects," Lisa Rofel (2007) examines how new sexual, material, and affective desires (from television melodramas to gay lifestyles and shopping sprees) are serving as arenas for negotiating questions about national belonging and China's place in a post–Cold War global order.

38. Looking beyond China to other late and post-socialist contexts, Elizabeth Dunn has examined how Polish factory workers are becoming "entrepreneurs of themselves" (2004, 22) in response to new management schemes seeking to maximize their capacities as "self-directed, self-activating, self-monitoring workers" (20). But she also documents how these women workers have invoked kinship claims and created gift relations with their supervisors in order to protect themselves from an objectifying market logic that ultimately treats them as interchangeable and expendable cogs.

CHAPTER 6: BORDERLINE TACTICS

1. Anthropologists have challenged the false teleology embedded in notions of "the transition" from socialism to capitalism (Hann, Humphrey, and Verdery 2002; Buyandelger 2008), offering instead critical perspectives grounded in the particular configurations of politics, economics, and cultures in the former Soviet bloc as well as post-socialist states in Africa, Asia, and Latin America. Health care has been a

particularly fertile ground for studying how these enduring socialist influences interact with emergent market logics. Challenging Western critiques of post-socialist health care as mired in corruption, Michele Rivkin-Fish (2005) has explored how Russian physicians and their female patients construct personalized and privatized forms of relationality inside state-sponsored clinics in order to create more trusting relationships. Jack Friedman (2009) has examined how psychiatrists in post-socialist Romania have deployed new diagnostic categories to protect their increasingly impoverished patients in the face of state efforts to deinstitutionalize publicly funded mental health care. Investigating the popularity of "placebo therapy" for alcohol addiction treatment and rehabilitation in Russia, Eugene Raikhel (2010) has traced how styles of clinical reasoning in Russian psychiatry have been affected by post-Soviet political and economic transformations. Sean Brotherton (2012) has mapped the effects of the Soviet collapse and subsequent loss of Soviet subsidies on Cuba's public health care system, exploring the ways in which bodily health and well-being are being transformed in the context of economic insecurity. My work builds on this anthropological scholarship by providing an ethnographic analysis of emerging (post)socialist practices at the margins of the urban Chinese health care system.

2. Social scientists working in China have documented this phenomenon in multiple arenas, most notably in housing (Forrest and Lee 2003; Fleischer 2010; Zhang 2010) and sexuality (Farquhar 2002; Farrer 2002; Friedman 2006; Rofel 2007).

3. Ethnographic studies of the Chinese state have recognized the importance of "disaggregating" this construct to examine the actions of cadres, bureaucrats, and policymakers at multiple levels of governance. Helen Siu (1989) recognized early on the agency, victimization, and ultimate complicity of local rural cadres who acted as brokers between peasants and the central government in the process of state involution. More recently, Matthew Kohrman (2005) has focused attention on the complex sociopolitical formation of various "biobureaucracies" involved in processes of state-building and embodied subject-making. Susan Greenhalgh (2008) has delved into the micropolitics of Chinese policymaking to document the ways in which aerospace engineers came to dominate the official discourse on population control with a strict one-child policy, while Susan Brownell (2008) has examined the role of state-sponsored sporting events, sports commissions, and training centers in creating and representing a modern nation-state.

4. My use of the term "tactics" is inspired by French theorist Michel de Certeau's analysis of everyday practices, in which he invoked the notion to describe the clandestine and makeshift "ways of operating" through which people craft meaningful lives for themselves. As "an art of the weak" that "insinuates itself into the other's place," a tactic must "seize on the wing the possibilities that offer themselves at any given moment. It must vigilantly make use of the cracks that particular conjunctions open in the surveillance of the proprietary powers" (1984, xviii–xix, 34–39). Challenging Michel Foucault's focus on the encompassing normative order produced by a diffuse "micro-physics of power," de Certeau engages in a very different project: "If it is true the grid of 'discipline' is everywhere becoming clearer and more extensive, it is all the more urgent to discover how an entire society resists being reduced to it" (1984, xiv). This analytical commitment is particularly important in

making sense of everyday life in contemporary China, as citizens navigate hegemonic ideologies of the state and the market.

5. The Ministry of Health utilizes a nationwide classification system to rank hospitals according to the following levels: Level 3 (三级 *sān jí*), Level 2 (二级 *èr jí*), and Level 1 (一级 *yī jí*). Within each level, hospitals are ranked as first class (甲等 *jiǎ děng*), second class (乙等 *yǐ děng*), or third class (丙等 *bǐng děng*) (although in practice these finer gradations are only used with higher-level hospitals). These rankings are intended to correspond to the quality and scope of services offered by the institutions, and they establish the fees that the institutions are allowed to charge. Thus the highest-ranked Level 3 First Class (三级甲等 *sān jí jiǎ děng*) hospitals offer the most comprehensive range and highest quality of medical services (with correspondingly higher prices). Often serving as teaching hospitals affiliated with key medical universities, these hospitals are nationally renowned flagship medical institutions administered directly by the national Ministry of Health or provincial-level departments of health. Lower-ranked hospitals offer fewer medical services and are generally administered by health bureaus at the township or municipal district level.

6. This designation was later expanded into "Economic and Technological Development Zone" (经济技术开发区 *jīngjì jìshù kāifā qū*), which emphasized the technonationalist underpinnings of this state development policy.

7. The Germans seized control of the city from the weakened Qing dynasty (during the suppression of the anti-imperialist Boxer Rebellion) at the end of the nineteenth century. They established the city as a strategic naval base, developed the urban infrastructure, and built the Tsingtao brewery, which now produces beer for a world market. Japanese forces subsequently occupied the city during both world wars. More recently, the city has experienced an influx of Koreans who have set up factories and other business enterprises (Kim 2013). The Chinese media reported in 2005 that the population of Korean expatriates living in Qingdao had "surged" to one hundred thousand (Xinhua News Agency 2005a).

8. This is a multimillion U.S. dollar radiosurgery system for treating brain disorders imported from Sweden.

9. This is a diagnostic technique for producing three-dimensional images of the body's functional processes.

CHAPTER 7: SEEKING TRUTH FROM FACTS

1. I would like to thank my colleague Robert Hegel for pointing out the eerie parallels between present-day Chinese clinicians (injecting their patients with saline solution in the name of scientific inquiry) and Lao She's 1930s medical entrepreneurs injecting hapless patients with hypodermic needles filled with jasmine and longjing tea.

2. A solvent used in antifreeze and brake fluid, this toxic but sweet-tasting compound was also found in toothpaste made in China and exported around the world.

3. Derived from the mucous membranes of pig intestines, raw materials for the drug are often produced by small, unregulated farms in rural China. Unscrupulous suppliers substituted a much cheaper chemical (oversulfated chondroitin sulfate).

4. After a wave of infants developed kidney stones during the summer of 2008, public health regulators detected that the popular Sanlu brand of baby formula was diluted with melamine, a chemical used in industrial plastic manufacturing that mimics protein. But, worried about generating negative publicity during the Beijing Olympics, officials waited until the fall to reveal the news. By then several infants had already died from kidney failure (Economist 2008; Jiang 2008). Nearly three hundred thousand infants had become ill by the time two Sanlu Dairy Group producers were sentenced to death in January 2009 for their role in selling hundreds of tons of adulterated milk powder (Sommerville 2009; Xinhua News Agency 2009). The contaminant was subsequently found in a whole host of other milk-based products, from White Rabbit candy and Koala March cookies to Pizza Hut cheese packets and Starbucks coffee.

5. Medical anthropologists who have examined questions of efficacy in medical practice have focused predominantly on traditional healing systems such as Chinese medicine (Hsu 1999; Zhan 2009), Ayurveda (Langford 2002), and Tibetan medicine (Adams 2002; Craig 2012; Saxer 2012). These ethnographic studies demonstrate how "traditional" or "indigenous" healing systems are thoroughly modernized phenomena shaped by transnational practices and global circulations of people, capital, and standards.

6. Chinese regulations for clinical trials have become even more stringent than the U.S. Food and Drug Administration's guidelines—at least on paper. Originally adopted in 1984 and revised in 2001 just before China's admittance as a formal member of the World Trade Organization, the Drug Administration Law of the People's Republic of China (中华人民共和国药品管理法) was enacted to "strengthen the governance of drug products, ensure drug quality and safety, and to protect the health of people and their legitimate rights and interests in the use of drugs" (为加强药品监督管理，保证药品质量，保障人体用药安全，维护人民身体健康和用药的合法权益，特制定本法 [Article 1]). The revised rules regulate all aspects of drug research, production, distribution, marketing, use, and administration by requiring drug manufacturers, distributors, and research institutions to obtain certification and follow specific practice guidelines. Thus all drug manufacturers are required to obtain official Drug Manufacturing Certificates (药品生产许可证) issued by the local drug regulatory department of the people's government by demonstrating that they will conduct production according to the Good Manufacturing Practice for Pharmaceutical Products (GMP) (药品生产质量管理规范) (Drug Administration Law, Articles 7 and 9). (Sienna Craig [2012] and Martin Saxer [2012] have analyzed the effects of Chinese GMP regulations on the production of Tibetan medicine.) Likewise, drug wholesalers and retailers are required to obtain Drug Supply Certificates (药品经营许可证) by demonstrating they will conduct business according to the Good Supply Practice for Pharmaceutical Products (GSP) (药品经营质量管理规范) (Drug Administration Law, Articles 14 and 16). Laboratories evaluating the safety of new drugs and medical institutions performing clinical studies of drug efficacy are required, respectively, to implement the Good Laboratory Practice for Non-Clinical Laboratory Studies (GLP) (药物非临床研究质量管理规范) and Good Clinical Practice (GCP) (药物临床试验质量管理规范) (Drug Administration Law, Article 30). The good-practice guidelines mandated by the Drug Administration

Law are based on globally recognized standards laid out by the International Conference on Harmonization of Technical Requirements for Registration of Pharmaceuticals for Human Use (ICH 1996).

7. An Investigational New Drug (IND) application applies to new drugs or biological products (U.S. FDA 2016). New medical devices deemed to pose significant risk are subject to the FDA's Investigational Device Exemption (IDE) regulations (U.S. FDA 2015). Notably, the FDA does not regulate new surgical procedures unless these employ devices or biological products (Spodick 1975; Deyo 2004). If Huang were operating in the United States, his procedure would come under the jurisdiction of the FDA since he is injecting a biological product (i.e., olfactory ensheathing glial cells).

8. Even within the biomedical community, there is a growing movement to examine the effectiveness of interventions—to assess whether new treatments work not just under the carefully controlled conditions of a randomized controlled trial (RCT) but also under "real-world" circumstances. The growing field of "comparative effectiveness research" is an example of this pushback against the narrow constraints of RCTs (IOM 2009).

9. These concerns harken back to a long tradition of anthropological scholarship on magic, science, and religion, which has engaged questions of rationality and efficacy in evaluating the status of knowledge claims produced by other societies (Malinowski 1948 [1922]; Evans-Pritchard 1976; Tambiah 1990; Good 1994; Nader 1996). Scholars of Chinese philosophy and religion have also examined notions of efficacy in the Chinese context, including French sinologist François Jullien's (1995) brilliant analysis of the Chinese term *shì* (势, variously translated as disposition or circumstance, power or potential) and anthropologist Steven Sangren's (1987) incisive dissection of *líng* (灵 magical efficacy) in the context of Chinese popular religion in Taiwan.

10. As Bruno Latour points out in his classic study of the pasteurization of France, the main challenge that Louis Pasteur faced in his research on the anthrax disease was how to make the activities inside the laboratory relevant to questions outside in the fields and on the animal farms. For Latour, this act of translation was Pasteur's crowning achievement: convincing the assorted farmers, veterinarians, politicians, and other groups that his laboratory was not only relevant but essential in solving the anthrax problem—or in Latour's terminology, making the laboratory the fulcrum or "obligatory point of passage" (1988, 43).

11. Prior to the establishment of the U.S. Food and Drug Administration, an unregulated drug and remedy market posed significant risks to the American public. As a groundbreaking report titled "The Great American Fraud" (Adams 1905) documented at the turn of the twentieth century, commonly available and widely advertised patent medicines not only involved deceptive marketing practices but also contained poisonous ingredients and addictive narcotics. The exposé of medical quackery by muckraking journalists such as Adams caused so much public outrage that Congress enacted the first of a series of food and drug laws in 1906, which eventually led to the establishment of the U.S. Food and Drug Administration (U.S. FDA 2014). Although the original act focused on the regulation of product labeling and prohibited false therapeutic claims for drugs, subsequent laws mandated

pre-market approval of all new drugs. After more than a hundred people died from taking Elixir of Sulfanilamide, a patent medicine for strep throat containing the poisonous antifreeze solvent diethylene glycol (Ballentine 1981), Congress passed the Federal Food, Drug, and Cosmetic Act of 1938. This act established a comprehensive system of drug regulation, with stringent requirements for manufacturers to prove that new drugs were safe before they could be sold (Geiger 1937; U.S. FDA 2014). RCTs became a key tool for clinicians and pharmaceutical manufacturers for proving the safety and efficacy of their products.

12. The Evidence-Based Medicine Working Group is a collaboration of clinicians, epidemiologists, and statisticians from Canada, the U.K., and the United States. The group is chaired by Gordon Guyatt, who first coined the term "evidence-based medicine" in 1991 (BMJ 2009). The EBM Working Group has published several editorials and clinical practice recommendations over the past two decades in the *Journal of the American Medical Association* (*JAMA*).

13. Byer has been an active advocate and spokesperson in the quest to find treatments for ALS, researching and publicizing the results of several promising therapies for the neurodegenerative disease. He has given public interviews to journalists (Shetty 2004), sent countless emails to people around the world interested in these therapies, and was featured in his son's award-winning documentary on ALS (Byer 2008). Since he is someone who has deliberately chosen to become a public spokesperson on experimental treatments for ALS, I have used Byer's actual name in this book. I should also note that while many PALS have only praise for Byer's tireless efforts, others have been less sanguine about their experiences with him. These complicated entanglements form a fascinating story that I must set aside for another book.

14. Named "BuNaoGao" (补脑膏 *bǔnǎogāo*, literally "mend brain ointment"), this herbal formulary was developed to treat neurodegenerative conditions by Xia Yongchao (夏永潮), a traditional Chinese medical practitioner at the Gansu Provincial TCM Hospital (甘肃省中医院 Gānsù Shěng Zhōngyī Yuàn). Stephen Byer discovered BNG in 2004 during the course of investigating possible treatments for his son Ben. Byer ultimately became a full-time volunteer liaison for Dr. Xia, making BNG available to hundreds of PALS outside of China. Byer helped develop a standardized protocol for non-Chinese PALS to prepare the herbal medication and monitor their long-term results in a systematic way. Ben Byer also recounted this story of discovery in his documentary *Indestructible*, which he completed before his death in July 2008.

15. Rilutek (generic name riluzole) is the first and currently only drug to be approved for the treatment of ALS (first by the European Commission, followed by the U.S. FDA in 1995). Although it does not cure the disease or improve symptoms, large-scale multicenter clinical trials have demonstrated that it extends the survival of patients by an average of three months (Bensimon et al. 1994; Lacomblez et al. 1996).

The financial costs are sobering, however. Without the prescription benefits of a health insurance plan or a manufacturer discount, the cost for sixty 50-milligram Rilutek tablets (a one-month supply) is $1,335.99 (price estimate as of May 2014 from goodrx.com, a website that enables consumers to compare prices among various pharmacies to obtain the best discounts). While U.S. neurologists have been quick to castigate Huang for charging $20,000 for the OEG procedure, few mainstream physicians have critiqued Sanofi (the pharmaceutical company that originally received exclusive marketing rights in the United States from the FDA to sell Rilutek) for charging $16,000 for a year's supply of Rilutek in spite of its arguably negligible benefits. The patent for Rilutek expired in June 2013, enabling other manufacturers to obtain approval from the U.S. FDA to market the generic riluzole (Madsen 2013). While the generic version has reduced the costs by a significant margin, all of the patients discussed in this book faced the challenge of much steeper brand-name pricing for the only FDA-approved treatment available for their disease.

16. Perhaps the most sensational example of this phenomenon was the ALS Ice Bucket Challenge, which went viral on social media in the summer of 2014 and inspired tens of thousands of people to dump buckets of ice water over their heads to raise money for ALS research. This grassroots effort ultimately raised over a hundred million dollars for ALS research and advocacy organizations. While scientists have welcomed these monetary donations, many have shown skepticism toward more active involvement by PALS to guide research initiatives.

17. "有的人只会说批评… OK Dobkin, 你说怎么做？你说需要做假手术对照, 你能做吗？你不能做。该手术要做非常不符合中国的医学伦理。

　　小宋, 我昨天已经说过这个问题, 如果说某个国家容许做这种为了所谓的科学伦理, 去做这种空白对照手术, 我非常鄙视这个国家, 它的医学伦理已经沦落到这个程度, 把人不当人, 把病人不当人, 而是作为一个机械, 当成一个动物来做实验, 非常不道德的！我觉得这种卑鄙的医学应该消除！…不顾病人的创伤, 不顾病人可能的危害, 可能的病发证, 甚至可能生命危险, 都不顾了。而就是要得到一个什么？得到一个所谓的科学结论。" (interview with the author, April 21, 2006).

18. This research report described the effectiveness of transplanted OEG cells in restoring motor function to adult Long-Evans hooded laboratory rats whose spines had been systematically contused by a weight-drop impactor device, according to the protocol Huang had learned as a postdoctoral researcher at New York University and fine-tuned later at Rutgers. Listing Wise Young and other Rutgers colleagues as coauthors, Huang documented functional improvements in the injured rats who had received OEG transplantation using a standardized locomotor rating scale (Basso, Beattie, and Bresnahan 1995). The two injured rats that had been injected only with saline solution did not have any weight-supporting ability, while the majority of rats that had received OEG transplantation (either immediately or two weeks following injury) demonstrated frequent to consistent weight-supported plantar steps and even occasional front-leg and hind-leg coordination.

19. The Chinese patients ranged from 2.5 to 55 years old and included both men and women with complete and incomplete injuries at varying levels of the spinal cord. Huang claimed that all twenty-three patients showed improvement in motor function as well as light touch and pin-prick sensation (according to the American Spinal Injury Association [ASIA] standardized assessment scale). The simple three-by-four cell table he used to showcase his data presented only pre- and post-surgical scores that were averaged across the entire group without listing standard deviations, making it impossible to assess whether results varied by age.

20. This paper attempted to assess the influence of age on the extent of functional recovery, breaking down the assessment scores by five separate age cohorts. Huang's report now listed the standard deviations along with each score, which revealed

large fluctuations that often overshadowed the purported point gains. According to Huang's reported data, the only statistically significant difference among the motor and sensory scores of the various age cohorts was in the sensory pin-prick scores of the oldest group. For these fourteen patients over age 51, their average post-surgical gain in pin-prick or *tòngjué* (痛觉 pain sensation) score was 25.4 points—but with a deviation from the mean of 24.3 points. As this suggests, the effect of the OEG transplantation was thus highly variable.

21. One exception was the online CareCure Community, whose members caught an early glimpse of Huang's clinical work through neuroscientist Wise Young. Wise had remained in touch with his former postdoctoral researcher via email and subsequently visited Naval General Hospital in December 2002. After observing Huang and his team perform two OEG transplantation operations and assessing Chinese patients who had undergone the procedure, Wise described Huang's efforts to the CareCure Community as a "credible phase 1 trial" that demonstrated the safety and feasibility of fetal OEG transplants (Wise Young 2002b). As we saw in chapter 3, Wise's preliminary assessment ignited a storm of interest among Care-Cure members. While some immediately began inquiring about the possibility of undergoing the experimental procedure themselves, others wanted to see more definitive evidence beyond the anecdotal online reports.

22. For ALS patients, New Century clinicians utilized the ALS Functional Rating Scale, which calculated patients' quality of function in four main areas: gross motor tasks, fine motor tasks, bulbar functions (e.g., speech and swallowing), and respiratory function (ALS CNTF Treatment Study [ACTS] Phase I–II Study Group 1996; Cedarbaum et al. 1999). Specific questions addressed a patient's ability to perform tasks related to speech, salivation, swallowing, handwriting, cutting food, dressing and hygiene, turning in bed, walking, climbing stairs, and breathing. While the original scale was designed "to track progression of patients' disability in ALS" (Cedarbaum et al. 1999, 18), Huang's staff adapted the scale to assess the possibility of improvement following the OEC transplantation.

23. Despite the push for universality as evidenced by the name change from "American" to "International," most of the hundreds of clinicians, patients, and family members I have interviewed over the past decade continue to refer to these standards as the "ASIA classification." Interestingly, the "ASIA" acronym itself erases the overt "Americanness" of the standards and even hints at an alternative geographical orientation rooted in the Far East.

24. As I discussed in chapter 4, Chinese patients were expected to procure the aborted fetus(es) for the experimental procedure. Despite his relative wealth and satisfaction with his earlier surgery, Lu found this requirement to be too onerous to undergo a second OEG fetal cell transplantation.

25. "以前我只能躺在床上看着天花板度日, 不能坐起来, 一坐起来就头晕眼花, 眼冒金星, 恶心。呕吐。做了手术, 现在能坐轮椅两个多小时了, 自己把着轮椅满院子转" (interview with the author, March 1, 2006).

26. "因大部分患者来医院检查行动不便, 需安排医生外出完成此工作" (Huang Hongyun, New Century neurosurgery department staff meeting, December 2005).

27. In 1980, around the time of Bird's birth, China had an overall Hepatitis B infection rate of 42.6 percent with perinatal transmission (transfer of a disease-causing

agent from mother to baby during the period immediately before and after birth) accounting for 35–50 percent of carriers (Yao 1996).

28. This involved finding donor cells that shared the same set of human leukocyte antigens (HLA) as those of the recipient. The more pairs of HLA antigens that match, the lower the chance of graft rejection, in which the recipient's immune system sees the transplanted cells as foreign and attacks the transplanted cells.

CHAPTER 8: I-WITNESSING

1. As the spouse of a physician, I can attest to the truth of Curt's remark. Given the increasing division of labor between various medical specialties and the proliferation of narrowly focused journals, it is not surprising that most general practitioners, emergency room doctors, and even orthopedic surgeons have trouble keeping up with the latest developments in neurobiology.

2. The paper Steven referred to contained the results of a study of 171 spinal-injured patients that Dr. Huang was trying to publish at the time. Rejected by several leading scientific journals with international reputations, the paper was eventually published at the end of the year by the *Chinese Medical Journal*, an English-language journal based in Beijing (Huang et al. 2003b).

3. To maintain her son's confidentiality, I have chosen to use pseudonyms for the entire family since I do not cite their public statements here. My purpose here is to illustrate another material pathway in the quest for evidence.

4. Laurence Kirmayer (1992) has highlighted the role of metaphor in giving meaning to illness experience that is grounded simultaneously in bodily experience and social interaction. As I have explored elsewhere (Song 2010), by describing himself as an "OEG pilgrim," Tim C. articulated a purposeful trajectory to his illness narrative steeped in an American idiom of self-reliance in the face of hardship. The pilgrimage metaphor gave meaningful shape to the suffering he endured in seeking treatment in an unfamiliar hospital in a foreign land. He lamented the hostile political climate in the United States under the Bush administration, blaming "the few 'righteous' decision makers in our government" for restricting stem cell research and driving him abroad to search for potential treatments (2003a). His use of pilgrimage evoked a metaphorical kinship with the early settlers of Plymouth Colony who left behind the familiarity of home to escape religious persecution and search out better opportunities in a new world. Tim C.'s special status as "OEG pilgrim" imbued him with a sense of purpose that extended beyond his own bodily concerns. He saw himself not only as an individual patient seeking to heal his own body but also as a contributor to the scientific enterprise. His industrial and agricultural metaphors (of building a Model-T and planting seeds) enacted a distinctly American tale of hard work and innovation in which his suffering played a leading role. As a self-declared pilgrim in the brave new world of experimental medicine, he interpreted the significance of his journey not just in terms of his own personal benefit but in terms of the future of the entire SCI community and scientific enterprise.

5. Many more individuals used CareCure to investigate the OEG procedure and contact Huang, without necessarily contributing back to the community in the form

of updates about their subsequent experiences. The "Soon-to-Be-Infamous Huang List" eventually included over five hundred inquiries directed to Dr. Huang about signing up for the OEG procedure, from as recently as 2012 (Sriram 2012).

EPILOGUE: ON THE CUTTING EDGE

1. "我随便拿一个东西给病人, 他就问消毒了吗? 这个东西是干净的吗? 在他的脑海里大概中国所有的东西都是不经过消毒的…我就感觉到很屈辱" (interview with author, March 14, 2006).

2. "我真的认为不是外国人都做得好, 我不相信外国医生都是好医生, 就像中国的所有医生不一定都是差医生一样, 中国确实有差医生, 但也确实有医术比较高明的医生, 在美国和欧洲也是一样, 他们的整体水平可能会高一点, 但是也有差的医生。因为我觉得在欧美这些发达国家, 他们的医生更多的依赖于器械, 因为他们的仪器非常发达, 他们更多的依赖于这些东西, 做什么检查之类的…他对原始的东西, 像捏皮球, 我想他不一定很顺手" (interview with author, March 14, 2006).

3. "可能在西班牙他们很少捏, 发达国家用机器用得很习惯, 而我们经常会自己捏, 他其实捏的时候没有什么技巧…我观察他, 他捏的完全和病人反的, 病人出气他捏, 病人吸气他放, 这样的话, 他每次捏的时候儿子就非常紧张的看着…不停地给他爸爸擦汗, 因为病人很辛苦…我不敢让他捏了, 我说算了, 我自己捏…我走的时候, 他们家人一直在说, 中国医生很好, 西班牙的医生不好" (interview with author, March 14, 2006).

4. Over a decade after Huang's pioneering work with fetal olfactory ensheathing glial cells, these cells continue to attract international attention for their potential to reverse spinal paralysis. Media outlets around the world have profiled Polish firefighter Darek Fidyka, who regained his ability to walk after an OEG cell transplantation procedure performed by a Polish British neurosurgical team in 2014 (Walsh 2014; Max 2016).

BIBLIOGRAPHY

ALL ONLINE SOURCES WERE VERIFIED in August 2016 unless otherwise noted.

Abkowitz, J. 2002. "Can Human Hematopoietic Stem Cells Become Skin, Gut, or Liver Cells?" *New England Journal of Medicine* 346(10): 770–72.

Abraham, Itty. 1998. *The Making of the Indian Atomic Bomb: Science, Secrecy and the Postcolonial State*. London: Zed Press.

Adams, Samuel Hopkins. 1905. "The Great American Fraud." *Collier's Weekly*, October 7. http://www.gutenberg.org/files/44325/44325-h/44325-h.htm.

Adams, Vincanne. 2002. "Randomized Controlled Crime: Postcolonial Sciences in Alternative Medicine Research." *Social Studies of Science* 32(5/6): 659–90.

Agamben, Giorgio. 1998. *Homo Sacer: Sovereign Power and Bare Life*. Translated by Daniel Heller-Roazen. Stanford, CA: Stanford University Press.

ALS CNTF Treatment Study (ACTS) Phase I–II Study Group. 1996. "The Amyotrophic Lateral Sclerosis Functional Rating Scale: Assessment of Activities of Daily Living in Patients with Amyotrophic Lateral Sclerosis." *Archives of Neurology* 53: 141–47. doi:10.1001/archneur.1996.00550020045014.

American Spinal Injury Association. 2015. "International Standards for Neurological Classification of Spinal Cord Injury." Revised 2011, updated 2015. http://asia-spinalinjury.org/wp-content/uploads/2016/02/International_Stds_Diagram_Worksheet.pdf.

Anagnost, Ann. 1995. "Surfeit of Bodies: Population and the Rationality of the State in Post-Mao China." In *Conceiving the New World Order: The Global Politics of Reproduction*, edited by Faye Ginsburg and Rayna Rapp, 22–41. Berkeley: University of California Press.

———. 2004. "The Corporeal Politics of Quality (Suzhi)." *Public Culture* 16(2): 189–208.

———. 2006. "Strange Circulations: The Blood Economy in Rural China." *Economy and Society* 35(4): 509–29.

Anderson, Benedict. 1991. *Imagined Communities: Reflections on the Origin and Spread of Nationalism*. Rev. ed. New York: Verso.

Anderson, D. J., F. H. Gage, and I. L. Weissman. 2001. "Can Stem Cells Cross Lineage Boundaries?" *Nature Medicine* 7: 393–95.

Andrews, Peter W. 2002. "From Teratocarcinomas to Embryonic Stem Cells." *Philosophical Transactions of the Royal Society B: Biological Sciences* 357(1420): 405–17.

Austrian Bioethics Commission. 2009. "Forschung an humanen embryonalen Stammzellen: Stellungnahme der Bioethikkommission" [Research on Human Embryonic

Stem Cells: Opinion of the Austrian Bioethics Commission]. http://www.bka.gv
.at/DocView.axd?CobId=34240.

Ballentine, Carol. 1981. "Taste of Raspberries, Taste of Death: The 1937 Elixir Sulfanilamide Incident." *FDA Consumer Magazine* (June). http://www.fda.gov/aboutfda/
whatwedo/history/productregulation/sulfanilamidedisaster/default.htm.

Banner, Olivia. 2014. "'Treat Us Right!': Digital Publics, Emerging Biosocialities, and
the Female Complaint." In *Identity Technologies: Constructing the Self Online*, edited
by Anna Poletti and Julie Rak, 198–216. Madison: University of Wisconsin Press.

Bardill, Jessica. 2014. "Native American DNA: Ethical, Legal, and Social Implications
of an Evolving Concept." *Annual Review of Anthropology* 43: 155–66.

Basso, D. Michele, Michael S. Beattie, and Jacqueline C. Bresnahan. 1995. "A Sensitive
and Reliable Locomotor Rating Scale for Open Field Testing in Rats." *Journal of
Neurotrauma* 12(1): 1–21. doi:10.1089/neu.1995.12.1.

BBC. 2001. "US Warned of Cloning 'Brain Drain.'" BBC News, August 2. http://news
.bbc.co.uk/2/hi/americas/1470155.stm.

Beijing Chaoyang Hospital 北京朝阳医院. 2012. "Běijīng chāoyáng yīyuàn " 北京朝
阳医院简介 [Beijing Chaoyang Hospital Introduction]. http://www.bjcyh.com.cn/
yygk/yyjj/2014/0629/3072.html.

Benjamin, Ruha. 2013. *People's Science: Bodies and Rights on the Stem Cell Frontier*.
Stanford, CA: Stanford University Press.

Bensimon, G., L. Lacomblez, V. Meininger, and the ALS/Riluzole Study Group. 1994.
"A Controlled Trial of Riluzole in Amyotrophic Lateral Sclerosis." *New England
Journal of Medicine* 330(9): 585–91.

Benson, Peter, and Stuart Kirsch. 2010. "Capitalism and the Politics of Resignation."
Current Anthropology 51(4): 459–86.

Bernal, Victoria. 2005. "Eritrea On-line: Diaspora, Cyberspace, and the Public Sphere."
American Ethnologist 32(4): 660–75.

———. 2014. *Nation as Network*. Chicago: University of Chicago Press.

Bharadwaj, Aditya. 2012. "Enculturating Cells: The Anthropology, Substance, and
Science of Stem Cells." *Annual Review of Anthropology* 41: 303–17.

BIONET. 2010. "Ethical Governance of Biological and Biomedical Research:
Chinese-European Co-operation. Final Report." BIOS Centre. London School
of Economics. http://www.lse.ac.uk/researchAndExpertise/units/BIONET/pdfs/
BIONET%20Final%20Report1.pdf.

Bjornson, C. R., R. L. Rietze, B. A. Reynolds, M. C. Magli, and A. L. Vescovi. 1999.
"Turning Brain into Blood: A Hematopoietic Fate Adopted by Adult Neural Stem
Cells in Vivo." *Science* 283: 534–37.

Bloch, Ernst. 1986 [1959]. *The Principle of Hope*. London: Blackwell.

Blumenthal, David, and William Hsiao. 2005. "Privatization and Its Discontents: The
Evolving Chinese Health Care System." *New England Journal of Medicine* 353(11):
1165–70.

BMJ. 2009. "BMJ Group Lifetime Achievement Award: Professor Gordon Guyatt."
BMJ 339: b5546.

Boellstorff, Tom. 2008. *Coming of Age in Second Life: An Anthropologist Explores the
Virtually Human*. Princeton: Princeton University Press.

Boellstorff, Tom, B. Nardi, C. Pearce, and T. L. Taylor. 2012. *Ethnography and Virtual
Worlds: A Handbook of Method*. Princeton: Princeton University Press.

Boer, Gerard J. 2005. "Niets te verliezen: ALS-patiënten ondergaan omstreden Chinese neurochirurgie" [Nothing to Lose: ALS Patients Undergoing Controversial Chinese Neurosurgery]. *Medisch Contact* 60(4): 150–51.

Bolnick, Deborah A., Duana Fullwiley, Troy Duster, Richard S. Cooper, Joan H. Fujimura, Jonathan Kahn, Jay S. Kaufman, Jonathan Marks, Ann Morning, Alondra Nelson, Pilar Ossorio, Jenny Reardon, Susan M. Reverby, and Kimberly TallBear. 2007. "The Science and Business of Genetic Ancestry Testing." *Science* 318: 399–400. doi:10.1126/science.1150098.

Bracken, Michael B., Mary Jo Shepard, William F. Collins, Theodore R. Holford, Wise Young, David S. Baskin, Howard M. Eisenberg, Eugene Flamm, Linda Leo-Summers, Joseph Maroon, et al. 1990. "A Randomized, Controlled Trial of Methylprednisolone or Naloxone in the Treatment of Acute Spinal Cord Injury." *New England Journal of Medicine* 323: 1209. doi:10.1056/NEJM199005173222001.

Bracken, Michael B., Mary Jo Shepard, Theodore R. Holford, Linda Leo-Summers, E. Francois Aldrich, Mahmood Fazi, Michael Fehlings, Daniel Herr, Patrick W. Hitchon, Lawrence F. Marshall, et al. 1997. "Administration of Methylprednisolone for 24 or 48 Hours or Tirilazad Mesylate for 48 Hours in the Treatment of Acute Spinal Cord Injury: Results of the Third National Acute Spinal Cord Injury Randomized Controlled Trial." *JAMA* 277(20): 1597–1604. doi:10.1001/jama.1997.03540440031029.

Brivanlou, Ali H., Fred H. Gage, Rudolf Jaenisch, Thomas Jessell, Douglas Melton, and Janet Rossant. 2003. "Setting Standards for Human Embryonic Stem Cells." *Science* 300(5621): 913–16. doi:10.1126/science.1082940.

Brooks, Jack. 1992. "Chinese Student Protection Act of 1992: Report to Accompany S. 1216 of the Committee on the Judiciary, House of Representatives, 102nd Congress, 2nd Session." http://files.eric.ed.gov/fulltext/ED351414.pdf.

Brotherton, P. Sean. 2012. *Revolutionary Medicine: Health and the Body in Post-Soviet Cuba*. Durham, NC: Duke University Press.

Brown, Nik. 2003. "Hope against Hype: Accountability in Biopasts, Presents and Futures." *Science Studies* 16(2): 3–21.

Brown, Phil, and Stephen Zavestoski, eds. 2004. "Special Issue: Social Movements in Health." *Sociology of Health & Illness* 26(6): 679–874.

Brownell, Susan. 2008. *Beijing's Games: What the Olympics Mean to China*. Lanham, MD: Rowman and Littlefield.

Bruijn, Lucie I., Timothy M. Miller, and Don W. Cleveland. 2004. "Unraveling the Mechanisms Involved in Motor Neuron Degeneration in ALS." *Annual Review of Neuroscience* 27: 723–49.

Buckley, Christopher. 1999. "How a Revolution Becomes a Dinner Party: Stratification, Mobility and the New Rich in Urban China." In *Culture and Privilege in Capitalist Asia*, edited by Michael Pinches, 208–29. London: Routledge.

Burawoy, Michael, and Katherine Verdery, eds. 1999. *Uncertain Transition: Ethnographies of Change in the Postsocialist World*. Lanham, MD: Rowman and Littlefield.

Burrell, Jenna, and Ken Anderson. 2008. "'I Have Great Desires to Look beyond My World': Trajectories of Information and Communication Technology Use among Ghanaians Living Abroad." *New Media & Society* 10(2): 203–24.

Bush, George W. 2001. "President Discusses Stem Cell Research." August 9. https://georgewbush-whitehouse.archives.gov/news/releases/2001/08/20010809-2.html.

Buyandelger, Manduhai. 2008. "Post-Post-Transition Theories: Walking on Multiple Paths." *Annual Review of Anthropology* 37: 235–50.

Byer, Ben. 2008. *Indestructible*. Directed, written, and produced by Ben Byer. New York: IndiePix Films, 2010. DVD.

Bynum, W. F. 2006. "The Rise of Science in Medicine, 1850–1913." In *The Western Medical Tradition 1800 to 2000*, edited by W. F. Bynum, Anne Hardy, Stephen Jacyna, Christopher Lawrence, and E. M. Tansey, 111–229. New York: Cambridge University Press.

CanDo.com. 2000a. "CanDo.com Merges with SpineWire.com to Unveil Premier Internet Gateway for the Mobility-Impaired Community: Partnership Brings Patent-Pending Proprietary Technology, Unique Business and Consumer Services, Top Management Team Expertise, Community Traffic, Special Advertising and Sponsorship Initiatives." Company Press Release. February 24. http://www.mult-sclerosis.org/news/Feb2000/CanDocomSpineWirecom.html.

———. 2000b. "CanDo.com Homepage" (December 2000 snapshot). http://web.archive.org/web/20001206101500/http://www.spinewire.com/.

Cao, Haidong, and Jianfeng Fu 曹海东, 傅剑锋. 2005. "Zhōngguó yīgǎi èrshí nián" 中国医改二十年." [Twenty Years of Health Reforms in China]. *Nánfāng Zhōumò* 南方周末 [Southern Weekend]. August 4. http://news.xinhuanet.com/health/2005-08/04/content_3308662.htm.

CareCure. 2016. "We Are the CareCure Community." http://sci.rutgers.edu/.

Cedarbaum, Jesse M., Nancy Stambler, Errol Malta, Cynthia Fuller, Dana Hilt, Barbara Thurmond, and Arline Nakanishi. 1999. "The ALSFRS-R: A Revised ALS Functional Rating Scale That Incorporates Assessments of Respiratory Function." [BDNF ALS Study Group (Phase III).] *Journal of the Neurological Sciences* 169: 13–21.

Chen, Changgui, Stanley Rosen, and David Zweig. 1995. *China's Brain Drain to the United States: Views of Overseas Chinese Students and Scholars in the 1990s*. Berkeley: Institute of East Asian Studies.

Chen, Haifeng 陈海峰. 1989. *Zhōngguó wèishēng bǎojiàn shi* 中国卫生保健史 [History of Chinese Health and Hygiene]. Shanghai: Shànghǎi Kēxué Jìshù Chūbǎn Shè 上海科学技术出版社 [Shanghai Science and Technology Press].

Chen, Lin, and Hongyun Huang 陈琳, 黄红云. 2009. "Shénjīng xiūfù xué xuékē tǐxì ruògān wèntí tàntǎo" 神经修复学学科体系若干问题探讨 [Neurorestoratology: New Concept and Bridge from Bench to Bedside]. *Zhōngguó Xiūfù Chóngjiàn Wàikē Zázhì* 中国修复重建外科杂志 [Chinese Journal of Reparative and Reconstructive Surgery] 23(3): 366–70.

Chen, Lin, Hongyun Huang, Hongmei Wang, Haitao Xi, Chengqing Gou, Jian Zhang, Feng Zhang, and Yancheng Liu 陈琳, 黄红云, 王洪美, 王洪美, 郗海涛, 苟成青, 张健, 张峰, 刘彦铖. 2006a. "Xiù qiào xìbāo yízhí zhìliáo wǎnqí jǐsuǐ sǔnshāng de cháng qī ānquán xìng píngjià: Cí gòngzhèn chéngxiàng sān nián suífǎng" 嗅鞘细胞移植治疗晚期脊髓损伤的长期安全性评价: 磁共振成像三年随访 [Long-Term Safety of Fetal Olfactory Ensheathing Glial Cell Transplantation in Treatment of Malignant Spinal Cord Injury: A Three-Year Follow-up with Magnetic Resonance Imaging]. *Zhōngguó Línchuáng Kāngfù* 中国临床康复 [Chinese Journal of Clinical Rehabilitation] 10(5): 28–29, 32.

Chen, Lin, Hongyun Huang, Yancheng Liu, Haotai Xi, Feng Zhang, Jian Zhang,

Hongmei Wang, Chengqing Gou, Ruiwen Liu, Chao Jiang, Zhao Jiang, Zixing Xie, and Chunyan Luo 陈琳; 黄红云; 刘彦铖; 郗海涛; 张峰; 张健; 王洪美; 苟成青; 刘瑞文; 姜超; 江昭; 谢自行; 罗春燕. 2006b. "Xiù qiào xìbāo yízhí zhìliáo jī wěisuō cè suǒ yìnghuà zhèng zhōngqí ānquán xìng píngjià" 嗅鞘细胞移植治疗肌萎缩侧索硬化症中期安全性评价 [Interim Safety Evaluation of Fetal Olfactory Ensheathing Cell Transplantation for Amyotrophic Lateral Sclerosis]. *Zhōngguó Línchuáng Kāngfu* 中国临床康复 [Chinese Journal of Clinical Rehabilitation] 10(25): 24–26.

Chen, Lin, Hongyun Huang, Jian Zhang, Feng Zhang, Yancheng Liu, Haitao Xi, Hongmei Wang, Zheng Gu, Yinglun Song, Yan Li, and Ke Tan 陈琳, 黄红云, 张健, 张峰, 刘彦铖, 郗海涛, 王洪美, 顾征, 宋英伦, 李荧, 谭可. 2007. "Pēitāi xiù qiào xìbāo yízhí zhìliáo jī wěisuō cè suǒ yìnghuà zhèng de jìnqí liáoxiào" 胚胎嗅鞘细胞移植治疗肌萎缩侧索硬化症的近期疗效 [Short-Term Outcome of Olfactory Ensheathing Cells Transplantation for Treatment of Amyotrophic Lateral Sclerosis]. *Zhōngguó Xiūfù Chóngjiàn Wàikē Zázhì* 中国修复重建外科杂志 [Chinese Journal of Reparative and Reconstructive Surgery] 9: 961–66.

Chen, Lin, Hongyun Huang, Haitao Xi, Zihang Xie, Ruiwen Liu, Zhao Jiang, Feng Zhang, Yancheng Liu, Di Chen, Qingmiao Wang, Hongmei Wang, Yushui Ren, and Changman Zhou. 2010. "Intracranial Transplant of Olfactory Ensheathing Cells in Children and Adolescents with Cerebral Palsy: A Randomized Controlled Clinical Trial." *Cell Transplantation* 19(2): 185–91.

Chen, Meei-Shia. 2001. "The Great Reversal: Transformation of Health Care in the People's Republic of China." In *The Blackwell Companion to Medical Sociology*, edited by William C. Cockerham, 456–82. Hoboken, NJ: Blackwell.

Chen, Nancy N. 2014. "Between Abundance and Insecurity: Securing Food and Medicine in an Age of Chinese Biotechnology." In *Bioinsecurity and Vulnerability*, edited by Nancy N. Chen and Lesley A. Sharp, 87–102. Santa Fe, NM: SAR Press.

Chew, Sheena, Alexander G. Khandji, Jacqueline Montes, Hiroshi Mitsumoto, and Paul H. Gordon. 2007. "Olfactory Ensheathing Glia Injections in Beijing: Misleading Patients with ALS." *Amyotrophic Lateral Sclerosis* 8: 314–16.

China Central Television (CCTV) 中国中央电视台. 2002. "Jǐsuǐ sǔnshāng zhìliáo yǒuwàng" 脊髓损伤治疗有望 [Hope for Spinal Cord Injury Treatment]. *Jiànkāng Zhī Lù* 健康之路 [Road to Health Program]. February 4. http://www.cctv.com/life/jiankangzhilu/benqi020204.html.

———. 2005. "Chéngbāo zhěnshì mài 'shén tiē'" 承包诊室卖 '神贴' [Renting a Diagnosis Room to Sell "Spirit Glue"]. *Jiāodiǎn Fǎngtán* 焦点访谈 [Focus Discussion]. March 20. http://www.cctv.com/health/20050320/100263.shtml.

Chu, Weihua 初卫华. 2001. "Zhìliáo wánquán xìng jǐsuǐ sǔnshāng yǒu jìnzhǎn: Xiùqiào xìbāo yízhí yìngyòng yú línchuáng" 治疗完全性脊髓损伤有进展: 嗅鞘细胞移植应用于临床 [Progress in the Treatment of Complete Spinal Cord Injury: Clinical Application of Olfactory Ensheathing Cell Transplantation]. *Jiànkāng Bào* 健康报 [Health News] December 22, p. 1.

Cochran, Sherman. 2006. *Chinese Medicine Men: Consumer Culture in China and Southeast Asia*. Cambridge, MA: Harvard University Press.

Cochrane, Archibald L. 1972. *Effectiveness and Efficiency: Random Reflections on Health Services*. London: Nuffield Provincial Hospitals Trust.

Cohen, Lawrence. 2001. "The Other Kidney: Biopolitics beyond Recognition." *Body & Society* 7(2–3): 9–29.

Coleman, E. Gabriella. 2010. "Ethnographic Approaches to Digital Media." *Annual Review of Anthropology* 39: 487–505.

Constable, Nicole. 2003. "Ethnography in Imagined Virtual Communities." In *Romance on a Global Stage: Pen Pals, Virtual Ethnography, and "Mail-order" Marriages*, 31–62. Berkeley: University of California Press.

Craig, Sienna. 2012. *Healing Elements: Efficacy and the Social Ecologies of Tibetan Medicine*. Berkeley: University of California Press.

Crapanzano, Vincent. 2004. *Imaginative Horizons: An Essay in Literary-Philosophical Anthropology*. Chicago: University of Chicago Press.

Cushing, Harvey. 1927. "Organization and Activities of the Neurological Service American Expeditionary Forces." In *The Medical Department of the United States Army in the World War*, edited by M. Ireland, 749–58. Washington, DC: GPO.

Cyranoski, David. 2005. "Paper Chase: Thousands of Patients Are Queueing to Be Treated by Hongyun Huang at His Beijing Clinic." News Feature, October 6. *Nature* 437: 810–11.

Cyranoski, David, and Apoorva Mandavilli. 2006. "People to Watch: Hongyun Huang, Yongzhang Luo, Hongkui Deng." *Nature Medicine* 12(3): 262.

Davis, Deborah, and Nancy E. Chapman. 2002. "Turning Points in Chinese Health Care: Crisis or Opportunity?" *Yale-China Health Journal* 1: 3–9.

De Certeau, Michel. 1984. *The Practice of Everyday Life*. Translated by Steven Rendall. Berkeley: University of California Press.

Dennis, Carina. 2002. "China: Stem Cells Rise in the East." *Nature* 419: 334–36.

Deyo, Richard A. 2004. "Gaps, Tensions, and Conflicts in the FDA Approval Process: Implications for Clinical Practice." *Journal of the American Board of Family Medicine* 17(2): 142–49.

Dobkin, Bruce H., Armin Curt, and James Guest. 2006. "Cellular Transplants in China: Observational Study from the Largest Human Experiment in Chronic Spinal Cord Injury." *Neurorehabilitation and Neural Repair* 20(1): 5–13.

Doucette, Ronald. 1984. "The Glial Cells in the Nerve Fiber Layer of the Rat Olfactory Bulb." *Anatomical Record* 210: 385–91.

———. 1990. "Glial Influences on Axonal Growth in the Primary Olfactory System." *Glia* 3: 433–49.

Duckett, Jane. 2011. *The Chinese State's Retreat from Health: Policy and the Politics of Retrenchment*. New York: Routledge.

Dumit, Joseph. 2000. "When Explanations Rest: 'Good-Enough' Brain Science and the New Socio-medical Disorders." In *Living and Working with the New Medical Technologies: Intersections of Inquiry*, edited by Margaret Lock, Allan Young, and Alberto Cambrosio, 209–32. Cambridge Studies in Medical Anthropology. New York: Cambridge University Press.

———. 2006. "Illnesses You Have to Fight to Get: Facts as Forces in Uncertain, Emergent Illnesses." *Social Science & Medicine* 62(3): 577–90.

Dunn, Elizabeth C. 2004. *Privatizing Poland: Baby Food, Big Business, and the Remaking of Labor*. Ithaca, NY: Cornell University Press.

Economist. 2003. "Chinese Entrepreneurs: On Their Way Back." *The Economist*, November 6. http://www.economist.com/node/2193704.

———. 2007. "China's Economy: How Fit Is the Panda?" *The Economist*, September 27. http://www.economist.com/node/9861591.

———. 2008. "China's Baby-Milk Scandal: Formula for Disaster. The Politics of an Unconscionable Delay." *The Economist*, September 18. http://www.economist.com/node/12262271.

———. 2013. "Looks Good on Paper: A Flawed System for Judging Research Is Leading to Academic Fraud." *The Economist*, September 28. http://www.economist.com/node/21586845.

Ellison, Peter. 1996. "Reproductive Ecology and 'Local Biologies.'" Paper presented at the Annual Meeting of the American Anthropological Association, Washington, DC.

———. 1999. "Reproductive Ecologies and Reproductive Cancers." In *Hormones, Health and Behavior: A Socio-ecological and Lifespan Perspective*, edited by Catherine Panter-Brick and Carol M. Worthman, 184–209. Cambridge: Cambridge University Press.

Epstein, Steven. 1996. *Impure Science: AIDS, Activism, and the Politics of Knowledge*. Berkeley: University of California Press.

———. 2007. *Inclusion: The Politics of Difference in Medical Research*. Chicago: University of Chicago Press.

———. 2008. "Patient Groups and Health Movements." In *The Handbook of Science and Technology Studies*, 3rd ed., edited by Edward J. Hackett, Olga Amsterdamska, Michael Lynch, and Judy Wajcman, 499–539. Cambridge, MA: MIT Press.

EuroStemCell. 2014. "Regulation of Stem Cell Research in Europe." http://www.eurostemcell.org/stem-cell-regulations.

Evans-Pritchard, E. E. 1976. *Witchcraft, Oracles, and Magic among the Azande*. Oxford: Clarendon Press.

Evidence-Based Medicine Working Group. 1992. "Evidence-Based Medicine: A New Approach to Teaching the Practice of Medicine." *Journal of the American Medical Association* 268(17): 2420–25.

Executive Order 13505 of March 9, 2009. "Removing Barriers to Responsible Scientific Research Involving Human Stem Cells." *Code of Federal Regulations*, Title 3. http://www.gpo.gov/fdsys/pkg/FR-2009-03-11/pdf/E9-5441.pdf.

Fairless, Richard, and Susan C. Barnett. 2005. "Olfactory Ensheathing Cells: Their Role in Central Nervous System Repair." *International Journal of Biochemistry & Cell Biology* 37(4): 693–99.

Farquhar, Judith B. 1996. "Market Magic: Getting Rich and Getting Personal in Medicine after Mao." *American Ethnologist* 23(2): 239–57.

———. 2002. *Appetites: Food and Sex in Post-Socialist China*. Durham, NC: Duke University Press.

Farrer, James. 2002. *Opening Up: Youth Sex Culture and Market Reform in Shanghai*. Chicago: University of Chicago Press.

Feigenbaum, Evan. 2003. *Chinese Techno-Warriors: National Security and Strategic Competition from the Nuclear Age to the Information Age*. Stanford, CA: Stanford University Press.

Fielding, Nigel, Raymond Lee, and Grant Blank, eds. 2008. *The SAGE Handbook of Online Research Methods*. Los Angeles: SAGE.

Fleischer, Friederike. 2010. *Suburban Beijing: Housing and Consumption in Contemporary China*. Minneapolis: University of Minnesota Press.

Fong, Vanessa. 2007. "Morality, Cosmopolitanism, or Academic Attainment? Discourses on 'Quality' and Urban Chinese-Only-Children's Claims to Ideal Personhood." *City & Society* 19(1): 86–113.

———. 2011. *Paradise Redefined: Transnational Chinese Students and the Quest for Flexible Citizenship in the Developed World.* Stanford, CA: Stanford University Press.

Forney, Matthew. 2004. "Giving Back Hope." *TIME*, August 16. http://www.time.com/time/magazine/article/0,9171,682348,00.html.

Forrest, R., and J. Lee, eds. 2003. *Chinese Urban Housing Reform.* New York: Routledge.

Fortun, M. 2008. *Promising Genomics: Iceland and deCODE Genetics in a World of Speculation.* Berkeley: University of California Press.

Foucault, Michel. 2008. *The Birth of Biopolitics: Lectures at the College de France, 1978–79.* Edited by Michel Senellart. Translated by Graham Burchell. New York: Palgrave MacMillan.

Fox, Susannah. 2010. "E-Patients, Cyberchondriacs, and Why We Should Stop Calling Names." Pew Research Center. http://www.pewinternet.org/2010/08/30/e-patients-cyberchondriacs-and-why-we-should-stop-calling-names/.

———. 2011. "The Social Life of Health Information, 2011." Pew Research Center. http://www.pewinternet.org/files/old-media//Files/Reports/2011/PIP_Social_Life_of_Health_Info.pdf.

Fox, Susannah, and Lee Rainie. 2000. "The Online Health Care Revolution: How the Web Helps Americans Take Better Care of Themselves." Pew Research Center. http://www.pewinternet.org/files/old-media//Files/Reports/2000/PIP_Health_Report.pdf.pdf.

Fox Keller, Evelyn. 2000. *The Century of the Gene.* Cambridge, MA: Harvard University Press.

Franklin, Sarah. 2007. *Dolly Mixtures: The Remaking of Genealogy.* Durham, NC: Duke University Press.

———. 2013. *Biological Relatives: IVF, Stem Cells, and the Future of Kinship.* Durham, NC: Duke University Press.

Franklin, Sarah, and Margaret Lock. 2003. *Remaking Life and Death: Towards an Anthropology of the Biosciences.* Santa Fe, NM: School of American Research.

Freed, C. R., P. E. Greene, R. E. Breeze, et al. 2001. "Transplantation of Embryonic Dopamine Neurons for Severe Parkinson's Disease." *New England Journal of Medicine* 344(10): 710–19.

Freeman, Carla. 2007. "The 'Reputation' of Neoliberalism." *American Ethnologist* 34(2): 252–67.

———. 2014. *Entrepreneurial Selves: Neoliberal Respectability and the Making of a Caribbean Middle Class.* Durham, NC: Duke University Press.

Freeman, T. B., D. E. Vawter, P. E. Leaverton, et al. 1999. "Use of Placebo Surgery in Controlled Trials of a Cellular-Based Therapy for Parkinson's Disease." *New England Journal of Medicine* 341: 988–92.

Friedman, Jack R. 2009. "The 'Social Case': Illness, Psychiatry, and Deinstitutionalization in Postsocialist Romania." *Medical Anthropology Quarterly* 23(4): 375–96.

Friedman, Sara. 2006. *Intimate Politics: Marriage, the Market, and State Power in Southeastern China.* Harvard East Asian Monographs 265. Cambridge, MA: Harvard University Press.

Fujimura, Joan. 1996. *Crafting Science: A Sociohistory of the Quest for the Genetics of Cancer*. Cambridge, MA: Harvard University Press.

Fullwiley, Duana. 2008. "The Biologistical Construction of Race." *Social Studies of Science* 38: 695–735.

Garcia, Angela. 2010. *The Pastoral Clinic: Addiction and Dispossession along the Rio Grande*. Berkeley: University of California Press.

Geertz, Clifford. 1988. *Works and Lives: The Anthropologist as Author*. Stanford, CA: Stanford University Press.

Geiger, J. C. 1937. "Concerning Elixir of Sulfanilamide." *California and Western Medicine* 47(5): 353. http://www.ncbi.nlm.nih.gov/pmc/articles/PMC1752690/pdf/calwestmed00381-0066b.pdf.

Germany Federal Law Gazette. 2002. "Gesetz zur Sicherstellung des Embryonenschutzes im Zusammenhang mit Einfuhr und Verwendung menschlicher embryonaler Stammzellen vom 28. Juni 2002 (BGBl. I S. 2277)" [Law for the Protection of Embryos in Connection with the Importation and Use of Human Embryonic Stem Cells, June 28, 2002 (Federal Law Gazette I p. 2277)]. http://www.gesetze-im-internet.de/bundesrecht/stzg/gesamt.pdf.

Gershon, Ilana. 2010. *The Breakup 2.0: Disconnecting over New Media*. Ithaca, NY: Cornell University Press.

Gieryn, Thomas F. 1983. "Boundary-Work and the Demarcation of Science from Non-Science: Strains and Interests in Professional Ideologies of Scientists." *American Sociological Review* 48(6): 781–95.

Giordana, Maria Teresa, Silvia Grifoni, Barbara Votta, Michela Magistrello, Marco Vercellino, Alessia Pellerino, Roberto Navone, Consuelo Valentini, Andrea Calvo, and Adriano Chiò. 2010. "Neuropathology of Olfactory Ensheathing Cell Transplantation into the Brain of Two Amyotrophic Lateral Sclerosis (ALS) Patients." *Brain Pathology* 20(4): 730–37.

Gladwell, Malcolm. 2000. *The Tipping Point: How Little Things Can Make a Big Difference*. New York: Little, Brown.

Glass, J. D., N. M. Boulis, K. Johe, S. B. Rutkove, T. Federici, M. Polak, C. Kelly, and E. L. Feldman. 2012. "Lumbar Intraspinal Injection of Neural Stem Cells in Patients with Amyotrophic Lateral Sclerosis: Results of a Phase I Trial in 12 Patients." *Stem Cells* 30: 1144–51.

Good, Byron. 1994. *Medicine, Rationality, and Experience*. New York: Cambridge University Press.

Good, Mary-Jo DelVecchio. 2001. "The Biotechnical Embrace." *Culture, Medicine and Psychiatry* 25: 395–410.

Good, Mary-Jo DelVecchio, Byron J. Good, Cynthia Schaffer, and Stuart E. Lind. 1990. "American Oncology and the Discourse on Hope." *Culture, Medicine and Psychiatry* 14: 59–79.

Goodman, David S. G., and Xiaowei Zang. 2008. "The New Rich in China: The Dimensions of Social Change." In *The New Rich in China: Future Rulers, Present Lives*, edited by David S. G. Goodman, 1–20. London: Routledge.

Greenhalgh, Susan. 1994. "Controlling Births and Bodies in Village China." *American Ethnologist* 21(1): 3–30.

———. 2003. "Planned Births, Unplanned Persons: 'Population' in the Making of Chinese Modernity." *American Ethnologist* 30(21): 196–215.

———. 2008. *Just One Child: Science and Policy in Deng's China*. Berkeley: University of California Press.

Greenhalgh, Susan, and Edwin A. Winckler. 2005. *Governing China's Population: From Leninist to Neoliberal Biopolitics*. Stanford, CA: Stanford University Press.

Gropp, M., V. Shilo, G. Vainer, M. Gov, Y. Gil, et al. 2012. "Standardization of the Teratoma Assay for Analysis of Pluripotency of Human ES Cells and Biosafety of Their Differentiated Progeny." *PLoS ONE* 7(9): e45532. doi:10.1371/journal .pone.0045532.

Grundner, T. M., and R. E. Garrett. 1986. "Interactive Medical Telecomputing: An Alternative Approach to Community Health Education." *New England Journal of Medicine* 314: 982–85.

Guest, James, L. P. Herrera, and T. Qian. 2006. "Rapid Recovery of Segmental Neurological Function in a Tetraplegic Patient Following Transplantation of Fetal Olfactory Bulb-Derived Cells." *Spinal Cord* 44: 135–42.

Gupta, Akhil. 1995. "Blurred Boundaries: The Discourse of Corruption, the Culture of Politics, and the Imagined State." *American Ethnologist* 22(2): 375–402. doi:10.1525/ae.1995.22.2.02a00090.

———. 2012. *Red Tape: Bureaucracy, Structural Violence, and Poverty in India*. Durham, NC: Duke University Press.

Gupta, Sanjey, and Joseph Walline. 2008. "The Education of and Utilization of Diagnostic and Therapeutic Procedures by Emergency Physicians in Beijing, China." *Annals of Emergency Medicine* 52(4): S68.

Guyatt, G., J. Cairns, D. Churchill, et al. 1992. "Evidence-Based Medicine: A New Approach to Teaching the Practice of Medicine." *Journal of the American Medical Association* 268(17): 2420–25.

Hakken, David. 1999. *Cyborgs@Cyberspace? An Ethnographer Looks to the Future*. New York: Routledge.

Hann, Chris, Caroline Humphrey, and Katherine Verdery. 2002. "Introduction: Postsocialism as a Topic of Anthropological Investigation." In *Postsocialism: Ideals, Ideologies and Practices in Eurasia*, edited by C. M. Hann, 1–28. London: Routledge.

Hanser, Amy. 2002. "The Chinese Enterprising Self: Young, Educated Urbanites and the Search for Work." In *Popular China: Unofficial Culture in a Globalizing Society*, edited by Perry Link, Richard P. Madsen, and Paul G. Pickowicz, 189–206. Lanham, MD: Rowman and Littlefield.

Harmon, Katherine. 2012. "How Has Stephen Hawking Lived Past 70 with ALS? An Expert on Lou Gehrig's Disease Explains What We Know about This Debilitating Condition and How Hawking Has Beaten the Odds." *Scientific American*, January 7. http://www.scientificamerican.com/article/stephen-hawking-als/.

Harris, Gardiner, and Walt Bogdanich. 2008. "Drug Tied to China Had Contaminant, F.D.A. Says." *New York Times*, March 6. http://www.nytimes.com/2008/03/06/health/06heparin.html.

HarrisInteractive. 2011. "The Growing Influence and Use of Health Care Information Obtained Online." The Harris Poll, September 15. http://media.theharrispoll.com/documents/HI-Harris-Poll-Cyberchondriacs-2011-09-15.pdf.

Health News 健康报. 2002. "Jiétǎn bìngrén zhìliáo yǒuwàng" 截瘫病人治疗有望 [Paraplegic Patients Have Hope for Treatment]. Editorial for Zhì Bìng Gùwèn 治病顾问

[Medical Treatment Consultation]. *Jiànkāng Bào* 健康报 [Health News], January 10, p. 7.

Heath, Deborah, Erin Koch, Barbara Ley, and Michael Montoya. 1999. "Nodes and Queries: Linking Locations in Networked Fields of Inquiry." *American Behavioral Scientist* 43(3): 450–63.

Helmreich, Stefan. 2008. "Species of Biocapital." *Science as Culture* 17(4): 463–78.

Henderson, Gail E., and Myron S. Cohen. 1984. *The Chinese Hospital: A Socialist Work Unit*. New Haven, CT: Yale University Press.

Henderson, Gail E., Larry R. Churchill, Arlene M. Davis, Michele M. Easter, Christine Grady, Steven Joffe, Nancy Kass, Nancy M. P. King, Charles W. Lidz, Franklin G. Miller, Daniel K. Nelson, Jeffrey Peppercorn, Barbra Bluestone Rothschild, Pamela Sankar, Benjamin S. Wilfond, and Catherine R. Zimmer. 2007. "Clinical Trials and Medical Care: Defining the Therapeutic Misconception." *PLoS Medicine* 4(11): e324. doi:10.1371/journal.pmed.0040324.

Herzfeld, Michael. 1992. *The Social Production of Indifference: Exploring the Symbolic Roots of Western Bureaucracy*. Chicago: University of Chicago Press.

Hesketh, Therese, and Wei Xing Zhu. 1997a. "Health in China: From Mao to Market Reform." *BMJ* 314(7093): 1543–45. doi:10.1136/bmj.314.7093.1543.

———. 1997b. "Health in China: The Healthcare Market." *BMJ* 314: 1616–18. doi:10.1136/bmj.314.7094.1616.

Higgins, Julian P. T., and Sally Green, eds. 2011. *Cochrane Handbook for Systematic Reviews of Interventions*. Version 5.1.0. The Cochrane Collaboration. http:// handbook.cochrane.org/.

Hine, Christine. 2000. *Virtual Ethnography*. London: Sage.

———. 2015. *Ethnography for the Internet: Embedded, Embodied and Everyday*. London: Bloomsbury Publishing.

Hoffman, Lisa. 2006. "Autonomous Choices and Patriotic Professionalism: On Governmentality in Late-Socialist China." *Economy and Society* 35(4): 550–70.

———. 2010. *Patriotic Professionalism in Urban China: Fostering Talent*. Philadelphia: Temple University Press.

Hogle, Linda F. 2010. "Characterizing Human Embryonic Stem Cells: Biological and Social Markers of Identity." *Medical Anthropology Quarterly* 24(4): 433–50.

Holmes, Tamara E. 2000. "Making the Net Work: Living with Disabilities on the Net." *USA Today*, July 21. http://www.usatoday.com/tech/columnist/cctam027.htm. Accessed September 16, 2007.

Horner, Philip J., and Fred H. Gage. 2000. "Regenerating the Damaged Central Nervous System." *Nature* 407(6807): 963–70.

Horst, Heather, and Daniel Miller, eds. 2012. *Digital Anthropology*. London: Berg.

Hsu, Elisabeth. 1999. *The Transmission of Chinese Medicine*. New York: Cambridge University Press.

Huang, Hongyun 黄红云. 2002. "Xiùqiào xìbāo yízhí zhìliáo jǐsuǐ sǔnshāng" 嗅鞘细胞移植治疗脊髓损伤 [Olfactory Ensheathing Cell Transplantation in the Treatment of Spinal Cord Injury]. Zhì Bìng Gùwèn 治病顾问 [Medical Treatment Consultation]. *Jiànkāng Bào* 健康报 [Health News], January 10, 7.

———. 2006. "Běijīng Xīn Shìjì Yīyuàn Shénjīng Jíbìng Yánjiū Zhìliáo Zhōngxīn Dì Yīgè Wǔ Nián (2006–2010 Nián) Fāzhǎn Gāngyào" 北京新世纪医院神经疾病研究治疗中心第一个五年 (2006–2010 发展纲要 [Beijing New Century Hospital

Neurological Disorders Research and Treatment Center First Five-Year Development Plan 2006–2010]. Self-published document, January 18.

———. 2014. "Information of Neurorestoratology." http://www.nrrfr.com/E/index.asp. Accessed May 29, 2014.

———. 2016. "What Is the Second Generation Comprehensive Neurorestoratology Therapy?" http://www.nrrfr.com/E/nr.asp?Bid=89&Id=261. Accessed February 8, 2016.

Huang, Hongyun, Lin Chen, and Paul R. Sanberg. 2012. "Clinical Achievements, Obstacles, Falsehoods, and Future Directions of Cell-Based Neurorestoratology." *Cell Transplantation* 21(S1): S3–S11.

Huang, Hongyun, Lin Chen, Hongmei Wang, Bo Xiu, Bingchen Li, Rui Wang, Jian Zhang, Feng Zhang, Zheng Gu, Ying Li, Yinglun Song, and Wei Hao 黄红云, 陈琳, 王洪美, 修波, 李炳辰, 王锐, 张建, 张峰, 顾征, 李荧, 宋英伦, 郝伟. 2003a. "Nián-líng duì xiùqiào xìbāo yízhí zhìliáo jǐsuǐ sǔnshāng liáoxiào de yǐngxiǎng" 年龄对嗅鞘细胞移植治疗脊髓损伤疗效的影响 [Age Influences on Recovery Outcome of Spinal Cord Injury Treated by Intraspinal Transplantation of OECs]. *Shoudu Yike Daxue Xuebao* 首都医科大学学报 [Journal of Capital University of Medical Sciences] 24(1): 56–59.

Huang, Hongyun, Lin Chen, Hongmei Wang, Bo Xiu, Bingchen Li, Rui Wang, Jian Zhang, Feng Zhang, Zheng Gu, Ying Li, Yinglun Song, Wei Hao, Shuyi Pang, and Junzhao Sun. 2003b. "Influence of Patients' Age on Functional Recovery after Transplantation of Olfactory Ensheathing Cells into Injured Spinal Cord Injury." *Chinese Medical Journal* 116(10): 1488–91.

Huang, Hongyun, Lin Chen, Hongmei Wang, Jian Zhang, Feng Zhang, Yancheng Liu, Haitao Xi, Ke Tan, Zheng Gu, Yinglun Song, and Ying Li 黄红云, 陈琳, 王洪美, 张建, 张峰, 刘彦铖, 郗海涛, 谭可, 顾征, 宋英伦, 李荧. 2006a. "Xiùqiào xìbāo yízhí zhìliáo jī wěisuō cè suǒ yìnghuà zhèng: 88 Lì jìnqí jiéguǒ bàogào" 嗅鞘细胞移植治疗肌萎缩侧索硬化症: 88 例近期结果报告 [Olfactory Ensheathing Cell Transplantation in the Treatment of Amyotrophic Lateral Sclerosis: Recent Result Report of 88 Cases]. *Zhongguo Linchuang Kangfu* 中国临床康复 [Chinese Journal of Clinical Rehabilitation] 10(1): 39–41.

Huang Hongyun, Lin Chen, Hongmei Wang, Haitao Xi, Chengqing Gou, Jian Zhang, Feng Zhang, and Yancheng Liu 黄红云; 陈琳; 王洪美; 郗海涛; 苟成青; 张健; 张峰; 刘彦铖. 2006b. "Xiùqiào xìbāo yízhí zhìliáo wǎnqí jǐsuǐ sǔnshāng ānquán xìng píngjià 38 gè yuè cí gòngzhèn suífǎng jiéguǒ" 嗅鞘细胞移植治疗晚期脊髓损伤安全性评价 38 个月磁共振随访结果 [Safety of Fetal Olfactory Ensheathing Cell Transplantation in Patients with Chronic Spinal Cord Injury: A 38-Month Follow-up with MRI]. *Zhongguo Xiufu Chongjian Waike Zazhi* 中国修复重建外科杂志 [Chinese Journal of Reparative and Reconstructive Surgery] 4: 439–43.

Huang, Hongyun, Lin Chen, Haitao Xi, Hongmei Wang, Jian Zhang, Feng Zhang, and Yancheng Liu. 2008. "Fetal Olfactory Ensheathing Cells Transplantation in Amyotrophic Lateral Sclerosis Patients: A Controlled Pilot Study." *Clinical Transplantation* 22: 710–18.

Huang, Hongyun, Lin Chen, Haitao Xi, Qingmiao Wang, Jian Zhang, Yancheng Liu, and Feng Zhang 黄红云; 陈琳; 郗海涛; 王庆苗; 张健; 刘彦铖; 张峰. 2009. "Xiùqiào xìbāo yízhí zhìliáo zhōngshū shénjīng xìtǒng jíbìng 1,255 lì línchuáng fēnxī" 嗅鞘细胞移植治疗中枢神经系统疾病1,255 例临床分析 [Olfactory Ensheathing Cells

Transplantation for Central Nervous System Diseases in 1,255 Patients]. *Zhong-guo Xiufu Chongjian Waike Zazhi* 中国修复重建外科杂志 [Chinese Journal of Reparative and Reconstructive Surgery] 23(1): 14–20.

Huang, Hongyun, Kai Liu, Wencheng Huang, Zonghui Liu, and Wise Young 黄红云, 刘凯,黄文成,刘宗惠. 2001. "Xiùqiào xìbāo cùshǐ jǐsuǐ cuò liè shāng hòu shénjīng zàishēng hé gōngnéng huīfù de yánjiū" 嗅鞘细胞促使脊髓挫裂伤后神经再生和功能恢复的研究 [Olfactory Ensheathing Glias Transplant Improves Axonal Regeneration and Functional Recovery in Spinal Cord Contusion Injury]. *Haijun Zong Yiyuan Xuebao* 海军总医院学报 [Naval General Hospital Journal] 14: 65–67.

Huang, Hongyun, Geoffrey Raisman, Paul R. Sanberg, Hari S. Sharma, and Lin Chen, eds. 2015a. *Neurorestoratology Volume 1: Theories and Techniques of Neurorestoratology.* Hauppauge, NY: Nova Science Publishers.

———, eds. 2015b. *Neurorestoratology Volume 2: Clinical Progress of Neurorestoratology.* Hauppauge, NY: Nova Science Publishers.

Huang, Hongyun, Hongmei Wang, Bo Xiu, Rui Wang, Ming Liu, Lin Chen, Shubin Qi, Zehua Zhang, Haiqing Wu, Chengqing Gou, Jianduo Cheng, Xiaobai Lu, and Zonghui Liu 黄红云,王洪美,修波,王锐,卢明,陈琳,亓树彬, 张泽华,武海青,苟成青,程建铎,陆晓白,刘宗惠. 2002. "Xiùqiào xìbāo yízhí zhìliáo jǐsuǐ sǔnshāng línchuáng shìyàn de chūbù bàogào" 嗅鞘细胞移植治疗脊髓损伤临床试验的初步报告 [Preliminary Report of Clinical Trial for Olfactory Ensheathing Cell Transplantation Treating Spinal Cord Injury]. *Haijun Zong Yiyuan Xuebao* 海军总医院学报 [Naval General Hospital Journal] 15: 18–21.

Hull, Matthew S. 2012. *Government of Paper: The Materiality of Bureaucracy in Urban Pakistan.* Berkeley: University of California Press.

Hvistendahl, Mara. 2015. "China Pursues Fraudsters in Science Publishing." *ScienceInsider*, November 20. doi:10.1126/science.aad7471.

Hwang, Seyoung, and Margaret Sleeboom-Faulkner. 2014. "Bioethical Governance in South Korea: Tensions between Bottom-up Movements and Professionalization and Scientific Citizenship." *East Asian Science, Technology and Society* 8(2): 209–28. doi:10.1215/18752160-2430586.

Ibrahim, Ahmed, Ying Li, Daqing Li, Geoffrey Raisman, and Wagih S El Masry. 2006. "Olfactory Ensheathing Cells: Ripples of an Incoming Tide?" *Lancet Neurology* 5(5): 453–57.

International Conference on Harmonisation of Technical Requirements for Registration of Pharmaceuticals for Human Use (ICH). 1996. "Guideline for Good Clinical Practice." http://www.ich.org/LOB/media/MEDIA482.pdf. Accessed October 27, 2010.

Institute of Medicine (IOM). 2009. *Initial National Priorities for Comparative Effectiveness Research.* Washington, DC: National Academies Press.

Jain, Kewal. 1973. *The Amazing Story of Health Care in New China.* Emmaus, PA: Rodale Press.

Janzen, John. 1978. *The Quest for Therapy in Lower Zaire.* Berkeley: University of California Press.

Jiang, Jessie. 2008. "China's Rage over Toxic Baby Milk." *TIME*, September 19. http://www.time.com/time/world/article/0,8599,1842727,00.html.

Johnson, Tim. 2004. "Paraplegics Grasping at Hope." *Edmonton Journal (Alberta)*, June 20, Sunday final edition. Knight Ridder Newspapers. LexisNexis Academic.

Judson, Horace Freeland. 2005. "The Problematical Dr. Huang Hongyun: Can an Experimental Technique Using Transplanted Fetal Cells Help Paralyzed Patients?" *MIT Technology Review*. http://www.technologyreview.com/news/405327/the-problematical-dr-huang-hongyun/.

Jullien, François. 1995. *The Propensity of Things: Toward a History of Efficacy in China*. New York: Zone Books.

Kahn, Jeffrey. 2001. "Stem Cells and a New Brain Drain." CNN.com Health, July 10. http://asia.cnn.com/2001/HEALTH/07/23/ethics.matters/index.html.

Karpf, D. 2012. "Social Science Research Methods in Internet Time." *Information, Communication & Society* 15(5): 639–61.

Kay, Lily. 2000. *Who Wrote the Book of Life? A History of the Genetic Code*. Stanford, CA: Stanford University Press.

Kendall, L. 2002. *Hanging Out in the Virtual Pub: Masculinities and Relationships Online*. Berkeley: University of California Press.

Kendzior, Sarah. 2011. "Digital Distrust: Uzbek Cynicism and Solidarity in the Internet Age." *American Ethnologist* 38(3): 559–75.

Kim, Jaesok. 2013. *Chinese Labor in a Korean Factory: Class, Ethnicity, and Productivity on the Shop Floor in Globalizing China*. Stanford, CA: Stanford University Press.

Kim, Syh, S. Frank, R. Holloway, et al. 2005. "Science and Ethics of Sham Surgery: A Survey of Parkinson Disease Researchers." *Archives of Neurology* 62: 1357–60.

Kipnis, Andrew. 2008. "Audit Cultures: Neoliberal Governmentality, Socialist Legacy, or Technologies of Governing?" *American Ethnologist* 35(2): 275–89.

Kirmayer, L. J. 1992. "The Body's Insistence on Meaning: Metaphor as Presentation and Representation in Illness Experience." *Medical Anthropology Quarterly*, n.s. 6(4): 323–46.

Kirshblum, Steven C., Stephen P. Burns, Fin Biering-Sorensen, William Donovan, Daniel E. Graves, Amitabh Jha, Mark Johansen, Linda Jones, Andrei Krassioukov, M. J. Mulcahey, Mary Schmidt-Read, and William Waring. 2011a. "International Standards for Neurological Classification of Spinal Cord Injury (Revised 2011)." *Journal of Spinal Cord Medicine* 34(6): 535–46. doi:10.1179/204577211X13207446293695.

Kirshblum, Steven C., William Waring, Fin Biering-Sorensen, Stephen P. Burns, Mark Johansen, Mary Schmidt-Read, William Donovan, Daniel E. Graves, Amitabh Jha, Linda Jones, M. J. Mulcahey, and Andrei Krassioukov. 2011b. "Reference for the 2011 Revision of the International Standards for Neurological Classification of Spinal Cord Injury." *Journal of Spinal Cord Medicine* 34(6): 547–54. doi:10.1179/107902611X13186000420242.

Kleinman, Arthur. 1978. *Patients and Healers in the Context of Culture*. Berkeley: University of California Press.

———. 1986. *Social Origins of Distress and Disease: Depression, Neurasthenia, and Pain in Modern China*. New Haven, CT: Yale University Press.

———. 1988. *The Illness Narratives: Suffering, Healing and the Human Condition*. New York: Basic Books.

———. 1999. "Experience and Its Moral Modes: Culture, Human Conditions, and Disorder." *Tanner Lectures on Human Values* 20: 355–420.

———. 2006. *What Really Matters: Living a Moral Life amidst Uncertainty and Danger*. New York: Oxford University Press.

Kleinman, Arthur, Yunxiang Yan, Jing Jun, Sing Lee, Everett Zhang, Tianshu Pan, Fei Wu, and Jinhua Guo. 2011. *Deep China: The Moral Life of the Person, What Anthropology and Psychiatry Tell Us about China Today*. Berkeley: University of California Press.

Klimanskaya, Irina, Young Chung, Sandy Becker, Shi-Jiang Lu, and Robert Lanza. 2006. "Human Embryonic Stem Cell Lines Derived from Single Blastomeres." *Nature* 444(23): 481–85.

Kluger, Jeffrey. 2001. "Spinal-Cord Research: Nerve Builder." America's Best Science and Medicine. *TIME*, August 20. http://content.time.com/time/magazine/article/0,9171,1000601,00.html.

Kohrman, Matthew. 2005. *Bodies of Difference: Experiences of Disability and Institutional Advocacy in the Making of Modern China*. Berkeley: University of California Press.

Krause, D. S., N. D. Theise, M. I. Collector, O. Henegariu, S. Hwang, R. Gardner, S. Neutzel, S. J. and Sharkis. 2001. "Multi-organ, Multi-lineage Engraftment by a Single Bone Marrow-Derived Stem Cell." *Cell* 105: 369–77.

Kwo, S., W. Young, and V. Decrescito. 1989. "Spinal Cord Sodium, Potassium, Calcium, and Water Concentration Changes in Rats after Graded Contusion Injury." *Journal of Neurotrauma* 6: 13.

Lacomblez, L., G. Bensimon, P. N. Leigh, P. Guillet, and V. Meininger. 1996. "Dose-Ranging Study of Riluzole in Amyotrophic Lateral Sclerosis: Amyotrophic Lateral Sclerosis/Riluzole Study Group II." *Lancet* 347(9013): 1425–31.

Lagasse, E., H. Connors, M. Al Dhalimy, M. Reitsma, M. Dohse, L. Osborne, X. Wang, M. Finegold, I. L. Weissman, and M. Grompe. 2000. "Purified Hematopoietic Stem Cells Can Differentiate into Hepatocytes in Vivo." *Nature Medicine* 6: 1229–34.

Lampton, David. 1977. *The Politics of Medicine in China: The Policy Process, 1949–1977*. Westview Special Studies on China and East Asia. Boulder, CO: Westview Press.

——— 1986. *A Relationship Restored: Trends in U.S.-China Educational Exchanges, 1978–1984*. Committee on Scholarly Communication with the People's Republic of China. Washington, DC: National Academy Press.

Lancet. 2010. "Scientific Fraud: Action Needed in China." *Lancet* 375(9709): 94. doi:10.1016/S0140-6736(10)60030-X.

Landecker, Hannah. 2007. *Culturing Life: How Cells Became Technologies*. Cambridge, MA: Harvard University Press.

Landzelius, Kyra. 2006. "Introduction: Patient Organization Movements and New Metamorphoses in Patienthood." *Social Science & Medicine* 62(3): 529–37.

Landzelius, Kyra, and Joseph Dumit, eds. 2006. "Special Issue: Patient Organisation Movements." *Social Science & Medicine* 62(3): 529–682.

Langford, Jean M. 2002. *Fluent Bodies: Ayurvedic Remedies for Postcolonial Imbalance*. Durham, NC: Duke University Press.

Lao, She 老舍. 2011. *Kāi Shì Dàjí: Lǎo Shě Xiǎoshuō Jīngdiǎn* 开市大吉: 老舍小说经典 [A Brilliant Beginning: Classic Short Stories by Lao She]. Beijing: Běijīng yànshān chūbǎnshè 北京燕山出版社 [Beijing Yanshan Press].

Latour, Bruno. 1988. *The Pasteurization of France*. Translated by Alan Sheridan and John Law. Cambridge, MA: Harvard University Press.

Lee, Sandra Soo-Jin, Joanna Mountain, and Barbara Koenig. 2001. "The Meanings of 'Race' in the New Genomics: Implications for Health Disparities Research." *Yale Journal of Health Policy, Law, and Ethics* 1: 33–75.

Lei, Sean Hsiang-lin. 2014. *Neither Donkey nor Horse: Medicine in the Struggle over China's Modernity*. Chicago: University of Chicago Press.

Lev, Michael A. 2004. "Chinese Doctor's Use of Unproven Fetal Cell Treatment Alarms U.S. Researchers." *Chicago Tribune*, August 27.

Lewis, John Wilson, and Xue Litai. 1988. *China Builds the Bomb*. Stanford, CA: Stanford University Press.

Li, Cheng. 2005a. "Introduction: Open Doors and Open Minds." In *Bridging Minds across the Pacific: U.S.-China Educational Exchanges, 1978–2003*, edited by Cheng Li, 1–24. Lanham, MD: Lexington Books.

———. 2005b. "Coming Home to Teach: Status and Mobility of Returnees in China's Higher Education." In *Bridging Minds across the Pacific: U.S.-China Educational Exchanges, 1978–2003*, edited by Cheng Li, 69–110. Lanham, MD: Lexington Books.

Li, Hongjun 李红军. 2004. "'Yuàn zhōng yuàn' nǎi yīliáo fǔbài de jízhōng yìngxiàn" '院中院' 乃医疗腐败的集中映现 ["Hospitals within Hospitals" Is the Focus of Medical Corruption]. *Sōuhú Xīnwén* 搜狐新闻 [Sohu News], October 27. http://news.sohu.com/20041027/n222720319.shtml.

Li, Ying, Pauline M. Field, and Geoffrey Raisman. 1997. "Repair of Adult Rat Corticospinal Tract by Transplants of Olfactory Ensheathing Cells." *Science* 277(5334): 2000–2002. doi:10.1126/science.277.5334.2000.

Li, Zhisui. 1994. *The Private Life of Chairman Mao*. New York: Random House.

Liao, Lianming, Lingsong Li, and Robert Chunhua Zhao. 2007. "Stem Cell Research in China." *Philosophical Transactions of the Royal Society B: Biological Sciences* 362(1482): 1107–12. doi:10.1098/rstb.2007.2037.

Lima, Carlos, J. Pratas-Vital, P. Escada, A. Hasse-Ferreira, C. Capucho, and J. D. Peduzzi. 2006. "Olfactory Mucosa Autografts in Human Spinal Cord Injury: A Pilot Clinical Study." *Journal of Spinal Cord Medicine* 29(3): 191–203, 204–6.

Lindgren, S. 2013. "The Potential and Limitations of Twitter Activism: Mapping the 2011 Libyan Uprising." *tripleC* 11(1): 207–20.

Liu, Kai, Ying Li, Hongmei Wang, Xiaorong Jiang, Yanting Zhao, Dongming Sun, Lin Chen, Wise Young, Hongyun Huang, and Changman Zhou. 2010. "The Immunohistochemical Characterization of Human Fetal Olfactory Bulb and Olfactory Ensheathing Cells in Culture as a Source for Clinical CNS Restoration." *Anatomical Record* 293(3): 359–69. doi:10.1002/ar.21030.

Liu, Li 刘莉. 2002. "Huáng Hóngyún: Gěi Sāng Lán men dài lái xīwàng" 黄红云: 给桑兰们带来希望 [Huang Hongyun: Giving Hope to Sang Lan]. *Kējì Rìbào* 科技日报 [Science and Technology Daily], August 26, 8.

Livingston, Julie. 2012. *Improvising Medicine: An African Oncology Ward in an Emerging Cancer Epidemic*. Durham, NC: Duke University Press.

Lock, Margaret. 1993. *Encounters with Aging: Mythologies of Menopause in Japan and North America*. Berkeley: University of California Press.

———. 2002. *Twice Dead: Organ Transplants and the Reinvention of Death*. Berkeley: University of California Press.

Longstaff, Holly, Vera Khramova, Marleen Eijkholt, Ania Mizgalewicz, and Judy Illes. 2013. "Hopes and Fears for Professional Movement in the Stem Cell Community." *Cell Stem Cell* 12: 517–19.

Lora-Wainwright, Anna. 2013. *Fighting for Breath: Living Morally and Dying of Cancer in a Chinese Village*. Honolulu: University of Hawaii Press.

Lowy, Ilana. 2000. "Trustworthy Knowledge and Desperate Patients: Clinical Tests for New Drugs from Cancer to AIDS." In *Living and Working with the New Medical Technologies: Intersections of Inquiry*, edited by M. Lock, A. Young, and A. Cambrosio, 49–81. New York: Cambridge University Press.

Lozada, Eriberto P. 1998. "A Hakka Community in Cyberspace: Diasporic Ethnicity and the Internet." In *On the South China Track: Perspectives on Anthropological Research and Teaching*, edited by Sidney C. H. Cheung, 149–82. Hong Kong: Hong Kong Institute of Asia-Pacific Studies, Chinese University of Hong Kong.

Lü, Xiaobo. 2000. "Booty Socialism, Bureau-Preneurs, and the State in Transition: Organizational Corruption in China." *Comparative Politics* 32(3): 273–94.

Ma, Hong 马红. 2003a. "Jiétān bìngrén yǒule xīn de zhìliáo fāngfǎ" 截瘫病人有了新的治疗方法 [Paraplegic People Have New Treatment Method]. Zònghé Xìnxī 综合信息 [Collected News]. *Jiànkāng Zīxún Bào* 健康咨询报 [Health Information News], March 3, p. 2.

———. 2003b. "Jiétān bìngrén zhìliáo yǒuwàng" 截瘫病人治疗有望 [Paraplegic Patients Have Hope for Treatment]. Yīyuàn Píngtái 医院平台 [Hospital Platform]. *Kējì Rìbào* 科技日报 [Science and Technology Daily], March 31.

Macbrayne, Rosaleen, and Juliet Rowan. 2005. "Speaking Again after Stem-Cell Transplant." *New Zealand Herald*, March 23. http://www.nzherald.co.nz/nz/news/article.cfm?c_id=1&objectid=10116758.

Maddox, Sam. 2000. "EWire Announcement: Merger with CanDo." February 28. http://www.dimenet.com/disculture/archive.php?mode=N&id=27. Accessed September 16, 2007.

Madsen, Amy. 2013. "Generic Riluzole on the Market." *MDA/ALS Newsmagazine*, June 21. http://alsn.mda.org/news/generic-riluzole-market.

Maienschein, Jane. 2009. "Regenerative Medicine in Historical Context." *Medicine Studies* 1: 33–40.

———. 2011. "Regenerative Medicine's Historical Roots in Regeneration, Transplantation, and Translation." *Developmental Biology* 358(2): 278–84.

Malinowski, Bronislaw. 1948 [1922]. *Magic, Science, and Religion and Other Essays*. Westport, CT: Greenwood Press.

Mao, Zedong 毛泽东. 1965. "Duì wèishēng gōngzuò de zhǐshì" 对卫生工作的指示 [Directive Regarding Health Work], June 26. In *Máo Zédōng Sīxiǎng Wànsuì (1961–1968)* 毛泽东思想万岁 (1961–1968) [Mao Zedong Thought (1961–1968)], 230–31. https://www.marxists.org/chinese/PDF/08/01210804.pdf.

"Mao Tse-Tung Dies in Peking at 82; Leader of Red China Revolution; Choice of Successor Is Uncertain." 1976. *New York Times*, September 9. http://www.nytimes.com/learning/general/onthisday/big/0909.html.

Markham, Annette. 1998. *Life Online: Researching Real Experience in Virtual Space*. Walnut Creek, CA: Altamira Press.

Marks, Harry. 1997. *The Progress of Experiment: Science and Therapeutic Reform in the United States, 1900–1990*. New York: Cambridge University Press.

Marshall, C. T., C. Lu, et al. 2006. "The Therapeutic Potential of Human Olfactory-Derived Stem Cells." *Histology and Histopathology* 21: 633–43.

Mattingly, Cheryl. 2010. *The Paradox of Hope: Journeys through a Clinical Borderland.* Berkeley: University of California Press.

Max, D. T. 2016. "One Small Step: A Paraplegic Undergoes Pioneering Surgery." *New Yorker,* January 25. http://www.newyorker.com/magazine/2016/01/25/one-small-step-annals-of-medicine-d-t-max.

McDonald, John, D. Becker, C. L. Sadowsky, J. A. Jane, T. E. Conturo, and L. M. Schultz. 2002. "Late Recovery Following Spinal Cord Injury: Case Report and Review of the Literature." *Journal of Neurosurgery* 97(2 Supplement): 252–65.

McGuire, Elizabeth. 2010. "Between Revolutions: Chinese Students in Soviet Institutes, 1948–1966." In *China Learns from the Soviet Union, 1949–Present,* edited by Thomas Bernstein and Hua-Yu Li, 359–89. Lanham, MD: Lexington Books.

Mediavilla, Daniel. 2006. "Thousands of Quadriplegics Make a Pilgrimage to Beijing after a Chinese Fairytale" [Miles de tetrapléjicos peregrinan a Pekín en pos de un cuento chino]. *ABC,* October 25. http://www.abc.es/hemeroteca/historico-25-10-2006/abc/Sociedad/miles-de-tetraplejicos-peregrinan-a-pekin-en-pos-de-un-cuento-chino_1423925375570.html.

Mehta, Paul, Vinicius Antao, Wendy Kaye, Marchelle Sanchez, David Williamson, Leah Bryan, Oleg Muravov, and Kevin Horton. 2014. "Prevalence of Amyotrophic Lateral Sclerosis—United States, 2010–2011." Centers for Disease Control and Prevention Morbidity and Mortality Weekly Report. *Surveillance Summaries* 63(7): 1–14. http://www.cdc.gov/mmwr/pdf/ss/ss6307.pdf.

Melton, Douglas. 2001. "Testimony on Stem Cell Research before the Senate Committee on Health, Education, Labor and Pensions (September 5, 2001)." http://www.ascb.org/testimony-on-stem-cell-research-before-the-senate-committee-on-health-education-labor-and-pensions/. Accessed October 5, 2015.

Miller, D., and D. Slater. 2000. *The Internet: An Ethnographic Approach.* New York: Berg.

Miller, F. G. 2003. "Sham Surgery: An Ethical Analysis." *American Journal of Bioethics* 3: 41–48.

Minkenberg, Michael. 2002. "Religion and Public Policy: Institutional, Cultural, and Political Impact on the Shaping of Abortion Policies in Western Democracies." *Comparative Political Studies* 35(2): 221–47.

Miyazaki, Hirokazu. 2004. *The Method of Hope: Anthropology, Philosophy, and Fijian Knowledge.* Stanford, CA: Stanford University Press.

Molina, Camilo A., Patricia L. Zadnik, Ziya L. Gokaslan, Timothy F. Witham, Ali Bydon, Jean-Paul Wolinsky, and Daniel M. Sciubba. 2013. "A Cohort Cost Analysis of Lumbar Laminectomy: Current Trends in Surgeon and Hospital Fees Distribution." *Spine Journal* 13(2013): 1434–37.

Montoya, Michael. 2008. "Bioethnic Conscription: Genes, Race, and Mexicana/o Ethnicity in Diabetes Research." *Cultural Anthropology* 22(1): 94–128.

———. 2011. *Making the Mexican Diabetic: Race, Science, and the Genetics of Inequality.* Berkeley: University of California Press.

Moreno-Flores, M. Teresa, Elizabeth J. Bradbury, M. Jesus Martin-Bermejo, Marta Agudo, Filip Lim, Erika Pastrana, Jesus Avila, Javier Diaz-Nido, Stephen B. McMahon, and Francisco Wandosell. 2006. "A Clonal Cell Line from Immortalized

Olfactory Ensheathing Glia Promotes Functional Recovery in the Injured Spinal Cord." *Molecular Therapy* 13(3): 598–608.

Nader, Laura, ed. 1996. *Naked Science: Anthropological Inquiry into Boundaries, Power, and Knowledge*. New York: Routledge.

Nardi, Bonnie. 2010. *My Life as a Night Elf Priest: An Anthropological Account of World of Warcraft*. Ann Arbor: University of Michigan Press.

———. 2015. "Virtuality." *Annual Review of Anthropology* 44: 15–31.

National Institutes of Health, U.S. Department of Health and Human Services. 2015. "Stem Cell Basics: Introduction." In *Stem Cell Information*. Bethesda, MD: National Institutes of Health, U.S. Department of Health and Human Services. http://stemcells.nih.gov/info/basics/pages/basics1.aspx.

National Spinal Cord Injury Association. 2005. "Spinal Cord Injury Hall of Fame." http://www.spinalcord.org/news.php?dep=9&page=41. Accessed August 2, 2007.

National Spinal Cord Injury Statistical Center. 2016. "Spinal Cord Injury Facts and Figures at a Glance." Birmingham: University of Alabama at Birmingham. https://www.nscisc.uab.edu/Public/Facts%202016.pdf.

Neff, Raymond. 1995. "The Cleveland Free-Net: Status as of June 1995." http://www.atarimax.com/freenet/common/html/freenet_status.php.

Nelkin, Dorothy and M. Susan Lindee. 2004 [1995]. *The DNA Mystique: The Gene as a Cultural Icon*. Ann Arbor: University of Michigan Press.

Novas, Carlos. 2006. "The Political Economy of Hope: Patients' Organizations, Science and Biovalue." *BioSocieties* 1: 289–305.

——— 2007. "Genetic Advocacy Groups, Science, and Biovalue: Creating Political Economies of Hope." In *New Genetics, New Identities*, edited by Paul Atkinson, Peter Glasner, and Helen Greenslade, 11–27. London: Routledge.

Novas, Carlos, and Nikolas Rose. 2000. "Genetic Risk and the Birth of the Somatic Individual." *Economy and Society* 29: 485–513.

Nuijten, Monique. 2003. *Power, Community and the State: The Political Anthropology of Organisation in Mexico*. London: Pluto.

Obama, Barack. 2009. "Remarks on Signing the Stem Cell Executive Order and Scientific Integrity Presidential Memorandum." Washington, DC, March 9. http://www.whitehouse.gov/the_press_office/Remarks-of-the-President-As-Prepared-for-Delivery-Signing-of-Stem-Cell-Executive-Order-and-Scientific-Integrity-Presidential-Memorandum.

Oglesby, Matthew, Steven J. Fineberg, Alpesh A. Patel, Miguel A. Pelton, and Kern Singh. 2013. "Epidemiological Trends in Cervical Spine Surgery for Degenerative Diseases between 2002 and 2009." *Spine* 38(14): 1226–32.

Oh, Jaimie. 2010. "50 Largest Hospitals in America." *Becker's Hospital Review*. http://www.beckershospitalreview.com/lists/50-largest-hospitals-in-america.html.

Ong, Aihwa. 1999. *Flexible Citizenship: The Cultural Logics of Transnationality*. Durham, NC: Duke University Press.

Ong, Aihwa, and Nancy Chen. 2010. *Asian Biotech: Ethics and Communities of Fate*. Durham, NC: Duke University Press.

Orleans, Leo S. 1988. *Chinese Students in America: Policies, Issues and Numbers*. Washington, DC: National Academy Press.

Osburg, John. 2013. *Anxious Wealth: Money and Morality among China's New Rich*. Stanford, CA: Stanford University Press.

Palmié, Stephan. 2007. "Genomics, Divination and 'Racecraft.'" *American Ethnologist* 34(2): 205–22.

Pang, Samantha Mei-che, Thomas Kwok-shing Wong, and Jacqueline Shukching Ho. 2002. "Changing Economics and Health Worker Training in Modern China." *Yale-China Health Journal* 1: 61–84.

Patra, Prasanna Kumar, and Margaret Sleeboom-Faulkner. 2013. "Discursive Dialects of Bioethics: Understanding the Institutional Embeddings of Human Stem Cell Experimentation in India." *BioSocieties* 8(1): 75–92. doi:10.1057/biosoc.2012.33.

Pearce, Celia, and Artemesia. 2009. *Communities of Play: Emergent Cultures in Multiplayer Games and Virtual Worlds*. Cambridge, MA: MIT Press.

People's Republic of China Communist Party Central Committee and State Council 中华人民共和国中共中央, 国务院. 1997. "Guānyú wèishēng gǎigé yǔ fāzhǎn de juédìng" 关于卫生改革与发展的决定 [Decision Concerning Health Reform and Development]. January 15. http://www.moh.gov.cn/wsb/pM30115/200804/18540.shtml.

People's Republic of China Ministry of Health 中华人民共和国卫生部. 1980. "Guānyú yǔnxǔ gètǐ kāiyè xíngyī wèntí de qǐngshì bàogào 1980 nián 8 yuè 24 rì guówùyuàn pīzhǔn" 关于允许个体开业行医问题的请示报告 1980 年 8 月 24 日国务院批准 [Report Concerning the Question of Allowing Individuals to Start Medical Practice Businesses Approved by the PRC State Council on August 24]. *Zhōnghuá rénmín gònghéguó guówùyuàn gōngbào* 中华人民共和国国务院公报 [PRC State Council Bulletin] 343(16) [December 1]: 514–17.

———. 1985. "Guānyú wèishēng gōngzuò gǎigé ruògān zhèngcè wèntí de bàogào" 关于卫生工作改革若干政策问题的报告 [Report Concerning Some Policy Questions in the Reform of Health Work]. *Zhōnghuá rénmín gònghéguó guówùyuàn gōngbào* 中华人民共和国国务院公报 [PRC State Council Bulletin] 465(13) [May 20]: 377–81.

———. 1992. "Guānyú shēnhuà wèishēng gǎigé de jǐ diǎn yìjiàn" 关于深化卫生改革的几点意见 [A Few Suggestions on Deepening the Health Reforms]. September 23. http://www.reformdata.org/content/19920923/25367.html.

———. 2004. "Yánlì dǎjí fēifǎ xíngyī zhuānxiàng zhěngzhì gōngzuò fāng'àn" 严厉打击非法行医专项整治工作方案 [Special Rectification Program to Crack Down on the Illegal Practice of Medicine]. http://www.law-lib.com/law/law_view.asp?id=84103.

People's Republic of China National People's Congress 中华人民共和国第九届全国人民代表大会常务委员会第二十次会议. 2001. "Zhōnghuá rénmín gònghéguó yàopǐn guǎnlǐ fǎ" 中华人民共和国药品管理法 [Drug Administration Law of the People's Republic of China]. Enacted 1984 and revised in 2001 by the 20th Session of the Standing Committee of the 9th National People's Congress. http://www.sda.gov.cn/WS01/CL0064/23396.html.

People's Republic of China State Council 中华人民共和国国务院. 1989. "Guānyú kuòdà yīliáo wèishēng fúwù yǒuguān wèntí de yìjiàn" 关于扩大医疗卫生服务有关问题的意见 [Suggestions on Questions Regarding the Expansion of Health Services]. http://www.china.com.cn/law/flfg/txt/2006-08/08/content_7057970.htm.

———. 1994. "Yīliáo jīgòu guǎnlǐ tiáolì" 医疗机构管理条例 [Regulation of Medical Institutions]. http://www.gov.cn/banshi/2005-08/01/content_19113.htm.

People's Republic of China State Council Development Research Center 中华人民共和国国务院发展研究中心. 2005. "Duì zhōngguó yīliáo wèishēng tǐzhì gǎigé de píngjià yú jiànyì" 对中国医疗卫生体制改革的评价与建议 [Appraisal and Suggestions on China's Health Care System Reforms]. http://www.china.com.cn/chinese/health/927874.htm.

Perkovich, George. 2002. *India's Nuclear Bomb: The Impact on Global Proliferation.* Berkeley: University of California Press.

Petryna, Adriana. 2002. *Life Exposed: Biological Citizens after Chernobyl.* Princeton: Princeton University Press.

———. 2005. "Ethical Variability: Drug Development and Globalizing Clinical Trials." *American Ethnologist* 32(2): 183–97.

———. 2009. *When Experiments Travel: Clinical Trials and the Global Search for Human Subjects.* Princeton: Princeton University Press.

Piepers, Sanne, and Leonard van den Berg. 2010. "No Benefits from Experimental Treatment with Olfactory Ensheathing Cells in Patients with ALS." *Amyotrophic Lateral Sclerosis* 11: 328–30.

Pierce, G. Barry. 1974. "Neoplasms, Differentiations, and Mutations." *American Journal of Pathology* 77(1): 103–18.

Pontifical Academy for Life. 2000. "Declaration on the Production and the Scientific and Therapeutic Use of Human Embryonic Stem Cells." http://www.vatican.va/roman_curia/pontifical_academies/acdlife/documents/rc_pa_acdlife_doc_20000824_cellule-staminali_en.html.

Prager, Joshua H. 1999. "People with Disabilities Are Next Consumer Niche." *Wall Street Journal*, December 15. http://www.wsj.com/articles/SB945213765959569213.

Rabeharisoa, Vololona, and Michel Callon. 2004. "Patients and Scientists in French Muscular Dystrophy Research." In *States of Knowledge: The Co-production of Science and Social order*, edited by Sheila Jasanoff, 142–60. London: Routledge.

Rabinow, Paul. 1996. "Artificiality and Enlightenment: From Sociobiology to Biosociality." In *Essays on the Anthropology of Reason*, 91–111. Princeton: Princeton University Press.

———. 1999. *French DNA: Trouble in Purgatory.* Chicago: University of Chicago Press.

Radin, Patricia. 2006. "'To Me, It's My Life': Medical Communication, Trust, and Activism in Cyberspace." *Social Science & Medicine* 62(3): 591–601.

Radtke, Christine, Masanori Sasaki, Karen L. Lankford, Peter M. Vogt, and Jeffery D. Kocsis. 2008. "Potential of Olfactory Ensheathing Cells for Cell-Based Therapy in Spinal Cord Injury." *Journal of Rehabilitation Research & Development* 45(1): 141–52.

Raikhel, Eugene. 2010. "Post-Soviet Placebos: Epistemology and Authority in Russian Treatments for Alcoholism." *Culture, Medicine and Psychiatry* 34(1): 132–68.

Raisman, Geoffrey. 1985. "Specialized Neuroglial Arrangement May Explain the Capacity of Vomeronasal Axons to Reinnervate Central Neurons." *Neuroscience* 14: 237–54.

———. 2001. "Olfactory Ensheathing Cells—Another Miracle Cure for Spinal Cord Injury." *Nature Reviews: Neuroscience* 2: 369–75.

Ramon-Cueto, A., and J. Avila. 1998. "Olfactory Ensheathing Glia: Properties and Function." *Brain Research Bulletin* 46: 175–87.

Ramon-Cueto, A., and M. Nieto-Sampedro. 1994. "Regeneration into the Spinal Cord of Transected Dorsal Root Axons Is Promoted by Ensheathing Glia Transplants." *Experimental Neurology* 127: 232–44.

Rapp, Rayna. 1999. *Testing Women, Testing the Fetus: The Social Impact of Amniocentesis in America*. New York: Routledge.

Rapp, Rayna, Deborah Heath, and Karen-Sue Taussig. 2001. "Genealogical Dis-ease: Where Hereditary Abnormality, Biomedical Explanation, and Family Responsibility Meet." In *Relative Values: Reconfiguring Kinship Studies*, edited by Sarah Franklin and Susan MacKinnon, 384–409. Durham, NC: Duke University Press.

Regalado, Antonio. 2004. "Buzz about Stem Cells Spurs Desperately Ill to Seek Help Overseas." *Wall Street Journal*, August 27, B1.

Rehabilitation Research and Training Center on Secondary Conditions of SCI. 2000. "Understanding Spinal Cord Injury and Functional Goals and Outcomes." Spinal Cord Injury InfoSheet #5. University of Alabama Spain Rehabilitation Center. Developed by Amie Jackson, Linda Lindsey, and Phil Klebine. http://images.main.uab.edu/spinalcord/pdffiles/info-5.pdf.

———. 2004. "Adjustment to Spinal Cord Injury." Spinal Cord Injury InfoSheet #20. Developed by Phil Klebine. http://images.main.uab.edu/spinalcord/pdffiles/20Adjust.pdf.

Reid, Brian. 2010. "It's Time to Retire 'Cyberchondriacs.'" *WCG: Common Sense*, August 12. http://blog.wcgworld.com/2010/08/its-time-to-retire-cyberchondriacs.

Rentz, E. Danielle, Lauren Lewis, Oscar J. Mujica, et al. 2008. "Outbreak of Acute Renal Failure in Panama in 2006: A Case-Control Study." *Bulletin of the World Health Organization* 86(10): 737–816.

Reston, James. 1971. "Now, about My Operation in Peking." *New York Times*, July 26, 1.

Reeve, Christopher. 1999. *Still Me*. Ballantine Books edition. New York: Random House.

Rivkin-Fish, Michele. 2005. *Women's Health in Post-Soviet Russia: The Politics of Intervention*. Bloomington: Indiana University Press.

Rofel, Lisa. 2007. *Desiring China: Experiments in Neoliberalism, Sexuality, and Public Culture*. Durham, NC: Duke University Press.

Rogaski, Ruth. 2004. *Hygienic Modernity: Meanings of Health and Disease in Treaty-Port China*. Berkeley: University of California Press.

Rose, Nikolas. 1992. "Governing the Enterprising Self." In *The Values of the Enterprise Culture: The Moral Debate*, edited by Paul Heelas and Paul Morris, 141–64. London: Routledge.

———. 2007. *The Politics of Life Itself: Biomedicine, Power, and Subjectivity in the Twenty-First Century*. Princeton: Princeton University Press.

Rosemann, Achim. 2013. "Medical Innovation and National Experimental Pluralism: Insights from Clinical Stem Cell Research and Applications in China." *BioSocieties* 8(1): 58–74.

Rosen, Stanley, and David Zweig. 2005. "Transnational Capital: Valuing Academic Returnees in a Globalizing China." In *Bridging Minds across the Pacific: U.S.-China Educational Exchanges, 1978–2003*, edited by Cheng Li, 111–32. Lanham, MD: Lexington Books.

Rosenberg, Charles E. 1987. *The Care of Strangers: The Rise of America's Hospital System*. New York: Basic Books.

Rothman, David. 1997. *Beginnings Count: The Technological Imperative in American Health Care*. New York: Oxford University Press.

Rotimi, Charles. 2003. "Genetic Ancestry Tracing and African Identity: A Double-Edged Sword?" *Developing World Bioethics* 3: 151–58.

Rowland, Lewis P., and Neil A. Shneider. 2001. "Medical Progress: Amyotrophic Lateral Sclerosis." *New England Journal of Medicine* 344(22): 1688–1700.

Salter, Brian, and Charlotte Salter. 2007. "Bioethics and the Global Moral Economy: The Cultural Politics of Human Embryonic Stem Cell Science." *Science, Technology & Human Values* 32(5): 554–81.

Sangren, P. Steven. 1987. *History and Magical Power in a Chinese Community*. Stanford, CA: Stanford University Press.

———. 2000. *Chinese Sociologics: An Anthropological Account of the Role of Alienation in Social Reproduction*. London School of Economics Monographs on Social Anthropology. Vol. 72. London: Athlone Press.

Sankar, Pamela. 2004. "Communication and Miscommunication in Informed Consent to Research." *Medical Anthropology Quarterly* 18(4): 429–46.

Saxer, Martin. 2012. *Manufacturing Tibetan Medicine: The Creation of an Industry and the Moral Economy of Tibetanness*. New York: Berghahn Books.

Schneider, Joseph W. 1993. "Family Care Work and Duty in a 'Modern' Chinese Hospital." In *Health and Health Care in Developing Countries*, edited by Peter Conrad and Eugene B. Gallagher. Philadelphia: Temple University Press.

Schwartz, R. S. 2006. "The Politics and Promise of Stem Cell Research." *New England Journal of Medicine* 355(12): 1189–91.

Sha Wenru 沙文茹. 2003. "Jiétān bìngrén chóngxīn zhànlì bù zài shì mèng" 截瘫病人重新站立不再是梦 [Paraplegic Patients Back on Their Feet Is No Longer a Dream]. *Zhōngguó Xiāofèizhě Bào* 中国消费者报 [China Consumer News], April 10.

Shamblott, Michael J., Joyce Axelman, Shunping Wang, Elizabeth M. Bugg, John W. Littlefield, Peter J. Donovan, Paul D. Blumenthal, George R. Huggins, and John D. Gearhart. 1998. "Derivation of Pluripotent Stem Cells from Cultured Human Primordial Germ Cells." *PNAS* 95(23): 13726–31. doi:10.1073/pnas.95.23.13726.

Shao, Jing. 2006. "Fluid Labor and Blood Money: The Economy of HIV/AIDS in Rural Central China." *Cultural Anthropology* 21(4): 535–69.

Shaw, Pamela J. 2005. "Molecular and Cellular Pathways of Neurodegeneration in Motor Neuron Disease." *Journal of Neurology, Neurosurgery & Psychiatry* 76: 1046–57. doi:10.1136/jnnp.2004.048652.

Sherman, Michael I., and Davor Solter, eds. 1975. *Teratomas and Differentiation*. New York: Academic Press.

Shetty, Raksha. 2004. "Fetal Cells Offer Hope in China." *CBS Evening News with Dan Rather*, July 27. http://www.cbsnews.com/news/fetal-cells-offer-hope-in-china/.

Shi, Lihong. 2011. "'The Wife Is the Boss': Sex-Ratio Imbalance and Young Women's Empowerment in Marriage in Rural Northeast China." In *Women and Gender in Contemporary Chinese Societies: Beyond Han Patriarchy*, edited by Shanshan Du and Ya-Chen Chen, 89–108. New York: Lexington Books.

———. 2014. "Micro-Blogs, Online Forums, and the Birth-Control Policy: Social Media and the Politics of Reproduction in China." *Culture, Medicine and Psychiatry* 38: 115–32.

Sidel, Victor, and Ruth Sidel. 1973. *Serve the People: Observations on Medicine in the People's Republic of China*. Boston: Beacon Press.

Simpson, Bob. 2000. "Imagined Genetic Communities: Ethnicity and Essentialism in the Twenty-First Century." *Anthropology Today* 16(3): 3–6.

Siu, Helen. 1989. *Agents and Victims in South China: Accomplices in Rural Revolution.* New Haven, CT: Yale University Press.

Sleeboom-Faulkner, Margaret, ed. 2010. *Frameworks of Choice: Predictive and Genetic Testing in Asia.* IIAS Publications Series. Amsterdam: Amsterdam University Press.

———. 2011. "Regulating Cell Lives in Japan: Avoiding Scandal and Sticking to Nature." *New Genetics and Society* 30(3): 227–40.

Sleeboom-Faulkner, Margaret, and Seyoung Hwang. 2012. "Governance of Stem Cell Research: Public Participation and Decision-making in China, Japan, South Korea, Taiwan and the UK." *Social Studies of Science* 42(5): 684–708.

Sleeboom-Faulkner, Margaret, Choon Chekar, Alex Faulkner, Carolyn Heitmeyer, Marina Marouda, Achim Rosemann, Nattaka Chaisinthop, Hung-Chieh Chang, Adrian Ely, Masae Kato, Prasanna K. Patra, Yeyang Su, Suli Sui, Wakana Suzuki, and Xinqing Zhang. 2016. "Comparing National Home-Keeping and the Regulation of Translational Stem Cell Applications: An International Perspective." *Social Science and Medicine* 153: 240–49.

Sommerville, Quentin. 2009. "Little Comfort in Milk Scandal Verdicts." BBC News, January 22. http://news.bbc.co.uk/2/hi/asia-pacific/7845545.stm.

Song, Priscilla. 2010. "Biotech Pilgrims and the Transnational Quest for Stem Cell Cures." *Medical Anthropology* 29(4): 384–402. doi:10.1080/01459740.2010.501317.

——— 2011. "The Proliferation of Stem Cell Therapies in Post-Mao China: Problematizing Ethical Regulation." *New Genetics and Society* 30(2): 141–53. doi:10.1080/14636778.2011.574375.

Southern Baptist Convention. 1992. "Resolution on Fetal Tissue Experimentation." Indianapolis. http://www.sbc.net/resolutions/552/resolution-on-fetal-tissue-experimentation.

——— 1999. "Resolution on Human Embryonic and Stem Cell Research." Atlanta. http://www.sbc.net/resolutions/620/resolution-on-human-embryonic-and-stem-cell-research.

——— 2000. "Resolution on Human Fetal Tissue Trafficking." Orlando, Florida. http://www.sbc.net/resolutions/553/on-human-fetal-tissue-trafficking.

Spence, Jonathan. 1990. *The Search for Modern China.* New York: W. W. Norton.

Spodick, David H. 1975. "Numerators without Denominators: There Is No FDA for the Surgeon." *JAMA* 232(1): 35–36. doi:10.1001/jama.1975.03250010017015.

Sui, Suli, and Margaret Sleeboom-Faulkner. 2015. "Governance of Stem Cell Research and Its Clinical Translation in China: An Example of Profit-Oriented Bionetworking." *East Asian Science, Technology, Society* 9(4): 397–414.

Sunder Rajan, Kaushik. 2006. *Biocapital: The Constitution of Postgenomic Life.* Durham, NC: Duke University Press.

Sung, Wen-Ching. 2010. "Chinese DNA." In *Asian Biotech: Ethics and Communities of Fate,* edited by Aihwa Ong and Nancy Chen, 263–92. Durham, NC: Duke University Press.

Sveningsson, Malin. 2003. "Ethics in Internet Ethnography." In *Readings in Virtual Research Ethics: Issues and Controversies,* edited by Elizabeth Buchanan, 45–61. Hershey, PA: IGI Global. doi:10.4018/978-1-59140-152-0.ch003.

Takahashi, Kazutoshi, and Shinya Yamanaka. 2006. "Induction of Pluripotent Stem Cells from Mouse Embryonic and Adult Fibroblast Cultures by Defined Factors." *Cell* 126(4): 663–76. doi:10.1016/j.cell.2006.07.024.

Takahashi, Kazutoshi, Koji Tanabe, Mari Ohnuki, Megumi Narita, Tomoko Ichisaka, Kiichiro Tomoda, and Shinya Yamanaka. 2007. "Induction of Pluripotent Stem Cells from Adult Human Fibroblasts by Defined Factors." *Cell* 131: 1–12. doi:10.1016/j.cell.2007.11.019.

TallBear, Kimberly. 2003. "DNA, Blood, and Racializing the Tribe." *Wicazo Sa Review* 18(1): 81–107.

——— 2013. *Native American DNA: Tribal Belonging and the False Promise of Genetic Science*. Minneapolis: University of Minnesota Press.

Tambiah, Stanley J. 1990. *Magic, Science, Religion, and the Scope of Rationality (Lewis Henry Morgan Lectures)*. Cambridge: Cambridge University Press.

Tang, Xianwu, Yuxiao Wang, and Er Ji 唐先武, 王宇晓, 吉尔. 2002. "Tā shìzhe ràng lúnyǐ rén zhàn qǐlái: Hǎijūn zǒng yīyuàn quán jūn shénjīng wàikē zhōngxīn zhǔrèn yīshī huáng hóngyún jiàoshòu tán zhì tān xīn sīlù" 他试着让轮椅人站起来：海军总医院全军神经外科中心主任医师黄红云教授谈治瘫新思路 [He Attempts to Let People in Wheelchairs Stand Up: Naval General Hospital PLA Neurosurgery Center Director Physician Professor Huang Hongyun Discusses a New Thought Path for Treating Paralysis]. *Kējì Rìbào* 科技日报 [Science and Technology Daily], January 29, 1.

Taussig, Karen-Sue, Rayna Rapp, and Deborah Heath. 2001. "Flexible Eugenics: Technologies of the Self in the Age of Genetics." In *Genetic Nature/Culture: Anthropology and Science beyond the Two-Culture Divide*, edited by Alan H. Goodman, Deborah Heath, and M. Susan Lindee, 58–76. Berkeley: University of California Press.

Taussig, Karen-Sue, Klaus Hoeyer, and Stefan Helmreich. 2013. "The Anthropology of Potentiality in Biomedicine: An Introduction to Supplement 7." *Current Anthropology* 54(S7): S3–S14.

Taylor, T. L. 2006. *Play between Worlds: Exploring Online Game Culture*. Cambridge, MA: MIT Press.

Thacker, Eugene. 2004. *Biomedia*. Minneapolis: University of Minnesota Press.

Thompson, Charis. 2013. *Good Science: The Ethical Choreography of Stem Cell Research*. Cambridge, MA: MIT Press.

Thomson, James A., Joseph Itskovitz-Eldor, Sander S. Shapiro, Michelle A. Waknitz, Jennifer J. Swiergiel, Vivienne S. Marshall, and Jeffrey M. Jones. 1998. "Embryonic Stem Cell Lines Derived from Human Blastocysts." *Science* 282(5391): 1145–47. doi:10.1126/science.282.5391.1145.

Tolkkinen, Karen. 2004. "ALS Treatment Creates Crisis of Faith for Two Baptist Families." *Baptist Standard*, October 29. https://www.baptiststandard.com/resources/archives/44-2004-archives/2645-als-treatment-creates-crisis-of-faith-for-two-baptist-families110104.

Tröhler, Ulrich. 2005. "Quantifying Experience and Beating Biases: A New Culture in Eighteenth Century British Clinical Medicine." In *Body Counts: Medical Quantification in Historical and Sociological Perspectives*, edited by Gerald Jorland, Annick Opinel, and George Weisz, 19–50. Montreal: McGill-Queen's University Press.

Tsing, Anna Lowenhaupt. 2005. *Friction: An Ethnography of Global Connection*. Princeton: Princeton University Press.

Tufekci, Zeynep, and Christopher Wilson. 2012. "Social Media and the Decision to Participate in Political Protest: Observations from Tahrir Square." *Journal of Communication* 62(2): 363–79. doi:10.1111/j.1460-2466.2012.01629.x

United Kingdom. 2008. "Human Fertilisation and Embryology Act 2008." Chapter 22. http://www.legislation.gov.uk/ukpga/2008/22/pdfs/ukpga_20080022_en.pdf.

U.S. Bureau of Oceans and International Environmental and Scientific Affairs. 2005. "U.S. China Science and Technology Cooperation (S&T Agreement): Report to Congress." http://www.state.gov/documents/organization/44816.pdf.

U.S. Food and Drug Administration (U.S. FDA). 2014. "Significant Dates in U.S. Food and Drug Law History." Last modified December 19, 2014. http://www.fda.gov/AboutFDA/WhatWeDo/History/Milestones/ucm128305.htm.

———. 2015. "Device Advice: Investigational Device Exemption (IDE)." Last modified September 4, 2015. http://www.fda.gov/MedicalDevices/DeviceRegulationandGuidance/HowtoMarketYourDevice/InvestigationalDeviceExemptionIDE/default.htm.

———.2016. "Information on Submitting an Investigational New Drug Application." Last modified June 2, 2016. http://www.fda.gov/BiologicsBloodVaccines/DevelopmentApprovalProcess/InvestigationalNewDrugINDorDeviceExemptionIDEProcess/ucm094309.htm.

U.S. National Institute of Neurological Disorders and Stroke (NINDS). 2013. "Spinal Cord Injury: Hope through Research." http://www.ninds.nih.gov/disorders/sci/detail_sci.htm.

U.S. National Institutes of Health. 2010. "Fact Sheet: Regenerative Medicine." http://report.nih.gov/nihfactsheets/Pdfs/RegenerativeMedicine(NIBIB).pdf.

Victor, Maurice, Allan H. Ropper, and Raymond D. Adams. 2000. *Adams and Victor's Principles of Neurology*. 7th ed. New York: McGraw-Hill Professional.

Vitzhum, Virginia. 2008. "Evolutionary Models of Women's Reproductive Functioning." *Annual Review of Anthropology* 37: 53–73.

——— 2009. "The Ecology and Evolutionary Endocrinology of Reproduction in the Human Female." *American Journal of Physical Anthropology* 140(S49): 95–136.

Vogel, Gretchen. 1999. "Breakthrough of the Year: Capturing the Promise of Youth." *Science* 286(5448): 2238–39.

Wagner, Sarah. 2008. *To Know Where He Lies: DNA Technology and the Search for Srebrenica's Missing*. Berkeley: University of California Press.

Waldby, Catherine, and Melinda Cooper. 2010. "From Reproductive Work to Regenerative Labor: The Female Body and the Stem Cell Industries." *Feminist Theory* 11(1): 3–22.

Walsh, Fergus. 2014. "Paralysed Man Walks Again after Cell Transplant." BBC News, October 21. http://www.bbc.com/news/health-29645760.

Wang, Lequan 王乐泉. 2006. "Zìzhìqū lǐngdǎo jiǎnghuà: Zài Xīnjiāng Yīkē Dàxué jiàn xiào wǔshí zhōunián qìngzhù dàhuì shàng de jiǎnghuà" 自治区领导讲话: 在新疆医科大学建校五十周年庆祝大会上的讲话 [Autonomous Region Party Secretary Speech at the Meeting Celebrating the Fiftieth Anniversary of the Founding of Xinjiang Medical University]. *Xīnjiāng Yīkē Dàxué Xuébào* 新疆医科大学学报 [Journal of Xinjiang Medical University] 29(10): 903.

Wang, Manqi 王漫琪. 2005. "Zhèngguī yīyuàn àn shè lìnglèi yàofáng; Jiēyáng cháfēng wéiguī zhěnshì" 正规医院暗设另类药房; 揭阳查封违规诊室 [Regular Hospital

Secretly Sets up Alternative Pharmacy; Jieyang City Inspects and Seizes Illegal Clinic]. *Yángchéng Wǎnbào* 羊城晚报 [Yang City (Guangzhou) Evening News], November 25. http://news.sohu.com/20051125/n227593609.shtml.

Wang, Shiping 王士平. 2006. "Nánwàng de jìyì shēnqiè de zhùfú" 难忘的记忆深切的祝福 [Deepest Blessings for Unforgettable Memories]. *Qìngzhù Xīnjiāng Yīkē Dàxué jiàn xiào wǔshí zhōunián jìniàn zhuānkān* 庆祝新疆医科大学建校五十周年纪念专刊 [Special Issue Celebrating the 50th Anniversary of the Founding of Xinjiang Medical University]. http://www.xjmu.edu.cn/xiaobaozaixian/document/308.doc. Accessed September 29, 2007.

Wang, Zhaoping 汪兆平. 2006. "Běijīng èr sān jí yīyuàn dà xǐ pái" 北京二三级医院大洗牌 [Big Shuffle for Beijing's Level 2 and 3 Hospitals]. *Zhōngguó Yīyuàn Yuànzhǎng* 中国医院院长 [Chinese Hospital Director], November 30. http://www.h-ceo.com/Article_Show.asp?ArticleID=1476. Accessed November 1, 2013.

Wank, David. 2001. *Commodifying Communism: Business, Trust, and Politics in a Chinese City*. Cambridge: Cambridge University Press.

Wasserstrom, Jeffrey. 1984. "Resistance to the One-Child Family." *Modern China* 10(3): 345–74.

Watt, Nicholas. 2006. "US Faces Science Brain Drain after Europe Backs Stem Cell Funding." *The Guardian*, July 24. http://www.theguardian.com/world/2006/jul/25/eu.genetics.

Watts, Jonathan. 2004. "'I Don't Know How It Works': Dr. Huang Hongyun Cultivates the Cells of Aborted Foetuses and Injects Them into the Brains and Spines of His Patients." *The Guardian*, November 30. http://www.theguardian.com/education/2004/dec/01/ highereducation.uk1. Accessed June 20, 2014.

Weber Max. 1978 [1968]. *Economy and Society: An Outline of Interpretive Sociology*, edited by Guenther Roth and Claus Wittich. Berkeley: University of California Press.

———. 2001 [1958]. *The Protestant Ethic and the Spirit of Capitalism*. Translated by Talcott Parsons. New York: Routledge.

Weijer, Charles. 2002. "I Need a Placebo Like I Need a Hole in the Head." *Journal of Law, Medicine and Ethics* 30: 69–72.

West, Cornell. 2008. *Hope on a Tightrope: Words and Wisdom*. Carlsbad, CA: Smiley Books.

White, Tyrene. 2006. *China's Longest Campaign: Birth Planning in the People's Republic, 1949–2005*. Ithaca, NY: Cornell University Press.

Wilson, Samuel, and Leighton Peterson. 2002. "The Anthropology of Online Communities." *Annual Review of Anthropology* 31: 449–67.

Wu, Lijuan, Youxin Wang, Xiaoxia Peng, Manshu Song, Xiuhua Guo, Hugh Nelson, and Wei Wang. 2014. "Development of a Medical Academic Degree System in China." *Medical Education Online* 19. doi:10.3402/meo.v19.23141.

Xi, Haitao, Lin Chen, Hongyun Huang, Feng Zhang, Yancheng Liu, Di Chen, and Juan Xiao. 2013. "Preliminary Report of Multiple Cell Therapy for Patients with Multiple System Atrophy." *Cell Transplantation* 22(S1): S93–S99.

Xinhua News Agency 新华通讯社. 2005a. "Shí wàn Hánguó rén yǒng xiàng Qīngdǎo: Chéng zuì shìyí Hánguó rén jūzhù de chéngshì" 十万韩国人涌向青岛：成最适宜韩国人居住的城市 [One Hundred Thousand Koreans Flock to Qingdao: The City Has Become the Most Suitable City for Koreans]. *Xīnhuá Tōngxùnshè* 新华通讯社

[Xinhua News Agency], February 2. http://news.xinhuanet.com/newscenter/2005-02/02/content_2539750.htm.

———. 2005b. "Nánkē ménzhěn yīshī zìbào hēimù: Bìngrén láile jiù yīdìng huì débìng" 男科门诊医师自爆黑幕: 病人来了就一定会得病 [Men's Medicine Department Doctor Exposes the Shady Truth: All Patients Will Be Diagnosed with an Illness]. *Xīnhuá Tōngxùnshè* 新华通讯社 [Xinhua News Agency], October 27. http://news.sohu.com/20051027/n227315727.shtml.

———. 2009. "Two Sentenced to Death for Roles in China Milk Scandal." Xinhua News Agency, January 22. http://news.xinhuanet.com/english/2009-01/22/content_10702487.htm.

Xiu, Jinlai 修金来. 2007. "Chíxùle liù nián; lìrùn xiàdié zhì jù'é kuīsǔn; Wànjié fúchén lù" 持续了六年利润下跌至巨额亏损 万杰浮沉录 [Lasted Six Years; Profits Fell with Huge Losses; A Record of Wanjie's Sinking and Floating]. *Zhōngguó Yīyuàn Yuànzhǎng* 中国医院院长 [Chinese Hospital Director], July 31. http://health.sohu.com/20070731/n251339994.shtml.

Yan, Lian 燕炼. 2006. Reply #46 to "Wǒ suǒ liǎojiě de Huáng Hóngyún jí tā de xiù qiào xìbāo yízhí shù" 我所了解的黄红云及他的嗅鞘细胞移植术 [My Understanding of Huang Hongyun and His Olfactory Ensheathing Glial Cell Transplant Surgery]. *Yànshān lùntán* 燕山论坛 [Yanshan Discussion Forum], June 21, 10:09 A.M. http://www.ysx2001.com/forum.php?mod=viewthread&tid=21036&page=2#pid95206.

Yan, Yunxiang. 1996. *The Flow of Gifts: Reciprocity and Social Networks in a Chinese Village*. Stanford, CA: Stanford University Press.

———. 2010. "The Chinese Path to Individualization." *British Journal of Sociology* 61(3): 489–512.

———. 2011. "The Changing Moral Landscape." In *Deep China: The Moral Life of the Person, What Anthropology and Psychiatry Tell Us about China Today*, edited by Arthur Kleinman et al., 36–77. Berkeley: University of California Press.

Yang, Jingqing. 2008. "Professors, Doctors, and Lawyers: The Variable Wealth of the Professional Classes." In *The New Rich in China: Future Rulers, Present Lives*, edited by David S. G. Goodman, 148–67. London: Routledge.

Yang, Mayfair. 1994. *Gifts, Favors, and Banquets: The Art of Social Relationships in China*. Ithaca, NY: Cornell University Press.

Yang, Nianqun 杨念群. 2006. *Zàizào "bìngrén": Zhōng xīyī chōngtú xià de kōngjiān zhèngzhì (1832–1985)* 再造"病人: 中西医冲突下的空间政治 (1832–1985) [Remaking Patients: The Spatial Politics Underlying the Conflict between Chinese and Western Medicine, 1832–1985]. Beijing: Zhōngguó Rénmín Dàxué Chūbǎnshè 中国人民大学出版社 [Remin University of China Press].

Yao, J. L. 1996. "Perinatal Transmission of Hepatitis B Virus Infection and Vaccination in China." *Gut* 38(Supplement 2): S37–S38.

Young, Wise. 1993. "Methods and Apparatus for Quantifying Tissue Damage, Determining Tissue Type, Monitoring Neural Activity, and Determining Hematocrit." United States Patent 5,200,345 (April 6). 28 pages and 11 figures.

——— 1997. "Fear of Hope." Editorial. *Science* 277(5334): 1907.

Zang, Xiaowei. 2008. "Market Transition, Wealth and Status Claims." In *The New Rich in China: Future Rulers, Present Lives*, edited by David S. G. Goodman, 53–70. London: Routledge.

Zhan, Mei. 2009. *Other-Worldly: Making Chinese Medicine through Transnational Frames*. Durham, NC: Duke University Press.

Zhang, Daqing 张大庆. 2006. *Zhōngguó jìndài jíbìng shèhuì shǐ, 1912–1937* 中国近代疾病社会史 1912–1937 [The Social History of Disease in Modern China, 1912–1937]. Jinan: Shāndōng Jiàoyù Chūbǎnshè 山东教育出版社 [Shandong Education Press].

Zhang, Hong. 2007. "From Resisting to 'Embracing'? The One-Child Policy: Understanding New Fertility Trends in a Central Chinese Village." *China Quarterly* 192: 855–75.

Zhang, Joy Yueyue. 2012. *The Cosmopolitanization of Science: Stem Cell Governance in China*. New York: Palgrave McMillan.

Zhang, Li. 2010. *In Search of Paradise: Middle Class Living in a Chinese Metropolis*. Ithaca, NY: Cornell University Press.

Zhang, Li, and Aihwa Ong, eds. 2008. *Privatizing China: Socialism from Afar*. Ithaca, NY: Cornell University Press.

Zhang, Zhihui 张智慧. 2006. "Běijīng yīgǎi xīnzhèng: 122 jiā èrjí yīyuàn shēngsǐ juézé" 北京医改新政: 122 家二级医院生死抉择 [Beijing Medical Reform's New Policy: 122 Level 2 Hospitals Face Life-or-Death Decision]. *Zhōngguó Yīliáo Qiányán* 中国医疗前沿 [China Healthcare Innovation; also translated as National Medical Frontiers of China], October 19. http://finance.people.com.cn/GB/1045/4936625.html.

Zhao, Shaohua 赵绍华. 2002. "Tānhuàn bìngrén shì zěnyàng zhàn qǐlái de" 瘫痪病人是怎样站起来的 [How Do People with Paralysis Stand Up]. *Jiànkāng Shíbào* 健康时报 [Health Times], January 17. http://www.people.com.cn/GB/paper503/5238/549351.html.

Zhengzhou University First Affiliated Hospital 郑州大学第一附属医院. 2015. "Yīyuàn jiǎnjiè" 医院简介 [Hospital Introduction]. http://fcc.zzu.edu.cn/s_lan1.htm.

Zhou, Tingyu 周婷玉. 2008. "Gāo Qiáng: Zhōngguó tèsè wèishēng fāzhǎn dàolù jùjué mángmù yǐnjìn guówài móshì" 高强: 中国特色卫生发展道路拒绝盲目引进国外模式 [Gao Qiang: Health Development Road with Chinese Characteristics Cannot Blindly Introduce Foreign Models]. *Xīnhuá tōngxùnshè* 新华通讯社 [Xinhua News Agency], January 9. http://politics.people.com.cn/GB/1027/6749971.html.

Zhu, Jianfeng. 2013. "Projecting Potentiality: Understanding Maternal Serum Screening in Contemporary China." *Current Anthropology* 54(S7). Potentiality and Humanness: Revisiting the Anthropological Object in Contemporary Biomedicine (October): S36–S44.

Zinberg, Dorothy. 1988. "PRC Science Students and Scholars Abroad." *Science* 239(4847): 1475.

CARECURE FORUM AND ALS BLOG CITATIONS

ANDY [PARAPLEGIC FROM CHICAGO INJURED IN 2002]

2003a. Reply to "Beijing—Brief Report of My China Trip" thread #16983 (June 17, 6:05 P.M.). Cure Forum, CareCure website. http://sci.rutgers.edu/forum/showpost.php?p=84411&postcount=183.

2003b. Reply to "Beijing—CJO's Big Trip" thread #18117 (September 20, 5:26 P.M.). Cure Forum, CareCure website. http://sci.rutgers.edu/forum/showpost.php?p=95020&postcount=8.

2003c. Reply to "Poll: Regarding what is happening in China" thread #32856 (September 20, 6:47 P.M.). Cure Forum, CareCure website. http://sci.rutgers.edu/forum/showpost.php?p=192597&postcount=7.

ANDY C [C5–6 COMPLETE TETRAPLEGIC FROM GREAT BRITAIN INJURED IN 1990]

2003. Reply to "Beijing—Brief Report of My China Trip" thread #16983 (January 21, 8:12 A.M.). Cure Forum, CareCure website. http://sci.rutgers.edu/forum/showpost.php?p=84293&postcount=66.

ANONYMOUS [T4–6 COMPLETE PARAPLEGIC]

2003. Reply to "Poll: Regarding what is happening in China" thread #32856 (September 20, 10:03 A.M.). Cure Forum, CareCure website, http://sci.rutgers.edu/forum/showpost.php?p=192593&postcount=3.

AO [C6 COMPLETE TETRAPLEGIC FROM SOUTH AFRICA INJURED IN 1996]

2003. Reply to "Poll: Regarding what is happening in China" thread #32856 (September 22, 9:24 A.M.). Cure Forum, CareCure website, http://sci.rutgers.edu/forum/showpost.php?p=192619 &postcount=28.

BCMOM [MOTHER OF A T4 COMPLETE PARAPLEGIC SON FROM ALABAMA]

2003. Reply to "the feeling that I cant stand this anymore" thread (November 16, 7:39 A.M.). Caregiving Forum, CareCure website, http://sci.rutgers.edu/forum/showpost.php?p=50868&postcount=11.

BEAKER [T4–5 PARAPLEGIC FROM OREGON INJURED IN 1978; LATER CHANGED SCREEN NAME TO SHANNON]

2003a. "Poll: Regarding what is happening in China" thread #32856 (September 20, 9:41 A.M.). Cure Forum, CareCure website, http://sci.rutgers.edu/forum/showthread.php?t=32856.

2003b. "Poll: Regarding what is happening in China" thread #32856 (September 20, 7:34 p.m.). Cure Forum, CareCure website, http://sci.rutgers.edu/forum/showpost.php?p=192600&postcount=10.

BETHENY [C5–6 INCOMPLETE TETRAPLEGIC FROM OKLAHOMA INJURED IN 2000]

2003. Reply to "Beijing—Tim C's OEG surgery report" thread #18083 (September 14, 12:32 P.M.). Cure Forum, CareCure website, http://sci.rutgers.edu/forum/showpost .php?p=93716&postcount=19.

BILL J. [T12 PARAPLEGIC AND FORMER FARMER FROM SOUTH DAKOTA]

2002. Reply to "Da cure is coming" thread #16779 (November 3, 6:03 P.M.). Cure Forum, CareCure website, http://sci.rutgers.edu/forum/showpost.php?p=82772 &postcount=15.

BOB CLARK [T4–6 COMPLETE PARAPLEGIC FROM FLORIDA INJURED IN 1979]

2005. Reply to "Please help with bowel program" thread #53751 (November 2, 6:14 A.M.) Care Forum, CareCure website, http://sci.rutgers.edu/forum/showpost.php?p =359723&postcount=19.

BOUTER, ARDI [DISABILITY ADVOCATE FROM THE NETHERLANDS DIAGNOSED WITH ALS IN 2003; UNDERWENT OEG SURGERY IN SEPTEMBER 2004]

2004. Fight Against ALS Together: 'Voor en Door ALS patienten' [For and by ALS patients]. Blog. http://www.ardibouter.com/index.html. Accessed June 14, 2006.

BRUNO S. [C3–C5 TETRAPLEGIC FROM AUSTRALIA]

2002. "cure, cure, cure here, this is a cure, might be, potential, cure" thread #16089 (June 23, 4:16 A.M.). Cure Forum, CareCure website, http://sci.rutgers.edu/forum/ showpost.php?p=77555&postcount=1.

CAROL [WIFE OF PARAPLEGIC FROM ALABAMA]

2003. Reply to "Beijing—CJO's Big Trip" thread #18117 (October 2, 10:33 A.M.). Cure Forum, CareCure website, http://sci.rutgers.edu/forum/showpost.php?p =95122&postcount=109.

CHIM-CHIM [WIFE OF A C6–7 INCOMPLETE TETRAPLEGIC FROM ATLANTA INJURED IN 2002]

2003. Reply to "Beijing—CJO's Big Trip" thread #18117 (September 20, 1:09 P.M.). Cure Forum, CareCure website, http://sci.rutgers.edu/forum/showpost.php?p =95014&postcount=2.

CHRISTOPHER PADDON [T7 PARAPLEGIC FROM NEW ZEALAND INJURED IN 1982]

2003. Reply to "Beijing—Brief Report of My China Trip" thread #16983 (January 23, 5:18 P.M.). Cure Forum, CareCure website, http://sci.rutgers.edu/forum/showpost .php?p=84299&postcount=72.

CJO [C5 TETRAPLEGIC COMPUTER INSTRUCTOR FROM SOUTH DAKOTA INJURED IN 2001; UNDERWENT OEG SURGERY IN SEPTEMBER 2003]

2003a. Reply to "Beijing—Brief Report of My China Trip" thread #16983 (January 20, 4:52 P.M.). Cure Forum, CareCure website, http://sci.rutgers.edu/forum/showpost .php?p=84289&postcount=62.

2003b. Reply to "Beijing—Brief Report of My China Trip" thread #16983 (February 8, 7:53 P.M.). Cure Forum, CareCure website, http://sci.rutgers.edu/forum/showpost .php?p=84306&postcount=79.

2003c. Reply to "Beijing—Brief Report of My China Trip" thread #16983 (February 9, 11:21 A.M.). Cure Forum, CareCure website, http://sci.rutgers.edu/forum/showpost .php?p=84316&postcount=89.

2003d. "Beijing—CJO's Big Trip" thread #18117 (September 20, 12:58 P.M.). Cure Forum, CareCure website, http://sci.rutgers.edu/forum/showpost.php?p=95013 &postcount=1.

2003e. Reply to "Beijing—CJO's Big Trip" thread #18117 (October 3, 1:47 A.M.). Cure Forum, CareCure website, http://sci.rutgers.edu/forum/showpost.php?p=95132 &postcount=119.

2007. "Home." http://www.chris-olson.com.

CLAY [T6 PARAPLEGIC ENGINEER FROM WISCONSIN INJURED IN 1999]

2003. Reply to "HandiBob/Bob's OEG surgery report" thread #18099 (September 23, 10:17 A.M.) Cure Forum, CareCure website, http://sci.rutgers.edu/forum/showpost .php?p=94227&postcount=51.

CURT LEATHERBEE [T4 PARAPLEGIC CARECURE MODERATOR FROM RHODE ISLAND INJURED IN 1981]

2003a. Reply to "Beijing—Brief Report of My China Trip" thread #16983 (January 20, 6:26 P.M.). Cure Forum, CareCure website, http://sci.rutgers.edu/forum/showpost .php?p=84291&postcount=64.

2003b. "More proof of OEG transplantation and its potential" thread #18055 (September 8, 7:59 P.M.). Cure Forum, CareCure website, http://sci.rutgers.edu/forum/ showthread.php?t=18055.

2003c. "OEG hype" thread #18058 (September 14, 12:09 P.M.). Cure Forum, CareCure website, http://sci.rutgers.edu/forum/showpost.php?p=93568&postcount=11.

2003d. Reply to "Beijing—CJO's Big Trip" thread #18117 (September 20, 6:28 P.M.). Cure Forum, CareCure website, http://sci.rutgers.edu/forum/showpost.php?p =95021&postcount=9.

2003e. Reply to "Poll: Regarding what is happening in China" thread #32856 (September 22, 11:04 A.M.). Cure Forum, CareCure website, http://sci.rutgers.edu/forum/showpost.php?p=192623 &postcount=32.

2003f. Reply to "Beijing—CJO's Big Trip" thread #18117 (October 2, 10:26 A.M.). Cure Forum, CareCure website, http://sci.rutgers.edu/forum/showpost.php?p=95121 &postcount=108.

DAHLIASINBLOOM [T12–L1 PARAPLEGIC FROM CALIFORNIA INJURED IN 1980]

2003. Reply to "Beijing –Read me—Help TIM" thread #18091 (September 15, 12:18 P.M.). Cure Forum, CareCure website, http://sci.rutgers.edu/forum/showpost.php?p=94032&postcount=5.

DOGGER [C5–6 TETRAPLEGIC FROM QUEENSLAND, AUSTRALIA, INJURED IN 1991]

2003. Reply #31 to "HandiBob/Bob's OEG surgery report" thread #18099 (September 19, 3:25 P.M.). Cure Forum, CareCure website, http://sci.rutgers.edu/forum/showthread.php?18099-Beijing-HandiBob-Bob-s-OEG-surgery-report&p=94207&viewfull=1#post94207.

DRNADER [T7 PARAPLEGIC PHARMACIST FROM EGYPT INJURED IN 1988]

2003. Reply to "HandiBob/Bob's OEG surgery report" thread #18099 (September 19, 3:37 P.M.). Cure Forum, CareCure website, http://sci.rutgers.edu/forum/showpost.php?p=94208&postcount=32.

DUKE [T12 INCOMPLETE PARAPLEGIC COMPUTER TECHNICIAN INJURED IN 2000]

2003. Reply to "Poll: Regarding what is happening in China" thread #32856 (September 21, 5:59 P.M.). Cure Forum, CareCure website, http://sci.rutgers.edu/forum/showpost.php?p=192616&postcount=25.

DURAMATER [NEUROSCIENCE NURSE AND CLINICAL CASE MANAGER FROM VIRGINIA; LATER CHANGED SCREEN NAME TO 1 FINE SPINE RN]

2002. "We had a great time together …" reply to "Travelling to the Open House" thread #43152 (December 14, 9:12 A.M.). Cure Forum, CareCure website, http://sci.rutgers.edu/forum/showpost.php?p=284213&postcount=6.

ERICBASTIAAN [SON OF DUTCH ALS PATIENT ARDI BOUTER, WHO UNDERWENT OEG SURGERY IN SEPTEMBER 2004]

2004. Reply #292 to "Beijing—Wish to contact Dr. Huang? Please post here!" thread #18100 (June 30, 2004, 9:26 A.M.). Cure Forum, CareCure website, http://sci .rutgers.edu/forum/showthread.php?18100-Beijing-Wish-to-contact-Dr-Huang -Please-post-here!&p=94751&viewfull=1#post94751.

FELPS [T12/L1 PARAPLEGIC INJURED IN 1992]

2002. "Wise—You have my attention," reply to "Beijing—Brief Report of My China Trip" thread #16983 (December 17, 9:10 P.M.). Cure Forum, CareCure website, http://sci.rutgers.edu/forum/showpost.php?p=84237&postcount=10.

2003. Reply to "HandiBob/Bob's OEG surgery report" thread #18099 (September 23, 8:45 P.M.). Cure Forum, CareCure website, http://sci.rutgers.edu/forum/showpost .php?p=94231&postcount=55.

GIAMBJJ [APPLIED SCIENCE PROFESSOR FROM ALABAMA WHOSE TETRAPLEGIC SON UNDERWENT OEG SURGERY IN JULY 2004]

2002. Reply to "Beijing—Brief Report of My China Trip" thread #16983 (December 17, 8:16 A.M.). Cure Forum, CareCure website, http://sci.rutgers.edu/forum/showpost .php?p=84228 &postcount=2.

GLOMAE [T12 PARAPLEGIC FROM TEXAS]

2003a. Reply to "Beijing—CJO's Big Trip" thread #18117 (October 2, 9:31 A.M.). Cure Forum, CareCure website, http://sci.rutgers.edu/forum/showpost.php?p=95123 &postcount=110.

2003b. Reply to "Beijing—CJO's Big Trip" thread #18117 (October 2, 7:50 P.M.). Cure Forum, CareCure website, http://sci.rutgers.edu/forum/showpost.php?p=95130 &postcount=117.

GOLANBENONI [BROTHER-IN-LAW OF ALS PATIENT FROM BROOKLYN, NEW YORK]

2004. Reply to "Seeking Alternatives for ALS Treatment" thread #20033 (September 11, 2004, 6:31 P.M.). Cure Forum, CareCure website, http://sci.rutgers.edu/forum/ showthread.php?20033-Seeking-Alternatives-for-ALS-Treatment&p=111818 &viewfull=1#post111818.

HANDIBOB [C5–6 INCOMPLETE TETRAPLEGIC FROM MICHIGAN; UNDERWENT OEG SURGERY IN SEPTEMBER 2003]

2003a. Reply to "HandiBob/Bob's OEG surgery report" thread #18099 (September 19, 12:47 A.M.). Cure Forum, CareCure website, http://sci.rutgers.edu/forum/showpost .php?p=94201&postcount=25.

2003b. Reply to "HandiBob/Bob's OEG surgery report" thread #18099 (September 20, 8:49 P.M.). Cure Forum, CareCure website, http://sci.rutgers.edu/forum/showpost .php?p=94211&postcount=35.

2003c. Reply to "HandiBob/Bob's OEG surgery report" thread #18099 (September 25, 11:04 P.M.). Cure Forum, CareCure website, http://sci.rutgers.edu/forum/showpost .php?p=94239&postcount=62.

2004a. Reply to "Beijing—HandiBob/Bob's OEG surgery report" thread #18099 (April 13, 7:35 A.M.). Cure Forum, CareCure website, http://sci.rutgers.edu/forum/showpost .php?p=94387&postcount=197.

2004b. Reply to "Beijing—HandiBob/Bob's OEG surgery report" thread #18099 (May 18, 8:13 A.M.). Cure Forum, CareCure website, http://sci.rutgers.edu/forum/showpost .php?p=94387&postcount=202.

2004c. Reply to "HandiBob/Bob's OEG surgery report" thread #18099 (June 15, 9:07 A.M.). Cure Forum, CareCure website, http://sci.rutgers.edu/forum/showpost.php?p =94387&postcount=209.

2005. Reply to "Beijing—HandiBob/Bob's OEG surgery report" thread #18099 (January 13, 12:19 P.M.). Cure Forum, CareCure website, http://sci.rutgers.edu/forum/ showthread.php?18099-Beijing-HandiBob-Bob-s-OEG-surgery-report&p =94420&viewfull=1#post94420.

2006. Reply to "Beijing—HandiBob/Bob's OEG surgery report" thread #18099 (July 20, 3:38 P.M.). Cure Forum, CareCure website, http://sci.rutgers.edu/forum/ showthread.php?18099-Beijing-HandiBob-Bob-s-OEG-surgery-report&p =499666&viewfull=1#post499666.

HONGYUN [NEUROSURGEON HUANG HONGYUN'S SCREEN NAME ON CARECURE]

2003a. Reply to "Beijing—Brief Report of My China Trip" thread #16983 (January 20, 8:01 A.M.). Cure Forum, CareCure website, http://sci.rutgers.edu/forum/showpost .php?p=84280&postcount=53.

2003b. Reply to "Beijing—Brief Report of My China Trip" thread #16983 (February 9:41 P.M.). Cure Forum, CareCure website, http://sci.rutgers.edu/forum/showpost .php?p=84308&postcount=81.

2005. Reply to "Dr. Hongyun Huang" thread #20890 (January 7, 9:20 P.M.). Cure Forum, CareCure website, http://sci.rutgers.edu/forum/showthread.php?20890-Dr -Hongyun-Huang&p=117794#post117794.

IP [C5–6 TETRAPLEGIC INJURED IN 1997]

2003a. Reply to "Beijing—Brief Report of My China Trip" thread #16983 (February 9, 11:21 A.M.). Cure Forum, CareCure website, http://sci.rutgers.edu/forum/showpost.php?p =84315&postcount=88.

2003b. Reply to "Beijing—Brief Report of My China Trip" thread #16983 (February 9, 11:34 A.M.). Cure Forum, CareCure website, http://sci.rutgers.edu/forum/showpost. php?p=84317&postcount=90.

2003c. Reply to "Beijing—Read me—Help TIM" thread #18091 (September 15, 12:00 P.M.). Cure Forum, CareCure website, http://sci.rutgers.edu/forum/showpost.php?p =94030&postcount=3.

2003d. Reply to "Beijing—Read me—Help TIM" thread #18091 (September 15, 1:11 P.M.). Cure Forum, CareCure website, http://sci.rutgers.edu/forum/showpost.php?p =94038&postcount=10.

IUBLONDIE25 [DAUGHTER-IN-LAW OF AN ALS PATIENT FROM CONNECTICUT WHO UNDERWENT OEG SURGERY IN APRIL 2004]

2004a. "I have just returned from Beijing…" thread #19206 (April 29, 2004, 5:44 P.M.). Cure Forum, CareCure website, http://sci.rutgers.edu/forum/showthread.php?19206 -I-have-just-returned-from-Beijing&p=105207&viewfull=1#post105207.

2004b. Reply #47 to "I have just returned from Beijing …" thread #19206 (August 10, 2004, 12:45 P.M.). Cure Forum, CareCure website, http://sci.rutgers.edu/forum/ showthread.php?19206-I-have-just-returned-from-Beijing&p=105254&viewfull =1#post105254.

2005. Reply #58 to "I have just returned from Beijing …" thread #19206 (September 26, 2004, 10:41 A.M.). Cure Forum, CareCure website, http://sci.rutgers.edu/forum/ showthread.php?19206-I-have-just-returned-from-Beijing&p=105267&viewfull =1#post105267.

JEFF [C6 TETRAPLEGIC SOFTWARE DEVELOPER FROM NEW JERSEY]

2002. "The Cure Rollercoaster," reply to "cure, cure, cure here, this is a cure, might be, potential, cure" thread #16089 (June 23, 9:24 A.M.). Cure Forum, CareCure website, http://sci.rutgers.edu/forum/showpost.php?p=77560&postcount=6.

2003a. Reply to "Poll: Regarding what is happening in China" thread #32856 (September 20, 5:30 P.M.). Cure Forum, CareCure website, http://sci.rutgers.edu/forum/ showpost.php?p=192595&postcount=5.

2003b. Reply to "Poll: Regarding what is happening in China" thread #32856 (September 21, 10:31 A.M.). Cure Forum, CareCure website, http://sci.rutgers.edu/forum/ showpost.php?p=192605&postcount=15.

2003c. Reply to "PARAS AND DR. HUANG" thread #18322 (November 3, 3:59 P.M.). Cure Forum, CareCure website, http://sci.rutgers.edu/forum/showpost.php?p =96820&postcount=4.

JERRY [PARAPLEGIC FROM FLORIDA INJURED IN 2002]

2006. "Welcome to My Life Journey: Jerry's Personal Site." Blog. http://web.archive.org/ web/20060412164723/; http://www.mylifejourney.net/letters.htm.

JIMNMS [C8/T1 COMPLETE TETRAPLEGIC FROM MISSISSIPPI INJURED IN 2002]

2003. Reply to "Poll: Regarding what is happening in China" thread #32856 (September 20, 7:06 P.M.). Cure Forum, CareCure website, http://sci.rutgers.edu/forum/showpost.php?p=192599&postcount=9.

JMUBLUEDUCK [C6–7 TETRAPLEGIC FROM VIRGINIA INJURED IN 1999; LATER CHANGED SCREEN NAME TO -SCOTT-]

2003a. Reply to "Beijing—Read me—Help TIM" thread #18091 (September 15, 2:27 P.M.). Cure Forum, CareCure website, http://sci.rutgers.edu/forum/showpost.php?p=94044&postcount=16.

2003b. Reply to "Beijing—Tim C's OEG surgery report" thread #18083 (September 26, 9:22 P.M.). Cure Forum, CareCure website, http://sci.rutgers.edu/forum/showpost.php?p=93842&postcount=143.

2003c. Reply to "Beijing—CJO's Big Trip" thread #18117 (October 2, 9:31 A.M.). Cure Forum, CareCure website, http://sci.rutgers.edu/forum/showpost.php?p=95119&postcount=106.

2003d. Reply to "Beijing—CJO's Big Trip" thread #18117 (October 2, 6:54 P.M.). Cure Forum, CareCure website, http://sci.rutgers.edu/forum/showpost.php?p=95129&postcount=116.

JSHOHAM [SON OF AN ALS PATIENT FROM CONNECTICUT WHO UNDERWENT OEG FETAL CELL SURGERY IN APRIL 2004]

2004. Reply #245 to "Beijing—Wish to contact Dr. Huang? Please post here!" thread #18100 (March 30, 2004, 10:19 P.M.). Cure Forum, CareCure website, http://sci.rutgers.edu/forum/showthread.php?18100-Beijing-Wish-to-contact-Dr-Huang-Please-post-here!&p=94703&viewfull=1#post94703.

KEWLCATKEZ [T8 PARAPLEGIC FROM ENGLAND INJURED IN 2005]

2007. Reply to "CareCure Forum" thread #5378 (November 16, 5:27 P.M.). Apparelyzed Spinal Cord Injury and Cauda Equina Syndrome Support Forum. http://www.apparelyzed.com/forums/topic/5378-carecure-forum/#entry45665.

LARWATSON [C5–6 TETRAPLEGIC LAWYER INJURED IN 1982]

2004. Reply to "China Bound! Leo" thread #19059 (April 14, 12:15 P.M.). Cure Forum, CareCure website, http://sci.rutgers.edu/forum/showpost.php?p=103786&postcount=36.

LEO [C4–5 TETRAPLEGIC FROM SOUTH DAKOTA INJURED IN 1976; UNDERWENT OEG SURGERY IN APRIL 2004]

2003a. Reply to "Beijing—Brief Report of My China Trip" thread #16983 (January 20, 4:43 P.M.). Cure Forum, CareCure website, http://sci.rutgers.edu/forum/showpost.php?p=84288&postcount=61.

2003b. Reply to "Beijing—Brief Report of My China Trip" thread #16983 (January 23, 8:33 A.M.). Cure Forum, CareCure website, http://sci.rutgers.edu/forum/showpost.php?p=84298&postcount=71.

2003c. Reply to "Beijing—CJO's Big Trip" thread #18117 (September 24, 6:45 P.M.). Cure Forum, CareCure website, http://sci.rutgers.edu/forum/showthread.php?18117-Beijing-CJO-s-Big-Trip&p=95047&viewfull=1#post95047.

2004. "Leo is China Bound!" thread #19024 (March 29, 9:59 A.M.). Cure Forum, CareCure website, http://sci.rutgers.edu/forum/showpost.php?p=103443&postcount=1.

LLAROSE2 [SISTER-IN-LAW OF A C5–6 INCOMPLETE TETRAPLEGIC WHO UNDERWENT OEG SURGERY IN SEPTEMBER 2003]

2003. Reply to "HandiBob/Bob's OEG surgery report" thread #18099 (September 25, 5:40 A.M.). Cure Forum, CareCure website, http://sci.rutgers.edu/forum/showpost.php?p=94236&postcount=59.

LOES CLAERHOUDT [NEWSPAPER COLUMNIST FROM THE NETHERLANDS DIAGNOSED WITH ALS IN 1999; UNDERWENT OEG SURGERY IN JANUARY 2005]

2005a. "Aangekomen" [Arriving]. Leven Met ALS [Living with ALS] blog (January 3). https://loesclaerhoudt.wordpress.com/2005/01/03/aangekomen/.

2005b. "Wachten 2…" [Wait 2…]. Leven Met ALS [Living with ALS] blog (January 11). https://loesclaerhoudt.wordpress.com/2005/01/11/wachten-2/.

2005c. "De grote dag" [The big day]. Leven Met ALS [Living with ALS] Blog (January 18). https://loesclaerhoudt.wordpress.com/2005/01/18/de-grote-dag/.

2005d. "Voor de laatste keer vanuit het ziekenhuis" [For the last time from the hospital]. Leven Met ALS [Living with ALS] Blog (February 1). https://loesclaerhoudt.wordpress.com/2005/02/01/voor-de-laatste-keer-vanuit-het-ziekenhuis-2/.

2005e. "Waar is de coach?" [Where is the coach?] Leven Met ALS [Living with ALS] Blog (March 21). https://loesclaerhoudt.wordpress.com/2005/03/21/waar-is-de-coach-2/.

2015a. "Loes Claerhoudt" Homepage. http://www.loesclaerhoudt.nl/index.htm.

2015b. "De rek is er wel zo'n beetje uit" [The rack is pretty much out]. Leven Met ALS [Living with ALS] blog (August 28). https://loesclaerhoudt.wordpress.com/2015/08/28/de-rek-is-er-wel-zon-beetje-uit/.

LUCAS [SON OF A WOMAN FROM ITALY DIAGNOSED WITH ALS IN FEBRUARY 2004]

2004. Reply #281 to "Beijing—Wish to contact Dr. Huang? Please post here!" thread #18100 (June 16, 2004, 2:28 A.M.). Cure Forum, CareCure website, http://sci .rutgers.edu/forum/showthread.php?18100-Beijing-Wish-to-contact-Dr-Huang -Please-post-here!&p=94739&viewfull=1#post94739.

MIKE C [C6–7 TETRAPLEGIC CARECURE MODERATOR INJURED IN 1996]

2003. Reply to "Poll: Regarding what is happening in China" thread #32856 (September 21, 4:00 A.M.). Cure Forum, CareCure website, http://sci.rutgers.edu/forum/ showpost.php?p=192603 &postcount=13.

MIMIN [MECHANICAL ENGINEER FROM ISRAEL INJURED IN 2005]

2007. Reply to "Policy Statement: Deletions of memberships, threads, and posts" thread #90943 (November 3, 3:18 P.M.). Cure Forum, CareCure website, http://sci.rutgers .edu/forum/showpost.php?p=745509&postcount=1.http://sci.rutgers.edu/forum/ showthread.php?90943-Policy-Statement-Deletions-of-memberships-threads-and -posts&p=745522&viewfull=1#post745522.

MJ [WIFE AND CAREGIVER OF T3–4 COMPLETE PARAPLEGIC INJURED IN 2001]

2002. Reply to "Online Now feature" thread #38288 (May 22, 8:39 P.M.). Announcements & Feedback Forum, CareCure website, http://sci.rutgers.edu/forum/showpost .php?p=239368&postcount=11.

MK99 [T4 PARAPLEGIC CARECURE MODERATOR FROM TORONTO; UNDERWENT OEG SURGERY IN NOVEMBER 2003]

2001. "why I chose Dr. Cheng," reply to "DR.CHENG" thread #14241 (October 2, 5:49 P.M.). Cure Forum, CareCure website, http://sci.rutgers.edu/forum/showpost .php?p=66691&postcount=4.

2002. "3 OEG procedures—any details?" thread #16197 (July 13, 6:31 P.M.). Cure Forum, CareCure website, http://sci.rutgers.edu/forum/showthread.php?t=16197.

2003a. Reply to "Beijing—Brief Report of My China Trip" thread #16983 (June 2, 6:22 P.M.).CureForum,CareCurewebsite,http://sci.rutgers.edu/forum/showpost.php?p =84395&postcount=167.

2003b. "Beijing—Wish to contact Dr. Huang? Please post here!" thread #18100 (September 17, 4:12 P.M.). Cure Forum, CareCure website, http://sci.rutgers.edu/forum/ showthread.php?18100-Beijing-Wish-to-contact-Dr-Huang-Please-post-here! &p=94457&viewfull=1#post94457.

2003c. Reply to "Poll: Regarding what is happening in China" thread #32856 (September 20, 1:46 P.M.). Cure Forum, CareCure website, http://sci.rutgers.edu/forum/ showpost.php?p=192594&postcount=4.

2003d. Reply to "When Huang operates C. Reeve" thread #18173 (October 1, 8:20 A.M.). Cure Forum, CareCure website, http://sci.rutgers.edu/forum/showpost.php?p =95727&postcount=27.

MKA [BROTHER OF A C6–5 INCOMPLETE TETRAPLEGIC FROM TURKEY]

2003. Reply to "Beijing—Tim C's OEG surgery report" thread #18083 (September 25, 2:17 A.M.). Cure Forum, CareCure website, http://sci.rutgers.edu/forum/showpost .php?p=93817&postcount=119.

MORGAN [T12 PARAPLEGIC FROM CALIFORNIA INJURED IN 1989]

2003a. Reply to "Beijing—CJO's Big Trip" thread #18117 (October 2, 9:02 A.M.). Cure Forum, CareCure website, http://sci.rutgers.edu/forum/showpost.php?p=95116 &postcount=103.

2003b. Reply to "Beijing—CJO's Big Trip" thread #18117 (October 2, 9:48 A.M.). Cure Forum, CareCure website, http://sci.rutgers.edu/forum/showpost.php?p=95120 &postcount=107.

2003c. Reply to "Beijing—CJO's Big Trip" thread #18117 (October 2, 2:26 P.M.). Cure Forum, CareCure website, http://sci.rutgers.edu/forum/showpost.php?p=95124 &postcount=111.

MVANDEMAR [PROGRAMMER AND CARECURE MEMBER]

2007. Reply to "Policy Statement: Deletions of memberships, threads, and posts" thread #90943 (November 5, 2:00 P.M.). Cure Forum, CareCure website, http://sci.rutgers .edu/forum/showthread.php?90943-Policy-Statement-Deletions-of-memberships -threads-and-posts&p=746449&viewfull=1#post746449.

PAULAMC [FAMILY FRIEND OF A C5–6 INCOMPLETE TETRAPLEGIC WHO UNDERWENT OEG SURGERY IN SEPTEMBER 2003]

2003. Reply #33 to "HandiBob/Bob's OEG surgery report" thread #18099 (September 19, 3:25 P.M.). Cure Forum, CareCure website, http://sci.rutgers.edu/forum/ showthread.php?18099-Beijing-HandiBob-Bob-s-OEG-surgery-report&p =94207&viewfull=1#post94209.

PAULSASK [C4–5 TETRAPLEGIC FROM CANADA INJURED IN 1992]

2003. "OEG hype" thread #18058 (September 9, 1:55 P.M.). Cure Forum, CareCure website, http://sci.rutgers.edu/forum/showpost.php?p=93558&postcount=1.

POONSUZANNE [MOTHER OF A T12 PARAPLEGIC SON FROM HONG KONG INJURED IN 2002]

2003. Reply to "PARAS AND DR. HUANG" thread #18322 (November 4, 12:09 A.M.). Cure Forum, CareCure website, http://sci.rutgers.edu/forum/showpost.php?p=96826 &postcount=10.

RAPID524 [C6 TETRAPLEGIC FROM TEXAS INJURED IN 2002]

2003. Reply to "Poll: Regarding what is happening in China" thread #32856 (September 21, 11:42 A.M.). Cure Forum, CareCure website, http://sci.rutgers.edu/forum/showpost.php?p=192606 &postcount=16.

RED_1 CANADA [T12 PARAPLEGIC FROM CANADA INJURED IN 2002]

2003. Reply to "Beijing—CJO's Big Trip" thread #18117 (September 20, 4:16 P.M.). Cure Forum, CareCure website, http://sci.rutgers.edu/forum/showpost.php?p=95018&postcount=6.

RUSTYREEVES [C4 SOFTWARE ENGINEER FROM MISSISSIPPI INJURED IN 1975]

2003a. Reply to "Beijing—Tim C's OEG surgery report" thread #18083 (September 14, 7:29 A.M.). Cure Forum, CareCure website, http://sci.rutgers.edu/forum/showpost.php?p=93706&postcount=9.

2003b. "Beijing—Read me—Help TIM" thread #18091 (September 15, 11:33 A.M.). Cure Forum, CareCure website, http://sci.rutgers.edu/forum/showpost.php?p=94028 &postcount=1.

2003c. Reply to "Beijing—Read me—Help TIM" thread #18091 (September 15, 12:25 P.M.). Cure Forum, CareCure website, http://sci.rutgers.edu/forum/showpost.php?p=94034&postcount=6.

2003d. Reply to "Beijing—Tim C's OEG surgery report" thread #18083 (September 15, 4:20 P.M.). Cure Forum, CareCure website, http://sci.rutgers.edu/forum/showpost.php?p=93737&postcount=39.

SCHMEKY [PARAPLEGIC ENGINEER FROM LOS ANGELES INJURED IN 2002]

2003a. Reply to "Beijing—Brief Report of My China Trip" thread #16983 (January 20, 2:55 P.M.). Cure Forum, CareCure website, http://sci.rutgers.edu/forum/showpost.php?p=84285&postcount=58.

2003b. Reply to "Beijing—Brief Report of My China Trip" thread #16983 (January 23, 6:50 P.M.). Cure Forum, CareCure website, http://sci.rutgers.edu/forum/showpost.php?p=84300&postcount=73.

2003c. Reply to "Beijing—Tim C's OEG surgery report" thread #18083 (September 14, 6:05 A.M.). Cure Forum, CareCure website, http://sci.rutgers.edu/forum/showpost.php?p=93702&postcount=5.

SCI PILOT [T12 PARAPLEGIC ENGINEER FROM CALGARY, CANADA, INJURED IN 2002]

2003. Reply to "Beijing—Brief Report of My China Trip" thread #16983 (January 20, 2:35 P.M.). Cure Forum, CareCure website, http://sci.rutgers.edu/forum/showpost.php?p=84283&postcount=56.

SENECA [C7–8 TETRAPLEGIC CARECURE MODERATOR; LATER CHANGED SCREEN NAME TO ANTIQUITY]

2003. Reply to "Poll: Regarding what is happening in China" thread #32856 (September 21, 8:16 P.M.). Cure Forum, CareCure website, http://sci.rutgers.edu/forum/showpost.php?p=192617&postcount=26.

2006. Reply to "Beijing—HandiBob/Bob's OEG surgery report" thread #18099 (July 26, 11:30 P.M.). Cure Forum, CareCure website, http://sci.rutgers.edu/forum/showthread.php?18099-Beijing-HandiBob-Bob-s-OEG-surgery-report&p=503504&viewfull=1#post503504.

SFAJT [T7 PARAPLEGIC FROM HOUSTON INJURED IN 2002]

2003. Reply to "Beijing—Brief Report of My China Trip" thread #16983 (March 24, 11:01 P.M.). Cure Forum, CareCure website, http://sci.rutgers.edu/forum/showpost.php?p=84355&postcount=127.

SRIRAM [PARAPLEGIC INJURED IN 2000]

2012. Reply to "Beijing—Wish to contact Dr. Huang? Please post here!" thread #18100 (September 17, 4:12 P.M.). Cure Forum, CareCure website, http://sci.rutgers.edu/forum/showthread.php?18100-Beijing-Wish-to-contact-Dr-Huang-Please-post-here!&p=1476441&viewfull=1#post1476441.

STEVEN EDWARDS [C3 TETRAPLEGIC COLUMNIST AND CARECURE ADMINISTRATOR FROM SOUTH CAROLINA INJURED IN 1996]

2003a. Reply to "Poll: Regarding what is happening in China" thread #32856 (September 20, 9:53 A.M.). Cure Forum, CareCure website, http://sci.rutgers.edu/forum/showpost.php?p=192592 &postcount=2.

2003b. Reply to "Poll: Regarding what is happening in China" thread #32856 (September 21, 11:44 A.M.). Cure Forum, CareCure website, http://sci.rutgers.edu/forum/showpost.php?p=192607 &postcount=17.

SWEET N SOUR [JOINT WEBSITE OF DUNCAN, A BRITISH SOLICITOR DIAGNOSED WITH ALS IN 2004 WHO UNDERWENT OEG SURGERY IN AUGUST 2005, AND HIS CARER GERALD]

2005a. "Welcome to [Duncan and Gerald's] Blog." Sweet N Sour Blog. http://www.sweet -n-sour.info/, accessed August 28, 2005.

2005b. "Our Departure, Arrival, and First Few Days in Beijing." Sweet N Sour Blog (August). http://www.sweet-n-sour.info/index.php?f=data_our_daily_journal&a=0, accessed December 28, 2006.

2005c. "Days Eleven to Fourteen." Sweet N Sour Blog (August). http://www.sweet-n-sour .info/index.php?f=data_our_daily_journal&a=2, accessed December 28, 2006.

THE MOM [MOTHER OF A C6–7 COMPLETE TETRAPLEGIC SON FROM TEXAS INJURED IN 2002]

2003a. Reply to "Beijing—Tim C's OEG surgery report" thread #18083 (September 21, 6:07 A.M.). Cure Forum, CareCure website, http://sci.rutgers.edu/forum/showpost .php?p=93794&postcount=96.

2003b. Reply to "Beijing—CJO's Big Trip" thread #18117 (September 28, 6:50 A.M.). Cure Forum, CareCure website, http://sci.rutgers.edu/forum/showpost.php?p=95079 &postcount=66.

TIM C. [C4–5 COMPLETE TETRAPLEGIC FROM NEW YORK WHO UNDERWENT OEG SURGERY IN SEPTEMBER 2003]

2003a. "Beijing—Tim C's OEG surgery report" thread #18083 (September 13, 7:49 P.M.). Cure Forum, CareCure website, http://sci.rutgers.edu/forum/showpost.php?p =93699&postcount=1.

2003b. Reply to "Beijing—Tim C's OEG surgery report" thread #18083 (September 15, 1:20 A.M.). Cure Forum, CareCure website, http://sci.rutgers.edu/forum/showpost .php?p=93732&postcount=34.

2003c. Reply to "Beijing—Tim C's OEG surgery report" thread #18083 (September 17, 5:42 A.M.). Cure Forum, CareCure website, http://sci.rutgers.edu/forum/showpost .php?p=93756&postcount=58.

2003d. Reply to "Beijing—Tim C's OEG surgery report" thread #18083 (September 17, 9:23 A.M.). Cure Forum, CareCure website, http://sci.rutgers.edu/forum/showpost .php?p=93771&postcount=73.

2003e. "THE REST OF THE STORY," reply to "Beijing—Wish to contact Dr. Huang? Please post here!" thread #18100 (September 18, 11:39 P.M.). Cure Forum, CareCure website, http://sci.rutgers.edu/forum/showpost.php?p=94500&postcount=44.

2003f. "Day Before Surgery," reply to "Beijing—Tim C's OEG surgery report" thread #18083 (September 21, 5:16 P.M.). Cure Forum, CareCure website, http://sci .rutgers.edu/forum/showpost.php?p=93792&postcount=94.

2003g. Reply to "Beijing—Tim C's OEG surgery report" thread #18083 (September 25, 1:49 A.M.). Cure Forum, CareCure website, http://sci.rutgers.edu/forum/showpost .php?p=93815&postcount=117.

2003h. Reply to "Beijing—Tim C's OEG surgery report" thread #18083 (September 26, 7:58 P.M.). Cure Forum, CareCure website, http://sci.rutgers.edu/forum/showpost .php?p=93840&postcount=141.

2003i. Reply to "Beijing—Read me—Help TIM" thread #18091 (September 26, 9:56 P.M.). Cure Forum, CareCure website, http://sci.rutgers.edu/forum/showpost.php?p =94096&postcount=68.

2003j. Reply to "Beijing—Tim C's OEG surgery report" thread #18083 (December 23, 8:17 P.M.). Cure Forum, CareCure website, http://sci.rutgers.edu/forum/showpost .php?p=93899&postcount=200.

2004a. "WOW, YES Merco, pain, so what's in it for me?," reply to "Beijing—Tim C's OEG surgery report" thread #18083 (June 20, 9:32 P.M.). Cure Forum, CareCure website, http://sci.rutgers.edu/forum/showpost.php?p=93940&postcount=240.

2004b. Reply to "Beijing—HandiBob/Bob's OEG surgery report" thread #18083 (March 8, 10:35 P.M.). Cure Forum, CareCure website, http://sci.rutgers.edu/ forum/showthread.php?18083-Beijing-Tim-C-s-OEG-surgery-report&p=93917 &viewfull=1#post93917.

2004c. Reply to "Beijing—HandiBob/Bob's OEG surgery report" thread #18083 (May 26, 11:49 P.M.). Cure Forum, CareCure website, http://sci.rutgers.edu/forum/ showthread.php?18083-Beijing-Tim-C-s-OEG-surgery-report&p=93927 &viewfull=1#post93927.

2004d. Reply to "Beijing—HandiBob/Bob's OEG surgery report" thread #18083 (April 2, 12:26 A.M.). Cure Forum, CareCure website, http://sci.rutgers.edu/forum/ showthread.php?18083-Beijing-Tim-C-s-OEG-surgery-report&p=93919 &viewfull=1#post93919.

2004e. Reply to "Beijing—HandiBob/Bob's OEG surgery report" thread #18083 (May 10, 7:59 P.M.). Cure Forum, CareCure website, http://sci.rutgers.edu/forum/showthread .php?45320-NEED-A-NEW-DRUG&p=293973&viewfull=1#post293973.

2004f. Reply to "Beijing—HandiBob/Bob's OEG surgery report" thread #18083 (May 26, 11:49 P.M.). Cure Forum, CareCure website, http://sci.rutgers.edu/ forum/showthread.php?18083-Beijing-Tim-C-s-OEG-surgery-report&p=93927 &viewfull=1#post93927.

2004g. Reply to "Beijing—HandiBob/Bob's OEG surgery report" thread #18083 (July 1, 10:35 P.M.). Cure Forum, CareCure website, http://sci.rutgers.edu/forum/ showthread.php?45375-Does-sitting-ever-stop-hurting&p=294356 &viewfull=1#post294356.

2004h. Reply to "Beijing—Tim C's OEG surgery report" thread #18083 (June 25, 8:21 P.M.). Cure Forum, CareCure website, http://sci.rutgers.edu/forum/showthread .php?18083-Beijing-Tim-C-s-OEG-surgery-report&p=93947&viewfull=1 #post93947.

2005. Reply to "To do or not to do" thread #49465 (August 2, 3:12 P.M.). Cure Forum, CareCure website, http://sci.rutgers.edu/forum/showpost.php?p=325577 &postcount=22.

2015. Reply to "It sure is frusterating with all the good things that seem to have been announced" thread #234673 (August 24, 2:00 P.M.). Cure Forum, CareCure website, http://sci.rutgers.edu/forum/showthread.php?234673-It-sure-is-frusterating -with-all-the-good-things-that-seem-to-have-been-announced&p=1776586 &viewfull=1#post1776586.

TROPHIC [AMERICAN EXPATRIATE LIVING IN MOSCOW DIAGNOSED WITH ALS IN 2003; UNDERWENT OEG SURGERY IN NOVEMBER 2004]

2004a. "How It All Started." Trophic Blog (August 4). http://trophic.blogspot.com/2004/08/how-it-all-started.html.

2004b. Reply to "Seeking Alternatives for ALS Treatment" thread #20033 (September 12, 5:22 A.M.). Cure Forum, CareCure website, http://sci.rutgers.edu/forum/showthread.php?20033-Seeking-Alternatives-for-ALS-Treatment&p=111821&viewfull=1#post111821.

2004c. "Beijing?" Trophic Blog (October 1). http://trophic.blogspot.com/2004/10/beijing.html.

2004d. "17–18 November 2004—The Beijing Workers' Sanatorium." Trophic Blog (November 18). http://trophic.blogspot.com/2004/11/17-18-november-2004-beijing-workers.html.

2004e. Reply to "OEG Treatment of ALS" thread #19598 (November 24, 5:47 A.M.). Cure Forum, CareCure website, http://sci.rutgers.edu/forum/showthread.php?19598-OEG-Treatment-of-ALS&p=108287&viewfull=1#post108287.

VGRAFEN [T6 COMPLETE PARAPLEGIC INJURED IN 1999 FROM CALIFORNIA]

2004. "Another step towards return, from the Prince of the run-on sentence" (February 15, 3:50 P.M.). Life forum, CareCure website, http://sci.rutgers.edu/forum/showpost.php?p=204411&postcount=1.

W. JUSTIN MARTIN [T12 PARAPLEGIC LAWYER FROM OHIO]

2006. Reply to "Beijing—HandiBob/Bob's OEG surgery report" thread #18099 (July 20, 3:38 P.M.). Cure Forum, CareCure website, http://sci.rutgers.edu/forum/showthread.php?18099-Beijing-HandiBob-Bob-s-OEG-surgery-report&p=503495&viewfull=1#post503495.

WILLIAMCRAIG [T11–12 APPARELYZED FORUM MEMBER FROM NEW ORLEANS]

2007. Reply to "CareCure Forum" thread #5378 (November 26, 12:23 A.M.). Apparelyzed Spinal Cord Injury and Cauda Equina Syndrome Support Forum. http://www.apparelyzed.com/forums/topic/5378-carecure-forum/#entry46318.

WISE YOUNG [FOUNDER OF CARECURE]

2001a. Update on Cando.com. http://carecure.rutgers.edu/Cando/Cando_Update.htm, accessed November 30, 2006.

2001b. Cure and Spinal Cord Injury in the Medical Literature. December 1. http://sci.rutgers.edu/index.php?page=viewarticle&afile=2_December_2001@CureSCI.htm.

2002a. The State of the CareCure Community. March 18. http://sci.rutgers.edu/index
.php?page=viewarticle&afile=18_March_2002@Community18Mar02.htm.

2002b. "Beijing—Brief Report of My China Trip" thread #16983 (December 17, 3:02 A.M.).
Cure Forum, CareCure website, http://sci.rutgers.edu/forum/showpost.php?p
=84227&postcount=1.

2003a. Reply to "Beijing—Brief Report of My China Trip" thread #16983 (February 14,
8:09 P.M.). Cure Forum, CareCure website, http://sci.rutgers.edu/forum/showpost
.php?p=84332&postcount=105.

2003b. "Welcome to the Acute SCI Forum" thread # 37268 (February 24, 1:22 P.M.).
New SCI Forum, CareCure website, http://sci.rutgers.edu/forum/showpost.php?p
=234969&postcount=1.

2003c. Reply to "Paras and Dr. Huang" thread #18164 (September 27, 11:07 A.M.). Cure
Forum, CareCure website, http://sci.rutgers.edu/forum/showpost.php?p=95635
&postcount=7.

2003d. Reply to "HandiBob/Bob's OEG surgery report" thread #18099 (September 28,
5:55 A.M.). Cure Forum, CareCure website, http://sci.rutgers.edu/forum/showpost
.php?p=94256&postcount=79.

2004. "OEG transplants: to have or not to have" thread #20714 (December 7, 12:47
P.M.). Cure Forum, CareCure website, http://sci.rutgers.edu/forum/showthread
.php?t=20714.

2007. "Policy Statement: Deletions of memberships, threads, and posts" thread #90943
(November 3, 3:59 P.M.). Cure Forum, CareCure website, http://sci.rutgers.edu/
forum/showpost.php?p=745509&postcount=1.

2010. "The Mission of CareCure" thread #13454 (May 2, 7:57 P.M.). Announcements
& Feedback Forum, CareCure website, http://sci.rutgers.edu/forum/showthread
.php?t=134543.

INDEX

Page numbers in italics refer to figures.